Cardiac
Resynchronization
Therapy

To my wife, Joan.
In her, I find joy, love and support that are beyond what the most beautiful marriage vows could have promised.
Cheuk-Man Yu

To my wife, Sharonne, and children, Sarah and Drew, for their tolerance.
David Hayes

To my wife, Heike, and my children for their silent, remarkable support through this endeavor.
In loving memory of my father, Luigi Auricchio.
Angelo Auricchio

Cardiac Resynchronization Therapy

EDITED BY

Cheuk-Man Yu
David L. Hayes
Angelo Auricchio

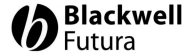

© 2006 by Blackwell Publishing

Blackwell Futura is an imprint of Blackwell Publishing
Blackwell Publishing, Inc., 350 Main Street, Malden, Massachusetts 02148–5020, USA
Blackwell Publishing Ltd, 9600 Garsington Road, Oxford OX4 2DQ, UK
Blackwell Science Asia Pty Ltd, 550 Swanston Street, Carlton, Victoria 3053, Australia

First published 2006

ISBN-13: 978–1-4051–4282–3
ISBN-10: 1–4051–4282–0

Library of Congress Cataloging-in-Publication Data
Cardiac resynchronization therapy / edited by Cheuk-Man Yu, David L. Hayes, Angelo Auricchio.
  p. ; cm.
  Includes bibliographical references and index.
  ISBN-13: 978-1-4051-4282-3 (alk. paper)
  ISBN-10: 1-4051-4282-0 (alk. paper)
1. Cardiac pacing. 2. Congestive heart failure. 3. Implantable cardioverter-defibrillators.
  [DNLM: 1. Cardiac Pacing, Artificial--methods. 2. Heart Failure, Congestive--therapy. 3. Defibrillators, Implantable. 4. Pacemaker, Artificial. WG 370 C2673 2006] I. Yu, Cheuk-Man. II. Hayes, David L. III. Auricchio, Angelo.

  RC685.C53C34 2006
  617.4'120645--dc22

                                                                           2005031755

A catalogue record for this title is available from the British Library

Commissioning Editor: Gina Almond
Development Editor: Vicki Donald
Set in 9.5/12 pt Minion by Sparks. Oxford – www.sparks.co.uk
Printed and bound in Singapore by Fabulous Printers Pte Ltd

For further information on Blackwell Publishing, visit our website:
www.blackwellcardiology.com

The publisher's policy is to use permanent paper from mills that operate a sustainable forestry policy, and which has been manufactured from pulp processed using acid-free and elementary chlorine-free practices. Furthermore, the publisher ensures that the text paper and cover board used have met acceptable environmental accreditation standards.

Blackwell Publishing makes no representation, express or implied, that the drug dosages in this book are correct. Readers must therefore always check that any product mentioned in this publication is used in accordance with the prescribing information prepared by the manufacturers. The author and the publishers do not accept responsibility or legal liability for any errors in the text or for the misuse or misapplication of material in this book.

Contents

Contributors

Editors

Angelo Auricchio MD PhD
Associate Professor of Cardiology
University Hospital Magdeburg
Magdeburg, Germany
Director Heart Failure Program
Fondazione Cardiocentro Ticino
Lugano, Switzerland

David L. Hayes MD
Chair, Division of Cardiovascular Diseases and Internal
Medicine, Mayo Clinic
Professor of Medicine, Mayo College of Medicine
Rochester, MN, USA

Cheuk-Man Yu MBChB(CUHK), MRCP(UK), MD(CUHK), FHKCP, FHKAM(Medicine), FRACP, FRCP (Edin)
Professor, Head of Division of Cardiology
Department of Medicine & Therapeutics
The Chinese University of Hong Kong
Prince of Wales Hospital
Hong Kong

Contributors

William T. Abraham MD, FACP, FACC
Professor of Medicine
Chief, Division of Cardiovascular Medicine
Associate Director, Davis Heart and Lung Research Institute
The Ohio State University
Columbus, OH, USA

Philip B. Adamson MD, FACC
Associate Professor, Director
The Heart Failure Institute at the Oklahoma Heart Hospital
Oklahoma City, OK, USA

Samuel Asirvatham MD
Assistant Professor of Medicine
Mayo Clinic College of Medicine
Rochester, MN, USA

Jeroen J. Bax MD, PhD
Leiden University Medical Center
Leiden
The Netherlands

Gabe B. Bleeker MD
Leiden University Medical Center
Leiden
The Netherlands

Ole-A. Breithardt MD
Assistant Professor of Cardiology
Klinikum Mannheim GmbH
University Hospital
Faculty of Clinical Medicine at the University of Heidelberg
Mannheim, Germany

J. Claude Daubert MD, FESC
Professor of Cardiology
Department of Cardiology
Centre Cardio-Pneumologique
CHU Pontchaillou
Rennes, France

Tammo Delhaas MD, PhD
Associate Professor
Maastricht University
Maastricht, The Netherlands

Joseph J. DeRose, Jr MD
Assistant Professor of Clinical Surgery
Columbia University College of Physicians and Surgeons
St. Luke's-Roosevelt Hospital Center
New York, NY, USA

Lieselot van Erven MD, PhD
Leiden University Medical Center
Leiden
The Netherlands

Cecilia Fantoni MD
Senior Cardiologist
Department of Cardiovascular Sciences
University of Insubria
Varese, Italy

Jeffrey W.H. Fung FRCP
Director of Cardiac Electrophysiology and Pacing Services
The Prince of Wales Hospital
The Chinese University of Hong Kong
Hong Kong, China

Stephane Garrigue MD
Director of Electrophysiology and Cardiac Pacing Department
Clinique Saint-Augustin
Bordeaux, France

Michael Glikson MD
Director of Pacing and Electrophysiology
Sheba Medical Center and Tel Aviv University
Tel-Hashomer, Israel

Osnat Gurevitz MD
Senior Cardiologist
Sheba Medical Center and Tel Aviv University
Tel-Hashomer, Israel

Garrie J. Haas MD, FACC
Associate Professor of Medicine
Director, Cardiovascular Clinical Research Unit
Heart Failure and Cardiac Transplant Program
Division of Cardiovascular Medicine
The Ohio State University
Columbus, OH, USA

Maren Jeffrey MD
Fellow
Hospital of the University of Pennsylvania
Philadelphia, PA, USA

Mariell Jessup MD
Hospital of the University of Pennsylvania
Philadelphia, PA, USA

Christophe Leclercq MD, PhD, FESC
Professor of Cardiology
Department of Cardiology
Centre Cardio-Pneumologique
CHU Pontchaillou
Rennes, France

David Luria MD
Senior Cardiologist
Sheba Medical Center and Tel Aviv University
Tel-Hashomer, Israel

Philippe Mabo MD
Professor of Cardiology
Department of Cardiology
Centre Cardio-Pneumologique
CHU Pontchaillou
Rennes, France

Frits W. Prinzen MD
Associate Professor
Maastricht University
Maastricht, The Netherlands

John E. Sanderson MD, FRCP, FACC
Professor of Cardiology
Keele University Medical School
University Hospital of North Staffordshire NHS Trust
Stoke on Trent, UK
(Previously Professor of Medicine & Therapeutics, The Chinese University of Hong Kong, Hong Kong)

Martin J. Schalij MD, PhD
Leiden University Medical Center
Leiden, The Netherlands

Jonathan S. Steinberg MD
Professor of Medicine
Columbia University College of Physicians and Surgeons
St. Luke's-Roosevelt Hospital Center
New York, NY, USA

Michael O. Sweeney MD
Cardiac Arrhythmia Service
Brigham and Women's Hospital
Assistant Professor of Medicine
Harvard Medical School
Boston, MA, USA

Qing Zhang BM, MM
Division of Cardiology
Department of Medicine and Therapeutics
Prince of Wales Hospital
The Chinese University of Hong Kong
Hong Kong

Foreword

This book is about a revolution in our thinking on heart failure. Over the past three or four decades a number of conceptual frameworks have been put forward in an attempt to explain the syndrome which is clinically recognizable as heart failure. Initial concepts emphasized salt and water retention through renal hypoperfusion. As more invasive measurement of hemodynamics became available, the importance of increased afterload and preload was appreciated and treatments evolved to reduce both of these, which did produce some symptomatic improvement and lower mortality. More recently the neurohormonal model has been fundamental in explaining the significant impact of blockade of the renin–angiotensin–aldosterone and sympathetic nervous systems. Success of these drugs focused attention onto the processes involved in ventricular remodeling, the gradual change in shape and increase in volume which lie behind the relentless progression of heart failure. Beta blockers in particular can induce reverse remodeling and this action may partly explain their major impact on mortality.

We are now moving into a new conceptual phase of heart failure management which could be called the "electrical-mechanical stage." Once again it is the application of a highly effective therapy which opens up new areas of potential mechanisms. It has been known for a long time that heart failure is often associated with abnormal electrical activation within the heart which leads to regional mechanical dyssynchrony. The most obvious and simplest marker of abnormal electrical activation is the presence of left bundle branch block (LBBB) on the surface ECG. However, this is only a marker; a LBBB pattern is not always associated with significant mechanical dyssynchrony and many patients with heart failure who have a narrow QRS can be shown to have mechanical dyssynchrony [1]. At the moment, the best and easiest way of detecting and quantifying the degree of mechanical dyssynchrony is by tissue Doppler imaging [2]. Many studies have shown, using these newer echocardiographic techniques, that mechanical dyssynchrony is common in the remodeled ventricle both in heart failure and also post-myocardial infarction [3].

The ability to correct electrical and mechanical dyssynchrony via simultaneous pacing of the left and right ventricles routinely has had to await the development of technology to place leads into the coronary sinus and thence into the left ventricular lateral wall cardiac vein, although probably the earliest proof of a benefit of biventricular pacing was in 1971 when Gibson and colleagues showed that simultaneous pacing of both ventricles or the left ventricle alone was superior to right ventricular pacing in patients following aorta valve replacement [4].

Recently the startling benefit of cardiac resynchronization therapy (CRT) that had been seen in many smaller studies has been confirmed in large-scale clinical trials [5]. CRT improves symptoms, reduces mortality and reverses ventricular remodeling. However, it is equally clear that not all patients benefit and there is a sub-set who fail to show the expected improvement. Much effort has been expended recently in trying to identify these patients and, at the moment, it appears that the best predictor of reverse remodeling is the definite presence of marked mechanical dyssynchrony pre-operatively. Whether using tissue Doppler imaging rather than the ECG for selection will reduce the numbers of non-responders remains to be proven. However, one of the most interesting aspects of CRT is how remarkable the degree of reverse remodeling can be in individual patients. This is of fundamental importance because it demonstrates that ventricular remodeling can be reversed quite quickly and to a major degree, which is extremely hopeful. It also illustrates what a powerful impact mechanical dyssynchrony by itself has on overall ventricular function and it is clearly a major factor, previously underestimated, in the whole remodeling process.

Although CRT is a major advance and is already bringing benefit to many patients with chronic heart failure, there are a number of questions and problems remaining. There are patient sub-groups where the benefit has not been clearly defined yet such as those with normal QRS duration and echocardiographic evidence of dyssynchrony. Others still debate the best echocardiographic measurements and whether selection based only on these parameters is justified, although recently the picture is becoming clearer. Should CRT be combined routinely with a cardioverter defibrillator? There are other technical problems remaining, such as correct positioning of the leads. At the moment in most centers the left ventricular lead is placed into the best available vein on the lateral wall. But, coronary venous anatomy is highly variable and this means that there is a certain degree of randomness to the position that the left ventricular lead is likely to find itself. Perhaps routine use of MRI to identify the presence of scar tissue that may hinder activation or quantifying more precisely the areas of latest activation and contraction will be useful in this regard. It may also be worth considering using epicardial leads more frequently for a more precise positioning.

All these questions are considered in this timely and excellent textbook on this important new development in heart failure. The Editors have collected an impressive group of authors who have enormous experience in this area and who write with authority. This book will, I am sure, prove extremely useful as it collates information from many different quarters of cardiology which have tended to become separate domains where individuals work in a rather isolated fashion. In fact, one of the good things about CRT is that it pulls together a rather

disparate group of sub-specialists: heart failure physicians, echocardiographic and imaging specialists, and electrophysiologists. Good teamwork is vital between these three groups to identify the most suitable patients, implant with optimal positioning of the leads, finetuning the pacemaker programmable features after surgery, and follow-up with careful titration of medical therapy. This book is likely, therefore, to become a classic in this very important new field of CRT which by its own success has illustrated the importance of abnormal activation in the pathophysiology of heart failure. We are making progress in the treatment of what was considered to be a progressive and highly lethal disease and CRT is another big step forward.

John E. Sanderson MA MD FRCP FACC

References

1 Yu CM, Lin H, Zhang Q, Sanderson JE. High prevalence of left ventricular systolic and diastolic asynchrony in patients with congestive heart failure and normal QRS duration. *Heart* 2003; **89**: 54–60.

2 Yu CM, Fung JWH, Zhang Q *et al.* Tissue Doppler imaging is superior to strain rate imaging and postsystolic shortening on the prediction of reverse remodeling in both ischemic and nonischemic heart failure after cardiac resynchronization therapy. *Circulation* 2004; **110**: 66–73.

3 Zhang Y, Chan AK, Yu CM *et al.* Left ventricular systolic asynchrony after acute myocardial infarction in patients with narrow QRS complexes. *Am Heart J* 2005; **149**: 497–503.

4 Gibson DG, Chamberlain DA, Coltart DJ, Mercer J. Effect of changes in ventricular activation on cardiac haemodynamics in man. Comparison of right ventricular, left ventricular and simultaneous pacing of both ventricles. *Br Heart J* 1971; **33**: 397–400.

5 Cleland JG, Daubert J-C, Erdmann E, Freemantle N, Gras D, Kappenberger L, Tavazzi L. Cardiac Resynchronization–Heart Failure (CARE–HF) Study Investigators. The effect of cardiac resynchronization on morbidity and mortality in heart failure. *N Engl J Med* 2005; 352: 1539–1549.

SECTION 1

Heart failure epidemiology and standard therapies

CHAPTER 1

The epidemiology of heart failure

Maren E. Jeffery, MD *& Mariell Jessup,* MD

Introduction

Heart failure is a clinical syndrome resulting from a structural or functional cardiac disorder that impairs the ability of the ventricle to fill with or eject blood commensurate with the needs of the body, or precludes it from doing so in the absence of increased filling pressures. This syndrome manifests primarily as dyspnea, fatigue, fluid retention, and decreased exercise tolerance. Heart failure may result from disorders of the pericardium, myocardium, endocardium or valvular structures, great vessels of the heart, or rhythm disturbances. However, because valvular disease, pericardial disorders and rhythm disturbances are usually easily amenable to effective surgical correction or other definitive treatment, heart failure is usually discussed primarily in terms of myocardial dysfunction.

From a practical standpoint, it is useful to divide patients with heart failure into those with primarily systolic dysfunction and those with diastolic dysfunction, which usually involves an assessment of the patient's ejection fraction. Patients with a low left ventricular (LV) ejection fraction, usually <40–45%, are classified as having systolic dysfunction. Such patients typically have dilatation of the LV cavity and a decreased cardiac output on the basis of diminished contractility of the myocardium. In contrast, patients with symptoms and exam findings consistent with heart failure but with a preserved ejection fraction are often said to have diastolic dysfunction, which is typically a disease of impaired ventricular filling.

Heart failure is a final common pathway of all diseases of the heart and is a major cause of morbidity and mortality. Approximately 4.9 million Americans carry the diagnosis of heart failure [1] and about 550 000 new cases occur each year in the US [2]. Hospital discharges for heart failure in the US have increased 155% between 1979 and 1999 to 962 000 per year [3]. Heart failure accounts for about 5% of annual hospital admissions, with more than 100 000 annual admissions in the UK and more than 2.5 million annual admissions in the US [4, 5]. Reports from several countries suggest that approximately 1–2% of the total health care budget is spent on the management of heart failure [6]. Yet, despite recent advances in the treatment of heart failure, the prognosis remains poor, with mortality data that are comparable with data for the worst forms of malignant disease.

Epidemiology of heart failure

Prevalence of heart failure

Population-based studies in heart failure are difficult to compare because of a lack of agreement on the definition of the disease from study to study. Studies investigating the prevalence of heart failure can generally be divided into those population studies based on physician records and prescriptions, studies based on clinical criteria, and those based on echocardiographic surveys. Not surprisingly, prevalence data may differ depending on the method of identifying subjects with disease. Likewise, data can vary widely in inpatient and outpatient population studies. Nonetheless, they have helped to shed light on the magnitude of the problem and have elicited several trends in the prevalence and etiology of the syndrome of heart failure.

Population studies based on physician records and prescriptions

Among the more recent reports, residents of

Rochester, Minnesota were screened for the diagnosis of heart failure in January 1982, using the resources of the Rochester Epidemiology Project. The age- and sex-adjusted prevalence was reported at 265.8 per 100 000 person-years. The prevalence rate was higher in men vs. women (327.3 vs. 213.6 per 100 000 person-years) and tended to increase with age. For example, rates increased from 74.4 per 100 000 among men 45–49 years old to 2595.5 per 100 000 among those 65–69 years old and 2765 per 100 000 among those 70–74 years old. A similar trend was seen among women (72.6 per 100 000 in those 45–49 years, increasing to 2743.8 per 100 000 among those 70–74 years) [7].

The REACH study (Resource Utilization Among Congestive Heart Failure) derived the incidence and prevalence of heart failure among 29 686 patients who had acquired an International Classification of Diseases (ICD) code for heart failure during an inpatient or two outpatient encounters within the Henry Ford Health System in Detroit, Michigan. In 1999, the age-adjusted prevalence of heart failure was found to be 14.5 per 1000 in men and 14.3 per 1000 in women. The higher prevalence of heart failure in this population may be attributable to the higher proportion of inpatients included in this study [8].

More recently, an extensive survey of the incidence and prevalence of heart failure in Scotland was done between April 1999 and March 2000. Using the continuous morbidity recording (CMR) in general practice scheme, data were collected from every face-to-face doctor–patient encounter for a total of 307 741 patients from 53 medical practices. Patients were identified by diagnostic codes for heart failure. The prevalence of heart failure among men aged 45–64 years of age was 4.3 per 1000 and 134 per 1000 in those over 85 years, again confirming the strong link between heart failure and increasing age. A similar trend was seen in women, in whom the prevalence rose from 3.2 in those 45–64 years to 85.2 in those over 85 years [9].

Population studies based on clinical criteria

Additional population studies involved clinical encounters with each study subject. Heart failure was identified based on various historical, physical exam, and laboratory findings. Among the best-known population studies, the Framingham Heart Study, for example, was a landmark longitudinal effort that established strict clinical criteria for diagnosing heart failure; the natural history of the disease in a defined population has been reported and has now been followed for over 50 years. The Framingham Heart Study was initiated in 1948 for the purpose of eliciting the etiology and natural history of cardiovascular diseases. Initially, 5209 residents between the ages of 30 and 62 years from Framingham, Massachusetts were enrolled in the study and followed for the development of cardiovascular disease with medical histories, physical exams, and laboratory tests every two years. Children and spouses of children of the original cohort were added to the study in 1971. A total of 9405 participants (47% male) were followed from September 1948 to June 1988. Congestive heart failure (CHF) developed in a total of 652 patients. The prevalence of CHF was found to dramatically increase with age, such that in men the prevalence jumped from 8 cases per 1000 patients in those aged 50–59 years to 66 cases per 1000 in those aged 80–89. Likewise in women, the prevalence increased from 8 cases per 1000 in those aged 50–59 to 79 cases per 1000 in those aged 80–89. During the 1980s, the age-adjusted prevalence of CHF was 7.4 cases/1000 men and 7.7 cases/1000 women [10, 11].

Another study done between 1960 and 1962 looked at 3102 residents from Evans County, Georgia between the ages of 40–74 years for whom medical histories, physical exams, ECGs and posterolateral chest X-rays were done as part of an epidemiologic survey. This study found a prevalence of 10 cases of heart failure per 1000 in residents aged 45–54 years, 28 cases per 1000 in those aged 55–64 years, and 35 cases per 1000 in those aged 65–74 years. The overall prevalence among all residents aged 45–74 years was 21 cases per 1000 [12].

In 2004, an update of the Rotterdam Study was published, giving a current account of the prevalence of heart failure in this population. The Rotterdam Study was a prospective cohort study of various cardiovascular, neurological, and ophthalmologic diseases in the elderly. A total of 7983 inhabitants of Ommoord (a suburb of Rotterdam in the Netherlands) who were aged 55 years or older were enrolled between July 1989 and 1993 and followed clinically until January 2000. The 1998 point prevalence of heart failure was 0.9% in subjects aged 55–64 years; 4% in those aged 65–74 years; 9.7% in those aged 75–84 years and 17.4% in those over the age of 85, again confirming the steep increase in the prevalence of heart failure with age [13].

Population studies based on clinical and echocardiographic criteria

To further examine the nature and prevalence of heart failure in the elderly population, the Helsinki Aging Study examined a randomly selected population of 501 Helsinki residents (367 females) who were born in 1904, 1909, and 1914 (aged 75–86 years). Heart failure was diagnosed on the basis of clinical criteria obtained by cardiologic assessment, including history, physical exam, ECG, and posterolateral chest X-ray. Participants also had a transthoracic echocardiogram to assess systolic and diastolic dysfunction. Of those enrolled in the study, 41 (8.2%) were diagnosed with heart failure. However, only 28% of these patients were found to have systolic dysfunction (defined as fractional shortening <25% and LV dilatation). The remainder had diastolic dysfunction or a preserved ejection fraction. The overall prevalence of LV systolic dysfunction in symptomatic and asymptomatic patients was 10.8% [14].

In 1997, a subset analysis of 1980 patients in the Rotterdam Study who had undergone echocardiographic study was published. Impaired LV function, defined as fractional shortening less than 25% (comparable to a LV ejection fraction of 42.5%), was reported in 3% of these subjects. Consistent with previous studies, the prevalence of LV systolic dysfunction was higher in those aged over 70 years (4.2%) [15].

More recently, the EPICA study was performed to estimate the prevalence of heart failure in mainland Portugal. Between April and October 1998, 551 patients (208 males, 343 females) out of a total 5434 subjects enrolled from various health care centers in the community were identified as having heart failure by a combination of clinical and echocardiographic criteria. Echocardiographic evidence of LV dysfunction was defined by LV fractional shortening below 28%, evidence of LV hypertrophy and/or chamber enlargement, moderate to severe valvular disease, or moderate to severe pericardial effusion. The estimated prevalence of all types of heart failure was 1.36% in those aged 25–49, 12.67% in ages 70–79, and 16.14% in those over 80 years of age. About 40% had preserved LV function, or a normal ejection fraction [16].

Table 1.1 summarizes the prevalence of heart failure as estimated from various population-based studies.

Table 1.1 Prevalence of heart failure

Study	Location	Study date	Overall prevalence rate	Prevalence rate in older population
Physician records/prescriptions				
Rodeheffer et al. [7]	Rochester, US	1981–1982	3/1000	–
REACH [8]	Southeast Michigan, US	1999	14.3/1000 (women) 14.5/1000 (men)	–
Murphy et al. [9]	Scotland	April 1999 to March 2000	7.1/1000	90.1/1000 (>85 years)
Clinical criteria				
Framingham [10, 11]	Framingham, US	1980–1989	7.7/1000 (women) 7.4/1000 (men)	79/1000 (80–89 years) 66/1000 (80–89 years)
Garrison et al. [12]	Georgia, US	1960–1962	21/1000	35/1000 (65–74 years)
Echocardiographic and clinical criteria				
Helsinki [14]	Helsinki, Finland	1990–1991	–	82/1000 (75–86 years)
Rotterdam [15]	Ommoord, Netherlands	1997	30/1000 (>55 years)	42/1000 (>70 years)
EPICA [16]	Portugal	1998	12.9/1000 (systolic dysfunction)	~30/1000 (>80 years)

Over the last decade, there has been a significant rise in the prevalence of heart failure. In the REACH study, for example, the prevalence rose from 3.7 per 1000 and 4.0 per 1000 in women and men, respectively, to 14.3 and 14.5 per 1000 between 1989 and 1999 [8]. This is likely attributable, in large part, to the increasing proportion of elderly people in the population, as these individuals have the highest incidence of coronary artery disease and hypertension, which are strongly correlated with the development of heart failure. In addition, the survival in those patients with coronary artery disease is improving. As myocardial infarction is the most powerful risk factor for heart failure, it follows that increasing survival post-myocardial infarction may lead to a higher prevalence of heart failure later in life. Improving mortality rates among patients with heart failure may also be playing a role [17].

Incidence of heart failure

Information on the incidence of heart failure and the change over time is much more limited than prevalence data. Results of some of the various studies on the incidence of heart failure are summarized in Table 1.2.

Similar to the prevalence data, several studies have documented the rising incidence of heart failure with age. The Framingham Heart Study, for example, showed that the annual incidence increased from 3 cases per 1000 in men aged 50–59 years to 27 cases per 1000 in men aged 80–89 years. A similar increase, from 2 to 22 cases per 1000 in the same age brackets, was seen among women. Furthermore, the incidence of heart failure was found to be one-third lower in women than men after adjustment for age. During the 1980s, the age-adjusted annual incidence of heart failure was 2.3 and 1.4 cases per 1000 in men and women, respectively [11].

Likewise, the Rotterdam study showed a jump in the incidence rate of heart failure from 1.4 cases per 1000 in those aged 50–59 to 47.4 per 1000 in those 90 years or older. The overall incidence of heart failure was 14.4 per 1000 person-years and was significantly higher in men (17.6 per 1000 man-years) compared with women (12.5 per 1000 woman-years) [13]. These age and gender trends were confirmed in a study of incident cases of heart failure in Olmstead County, Minnesota in 1991 [18] and another study of 696 884 people in a general practice population in the UK [19].

Of great debate recently is whether the incidence of heart failure is decreasing in response to advances in medical treatment for heart failure. Data from the Framingham Heart Study were published in 2002 and suggested that over the last 50 years the incidence of heart failure amidst a cohort of 10 311 subjects has declined among women but not among men. In men, for example, the age-adjusted inci-

Table 1.2 Incidence of heart failure

Study	Location	Study date	Overall incidence rate	Incidence rate in older population
Framingham [10, 11]	Framingham, US 1.4/1000 (women) 22/1000 (women ≥80 years)	1980–1989	2.3/1000 (men)	27/1000 (men ≥80 years)
Rodeheffer et al. [7]	Minnesota, US	1981–1982	1.6/1000 (men)	9.4/1000 (men 70–74 years)
			0.7/1000 (women)	9.8/1000 (women 70–74 years)
Senni et al. [18]	Minnesota, US	1991	2/1000	
De Giuli et al. [19]	UK	1991	9.3/1000	45/1000 (≥85 years)
Rotterdam [13]	Ommoord, Netherlands	1997–1999	17.6/1000 (men ≥55 years)	47.4/1000 (≥90 years)
			12.5/1000 (women ≥55 years)	
Roger et al. [1]	Minnesota, US	1979–2000	3.8/1000 (men)	
			2.9/1000 (women)	

dence of heart failure from 1950 to 1969 was 627 cases/100 000 person-years (95% confidence interval (CI) 475–779), as compared with 564 (95% CI 463–665) cases/100 000 person-years between 1990 and 1999 (rate ratio 0.93, 95% CI 0.71–1.23). In contrast, for women the age-adjusted incidence of heart failure fell from 420 cases/100 000 person-years (95% CI 336–504) to 327 cases/100 000 person-years (95% CI 266–388, rate ratio 0.69 [95% CI 0.51–0.93]) over the same period [2]. However, a recent population-based cohort study conducted in Olmstead County, Minnesota was not able to corroborate these findings. Among 4537 residents (57% women, mean age 74 years) with a diagnosis of heart failure identified between 1979 and 2000, the incidence of heart failure did not change over time in either gender [1].

Mortality of heart failure

The mortality of heart failure is alarmingly high. Data derived from the Framingham cohort published in 1993, for example, suggested that the overall one-year survival rates in men and women were 57% and 64% respectively. The overall five-year survival rates were 25% in men and 38% in women. In comparison, five-year survival for all cancers among men and women in the United States during that same period was about 50% [11]. Survival tends to be better in women. Furthermore, the mortality of heart failure appears to increase with age. For example, a Scottish study examining 66 547 patients admitted with heart failure between January 1986 and December 1995 reported the 30-day mortality rate in patients less than 55 years of age to be 10.41% and the five-year mortality rate to be 46.75%. In contrast, the 30-day and five-year mortality in patients 75–84 years of age was 22.18% and 88% respectively [20]. The underlying cause of heart failure also appears to influence prognosis, as patients with ischemic cardiomyopathy suffer an overall higher mortality.

Recent studies, however, suggest that with the advent of improved medical therapies, survival in patients with heart failure may be improving. Among subjects in the Framingham Heart Study cohort, for example, the 30-day, one-year, and five-year age-adjusted mortality rates among men declined from 12%, 30%, and 70%, respectively, in the period from 1950 to 1969 to 11%, 28%, and 59%, respectively, in the period from 1990 to 1999. The corresponding rates among women were 18%, 28%, and 57% for the period from 1950 to 1969 and 10%, 24%, and 45% for the period from 1990 to 1999. Overall, there was an improvement in the survival rate after the onset of heart failure of 12% per decade [2]. These data were corroborated by a study conducted in Olmsted County, Minnesota in which the five-year age-adjusted survival was found to be 43% during the period from 1979 to 1984 as compared with 52% in the period from 1996 to 2000 [1].

Though the reasons for the decline in heart failure mortality over time are not completely understood, the advent of improved medical therapies has almost certainly played a central role. Angiotensin-converting enzyme (ACE) inhibitors, beta-blockers, and spironolactone, for example, have significantly reduced mortality and morbidity in New York Heart Association (NYHA) class II–IV patients while improving their quality of life [22–24]. The benefits of drug therapy are limited, however, and despite aggressive medical treatment for heart failure many are left with grave debilitation. This has spawned great interest in a variety of non-pharmacologic treatments for patients with drug-refractory heart failure. Heart transplant remains the best solution, but it can only be applied to a restricted number of patients and the supply of donor hearts is limited. Thus investigation has continued, searching for other therapies to improve symptoms and/or survival in patients with end-stage cardiomyopathies.

Permanent dual-chamber pacing with a short atrioventricular delay, for example, had been proposed over a decade ago as an adjuvant treatment for advanced heart failure based on the observation of prolonged PR intervals in patients with chronic symptoms of the syndrome. However, the initially encouraging data from early studies were not substantiated with long-term follow-up during prospective studies. Perhaps one of the major reasons for the failure of standard dual-chamber pacing is that in patients with chronic LV dysfunction, although it corrects (at least in part) atrioventricular asynchrony of the left heart, it also enhances the electromechanical consequences of intraventricular conduction delay which are often found in such patients.

Indeed, a wide QRS complex is frequently observed in patients with chronic heart failure associated with LV systolic dysfunction and has been associated with a significantly higher mortality in this population. This is likely in part due to the deleterious effects that intraventricular conduction delay (IVCD) has on both systolic function and LV filling, as well as its propensity to aggravate functional mitral regurgitation. Together, these factors have made IVCD an attractive target for heart failure therapy.

Epidemiology of intraventricular conduction delay

Data on the prevalence and prognosis of intraventricular conduction delay, manifesting as either right bundle branch block (RBBB) or left bundle branch block (LBBB), are difficult to compare, as patient populations (and associated comorbidities) vary widely from one study to another. Nevertheless, taken collectively, these studies suggest that IVCD in the general population becomes more common with advancing age and is often associated with hypertension, diabetes, coronary artery disease, or cardiomegaly; heart failure is also often found. As a frequent marker of underlying cardiovascular disease, both LBBB and RBBB have been shown to be associated with higher mortality, though the data on mortality with BBB in the general population are conflicting.

Intraventricular conduction delays are much more common in patients with heart failure, and in this setting carry a much more ominous prognosis. Several studies have documented the link between IVCD and symptomatic heart failure and have identified a trend between progressive widening of the QRS interval and higher mortality.

Prevalence of intraventricular conduction delay

Table 1.3 summarizes some of the various studies on the prevalence of IVCD.

The prevalence of IVCD in the general population is fairly low, but seems to increase with age. Both points are illustrated in a study of the community of Tecumseh, Michigan performed between 1959 and 1960. Subjects ranged in age from 16 to greater than 80 years. In this cohort, the prevalence of BBB was found to be quite low. Out of 8541 subjects, 18 (12 women, 6 men) were found to have LBBB (0.2%) and 18 (6 women, 12 men) were found to have RBBB (0.2%). Over 67% of those with BBB were older than 67 years [25]. The relatively low frequency of BBB in a healthy population was again seen in a study by Rotman et al., looking at a series of over 237 000 ECGs on US Air Force flying personnel or training applicants. The prevalence of RBBB and LBBB was 0.16% (394 men) and 0.05% (125 men), respectively [26].

Table 1.3 Prevalence of intraventricular conduction delay

Study	Location	Study date	Overall prevalence rate	Prevalence rate in older population
In the general population:				
Ostrander [25]	Michigan, US	1959–1960	2/1000 (RBBB) 2/1000 (LBBB)	RBBB: 29/1000 (≥60 years) LBBB: 6/1000 (≥60 years)
Rotman and Triebwasser [26]	Texas, US	1957–1972	1.6/1000 (RBBB) 0.5/1000 (LBBB)	–
Edmands [27]	California, US	1962–1966	–	RBBB: 24/1000 (≥52 years) LBBB: 12/1000 (≥52 years)
Study of Men Born 1913 [28]	Goteborg, Sweden	1963–1993	7/1000 (RBBB) 4/1000 (LBBB)	RBBB: 113/1000 (80 years) LBBB: 57/1000 (80 years)
In patients with heart failure:				
Shanim et al. [32]	London, UK	1993–1996	369/1000 (QRS>120 ms)	–
IN-CHF [31]	Italy	1995–2000	61/1000 (RBBB) 252/1000 (LBBB)	–

LBBB, left bundle branch block; RBBB: right bundle branch block.

Edmands, who looked at BBB in a retirement community of residents over the age of 52 in Seal Beach, California found the prevalence of BBB to be 3.7% (57 out of 1560 patients). Nineteen residents (1.2%) had LBBB (8 men, 11 women) and another 38 residents (2.4%) had RBBB (24 men, 14 women). A total of 18 (94.7%) of those with LBBB and 32 (84%) of those with RBBB were 65 years or older, again confirming the association of IVCD with increasing age. About 50% of those with LBBB had cardiomegaly on chest X-ray compared with 16% of controls [27]. The prevalence of BBB was slightly higher in another study of the population of men born in 1913. Of 855 men examined, 82 (9.6%) had BBB. The prevalence of BBB increased from 1% at age 50 years to 17% at age 80 [28].

In contrast, the prevalence of IVCD among patients with heart failure has been found to be markedly higher than in the general population. In a study of 34 patients with serial ECGs performed before death secondary to necropsy-proven idiopathic dilated cardiomyopathy, for example, 13 (38%) were found to have BBB. Of these 13 patients, 10 had LBBB [29]. Later, Xiao *et al.* examined the prevalence of IVCD in 58 patients with dilated cardiomyopathy. A QRS duration of >160 ms was seen in 19 (33%) of these patients [30]. Another study of 5517 patients with heart failure selected from the Italian Network on CHF (IN-CHF) registry between 1995 and January 2000 also demonstrated a high prevalence of IVCD in heart failure patients. A total of 1391 patients (25.2%) were found to have complete LBBB; 336 (6.1%) had complete RBBB. Other forms of IVCD were diagnosed in 339 (6.1%) of patients [31]. Yet another study examined 241 patients with systolic heart failure admitted to the Royal Bromptom Hospital between July 1993 and March 1996. From these 241 patients, 89 (37%) were diagnosed with IVCD (defined as QRS duration >120 ms). Of these, 52 had a QRS duration of 120–160 ms, and the remaining 37 had a QRS >160 ms [32].

Prognosis of intraventricular conduction delay

The mortality data on IVCD among the general population is somewhat conflicting. Smith *et al.*, for example, who looked at 29 naval aviators whose ECGs changed from a normal pattern to that of a BBB, found no significant increase in mortality when compared with a control cohort of 666 men [33]. Likewise, in the study of men born in 1913, there was no correlation found between the development of BBB and either (1) risk factors for coronary artery disease at age 50 years, (2) incidence of myocardial infarction during follow-up, or (3) cardiovascular deaths [28].

However, the Framingham Study found a significant correlation between LBBB and increased mortality and the development of heart disease. A total of 55 people (31 men, 24 women) who developed LBBB after the initial study examination were identified among the 5209 people enrolled. Before the onset of LBBB, case subjects had a statistically significant excess of most of the designated cardiovascular abnormalities (65% had hypertension, 44% had cardiomegaly on chest X-ray, 20% had known coronary artery disease; only 27% had no cardiovascular disease). One-third of those case subjects who were free from clinical coronary disease before the onset of LBBB developed one of its manifestations coincident with or after the first appearance of LBBB. At each two-year interval after the onset of LBBB the cumulative mortality rate from cardiovascular disease was approximately five times greater in the case subjects than in controls. About 50% of those with LBBB died of cardiovascular disease within 10 years of onset of LBBB, compared with only 11.6% of similar-aged controls. After correcting for the influence of diabetes, systolic blood pressure, age, coronary artery disease, and heart failure, the relationship between LBBB and risk of cardiovascular mortality was still statistically significant in men (but not women) [34].

Likewise, in a study of 146 patients with LBBB who had been admitted to the University of Kansas Medical Center or Kansas City Veterans Administration Hospital between 1954 and 1963, the average duration of survival after the conduction disturbance had been diagnosed was 36 months [35]. Similar survival data (3.3 years) were found in a study of 555 patients with LBBB who had been admitted to the Massachusetts General Hospital between 1937 and 1948. Almost one-half of the case subjects in this study whose QRS duration exceeded 160 ms had marked cardiac enlargement. Heart size correlated to survival; patients without cardiac enlargement survived 4.3 years compared with 2.5 years in those with marked cardiomegaly. A total of

429 patients (77%) had either hypertension, coronary artery disease or both. Of the 357 deaths that had occurred at the end of the study, 255 (71%) were attributed to heart disease, with the majority having either heart failure or myocardial infarction [36]. The higher mortality and stronger association of LBBB with cardiovascular disease is perhaps a reflection of bias imposed by selecting an inpatient population with clinical indication for ECG.

In patients with cardiomyopathy, strong evidence exists to suggest that LBBB is associated with a significantly higher mortality. In the study by Xiao and his colleagues, for example, a QRS duration of >160 ms was found in 8 out of 10 patients who died (80%), but only 5 of the 39 stable patients (12.8%). QRS duration tended to widen over time [30]. Another study by Shamim *et al.* took 241 heart failure patients and divided them into three groups: those with QRS <120 ms, those with QRS 120–160 ms, and those with QRS duration exceeding 160 ms. All patients were then followed to determine their 36-month mortality rates. Of the 141 patients with QRS <120 ms, 27 (20%) had died at 36 months, compared with 18/52 patients (36%) with QRS 120–160 ms and 19/37 patients (58.3%) with IVCD of greater than 160 ms. Thus, IVCD was shown to have negative prognostic value in patients with heart failure, with a stepwise increase in mortality as a graded increase in the IVCD occurs [32]. The deleterious effect of LBBB was further demonstrated in a study of patients with heart failure from the IN-CHF registry. Of the 659 patients (from a total 5517 enrolled, 11.9%) who died during the one-year follow-up period, the one-year all-cause mortality rate for patients with LBBB was 16.1% (224 of 1391). This rate was 11.9% (40 of 336) for patients with RBBB. All-cause mortality and mortality rates as the result of sudden death were significantly greater among patients with LBBB. Increased mortality rates were not seen in patients with RBBB [31, 37].

In summary, LBBB results in significant intraventricular (LV) and interventricular dyssynchrony. Clinical consequences include significant impairment in systolic and diastolic function and functional mitral regurgitation. Dyssynchrony decreases cardiac efficiency and increases sympathetic activity. In patients with normal LV function, these changes are generally well-tolerated. However, in patients with severe LV dysfunction and symptomatic heart failure the results can be more profound and can contribute significantly to the increased morbidity and mortality observed in patients with IVCD and heart failure. These factors made IVCD a reasonable target for adjuvant therapy in this population. Biventricular pacing, by partially restoring intra- and interventricular synchrony, has the potential to mitigate the deleterious hemodynamic consequences of IVCD described above.

Summary

- Heart failure is a major public health problem in industrialized countries, the prevalence of which appears to be rising over the last decade.
- The incidence and prevalence of heart failure seem to increase with age.
- The prognosis in heart failure patients remains poor, with mortality data similar to the worse forms of malignant disease. Recent studies, however, suggest that survival in heart failure may be improving, concurrent with the advent of improved medical therapy.
- IVCD is frequently seen in patients with heart failure and is a marker of higher mortality in this population. Thus IVCD has become an attractive target for heart failure therapy.
- IVCD, particularly LBBB, results in significant intra- and interventricular dyssynchrony, with clinical consequences that include impairment of systolic and diastolic function and aggravation of functional mitral regurgitation.
- Biventricular pacing, by partially restoring intra- and interventricular synchrony, has the potential to mitigate the deleterious consequences imposed by IVCD.

References

1 Roger VL, Weston SA, Redfield MM *et al.* Trends in heart failure incidence and survival in a community-based population. *JAMA* 2004; **292**: 344–350.
2 Levy D, Kenchaiah S, Larson MG *et al.* Long-term trends in the incidence of and survival with heart failure. *N Engl J Med* 2002; **347**: 1397–1402.
3 Lloyd-Jones DM, Larson MG, Leip EP *et al.* Lifetime risk for developing congestive heart failure: The Framingham Heart Study. *Circulation* 2002; **106**: 3068–3072.
4 Haldeman GA, Croft JB, Giles WH *et al.* Hospitalization

of patients with heart failure: National Hospital Discharge Survey, 1985 to 1995. *Am Heart J* 1999; **137**: 352–360.

5 Davis RC, Hobbs FDR, Lip GYH. History and epidemiology. (Clinical Review: ABC of heart failure). *BMJ* 2000; **320**: 39–42.

6 Cleland JGF. Health economic consequences of the pharmacologic treatment of heart failure. *Eur Heart J* 1998; **19**: P32–39.

7 Rodeheffer RJ, Jacobsen SJ, Gersh BJ *et al.* The incidence and prevalence of congestive heart failure in Rochester, Minnesota. *Mayo Clin Proc* 1993; **68**: 1143–1150.

8 McCullough PA, Philbin EF, Spertus JA *et al.* Confirmation of a heart failure epidemic: Findings from the Resource Utilization Among Congestive Heart Failure (REACH) study. *J Am Coll Cardiol* 2002; **39**: 60–69.

9 Murphy NF, Simpson CR, McAlister FA *et al.* National Survey of the prevalence, incidence, primary care burden, and treatment of heart failure in Scotland. *Heart* 2004; **90**: 1129–1136.

10 McKee PA, Castelli WP, McNamara PM *et al.* The natural history of congestive heart failure: The Framingham Study. *N Engl J Med* 1971; **285**: 1441–1446.

11 Ho KKL, Pinsky JL, Kannel WB, *et al.* The epidemiology of heart failure: The Framingham Study. *J Am Coll Cardiol* 1993; **22**: 6A–13A.

12 Garrison GE, McDonough JR, Hames CG *et al.* Prevalence of chronic congestive heart failure in the population of Evans County, Georgia. *Am J Epidemiol* 1966; **83**: 338–344.

13 Bleumink GS, Knetsch AM, Sturkenboom MCJM *et al.* Quantifying the heart failure epidemic: prevalence, incidence rate, lifetime risk and prognosis of heart failure: The Rotterdam Study. *Eur Heart J* 2004; **25**: 1614–1619.

14 Kupari M, Lindroos M, Ilvanainen AM *et al.* Congestive heart failure in old age: prevalence, mechanisms and 4-year prognosis in the Helsinki Ageing Study. *J Intern Med* 1997; **241**: 387–394.

15 Mosterd A, de Bruijne MC, Hoes AW *et al.* Usefulness of echocardiography in detecting left ventricular dysfunction in population-based studies: The Rotterdam Study. *Am J Cardiol* 1997; **79**: 103–104.

16 Ceia F, Fonseca C, Mota T *et al.* Prevalence of chronic heart failure in Southwestern Europe: the EPICA study. *Eur J Heart Failure* 2002; **4**: 531–539.

17 Stewart S, MacIntyre K, Capewell S *et al.* Heart failure and the aging population: an increasing burden in the 21st century? *Heart* 2003; **89**: 49–53.

18 Senni M, Tribouilloy CM, Rodeheffer RJ *et al.* Congestive heart failure in the community: A study of all incident cases in Olmstead County, Minnesota, in 1991. *Circulation* 1998; **98**: 2282–2289.

19 De Giuli F, Khaw K, Cowie MR *et al.* Incidence and outcome of persons with a clinical diagnosis of heart failure

in a general population of 696,884 in the United Kingdom. *Eur J Heart Failure* 2005; **7**: 295–302.

20 Ho KKL, Anderson KM, Kannel WB *et al.* Survival after the onset of congestive heart failure in Framingham Heart Study patients. *Circulation* 1993; **88**: 107–115.

21 MacIntyre K, Capewell S, Stewart S *et al.* Evidence of improving prognosis in heart failure: trends in case fatality in 66,547 patients hospitalized between 1986 and 1995. *Circulation* 2000; **102**: 1126–1131.

22 The CONSENSUS Trial Study Group. Effects of enalapril on mortality in severe congestive heart failure: Results of the Cooperative North Scandinavian Enalapril Survival Study (CONSENSUS). *N Engl J Med* 1987; **316**: 1429–1435.

23 Bristow MR. B-Adrenergic receptor blockade in chronic heart failure. *Circulation* 2000; **101**: 558–569.

24 Pitt B, Zannad F, Remme WJ *et al.* The effect of spironolactone on morbidity and mortality in patients with severe heart failure. *N Engl J Med* 1999; **341**: 709–717.

25 Ostrander LD. Bundle-branch block. *Circulation* 1964; **30**: 872–881.

26 Rotman M, Triebwasser JH. A clinical follow-up study of right and left bundle branch block. *Circulation* 1975; **51**: 477–483.

27 Edmands RE. An epidemiologic assessment of bundle-branch block. *Circulation* 1966; **34**: 1081–1087.

28 Eriksson P, Hansson P, Eriksson H *et al.* Bundle-branch block in a general male population: The Study of Men Born 1913. *Circulation* 1998; **98**: 2494–2500.

29 Wilensky RL, Yudelman P, Cohen AI *et al.* Serial electrocardiographic changes in idiopathic dilated cardiomyopathy confirmed at necropsy. *Am J Cardiol* 1988; **62**: 276–283.

30 Xiao HB, Roy C, Fujimoto S *et al.* Natural history of abnormal conduction and its relation to prognosis in patients with dilated cardiomyopathy. *Int J Cardiol* 1996; **53**: 163–170.

31 Baldasseroni S, Opasich C, Gorini M *et al.* Left bundle branch block is associated with increased 1-year sudden and total mortality rate in 5517 outpatients with congestive heart failure: A report from the Italian Network on Congestive Heart Failure. *Am Heart J* 2002; **143**: 398–405.

32 Shamim W, Francis DP, Yousufuddin M *et al.* Intraventricular conduction delay: a prognostic marker in chronic heart failure. *Int J Cardiol* 1999; **70**: 171–178.

33 Smith RF, Jackson DH, Harthorne *et al.* Acquired bundle branch block in a healthy population. *Am Heart J* 1970; **6**: 746–751.

34 Schneider JF, Thomas HE, Kreger BE *et al.* Newly acquired left bundle-branch block: The Framingham Study. *Ann Intern Med* 1979; **90**: 303–310.

35 Smith S, Hayes WL. The prognosis of complete left bun-

dle branch block. *Am Heart J* 1965; **70**: 157–159.

36 Johnson RP, Messer AL, Shreenivas *et al.* Prognosis in bundle branch block II. Factors influencing the survival period in left bundle branch block. *Am Heart J* 1951; **41**: 225–238.

37 Baldasseroni S, Gentile A, Gorini M *et al.* Intraventricular conduction defects in patients with congestive heart failure: left but not right bundle branch block is an independent predictor of prognosis: A report from the Italian Network on Congestive Heart Failure (IN-CHF database). *Ital Heart J* 2003; **4**: 607–613.

38 Bramlet DA, Morris KG, Coleman RE *et al.* Effects of rate-dependent left bundle branch block on global and regional left ventricular function. *Circulation* 1983; **67**: 1059–1065.

39 Curry CW, Nelson GS, Wyman BT *et al.* Mechanical dyssynchrony in dilated cardiomyopathy with intraventricular conduction delay as depicted by 3D tagged magnetic resonance imaging. *Circulation* 2000; **101**: e2.

40 Grines CL, Bashore TM, Boudoulas H *et al.* Functional abnormalities in isolated left bundle branch block: The effect of interventricular asynchrony. *Circulation* 1989; **79**: 845–853.

41 Breithardt OA, Sinha AM, Schwammenthal E *et al.* Acute effects of cardiac resynchronization therapy on functional mitral regurgitation in advanced systolic heart failure. *J Am Coll Cardiol* 2003; **41**: 765–770.

CHAPTER 2

Comprehensive pharmacologic management strategies for heart failure

Garrie J. Haas, MD, FACC *& William T. Abraham,* MD, FACP, FACC

Introduction

Over the past two decades, we have seen significant advances in the pharmacologic approach to heart failure management. The results from large multicenter clinical trials have identified the benefit of polypharmacy directed primarily at neurohormonal antagonism. The development of treatment strategies based on these results now forms the foundation of therapy for all classes and stages of heart failure due to systolic left ventricular (LV) dysfunction. The recently published 2005 American College of Cardiology/American Heart Association (ACC/AHA) Guidelines for the Management of Chronic Heart Failure provide the best template to facilitate medical therapy [1]. Major efforts are underway to assure adherence to these guidelines in clinical practice [2].

While there has been a significant positive impact on heart failure outcomes with the advent of new pharmacologic approaches to treatment, the disease remains burdensome concerning quality of life, hospitalizations, and mortality while producing major economic stress on the health care system. Even though we have observed a significant annual mortality improvement in some of our more rigorously controlled clinical trials, observational data from large heart failure populations continue to report unacceptably high one- and five-year age-adjusted mortality rates, thus reinforcing the fact that there is still much progress to be made in the treatment of this chronic disorder [3].

Pharmacologic modulation of the neurohormonal system in heart failure provides the foundation for our therapeutic approach in all patients with the disease. The goal of this treatment is to retard the pathologic remodeling process that, if left unchecked, leads to progressive ventricular dysfunction, disease progression, and irreversible myocardial injury (Fig. 2.1). While the era of device therapy for heart failure is currently expanding at a tremendous rate, the clinician should be aware of the importance of achieving specific pharmacologic goals in their heart failure patients. It should be recognized that in most clinical situations, a comprehensive pharmacologic strategy is desired prior to advancing to devices designed to treat heart failure.

In this chapter, the role for neurohormonal antagonism and additional medical therapies for treating chronic heart failure due to LV systolic dysfunction will be reviewed and a practical pharmacologic strategy for treatment will be presented. Treatment concepts will parallel the heart failure staging nomenclature initially put forth by the 2001 ACC/AHA Guidelines [4]. This staging system emphasizes both the evolution and progression of heart failure and is complementary to the traditional New York Heart Association (NYHA) classification scheme, which is based on subjective symptomatic status. Both classification systems are clinically useful, particularly with respect to treatment strategies.

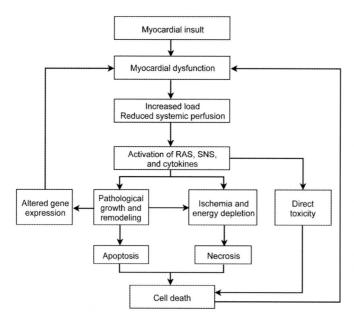

Figure 2.1 The mechanisms of heart failure progression are triggered by neurohormonal activation following myocardial insult leading to ventricular dysfunction. RAS, renin angiotensin system; SNS, sympathetic nervous system. From Cohn JN, Johnson GR, Shabetai R, *et al*. Ejection fraction, peak exercise oxygen consumption, cardiothoracic ratio, ventricular arrhythmias, and plasma norepinephrine as determinants of prognosis in heart failure. *Circulation* 1993; **87** (suppl V1): 5–16 with permission.

The ACC/AHA staging system (stages A–D) allows for an improved matching of therapies based on disease progression and also emphasizes the importance of aggressively managing diseases that place patients at risk for heart failure [5]. Stage A patients have multiple risk factors for heart failure, such as diabetes, coronary artery disease, and hypertension but do not manifest cardiac structural abnormalities. Stage B patients have LV structural abnormalities but do not have symptoms of heart failure. In other words, these patients have asymptomatic LV dysfunction. Stages C and D represent those patients with current or prior symptomatic heart failure that

responds to (stage C) or is refractory to (stage D) maximal medical therapy (Fig. 2.2). This chapter will focus primarily on stage B and C patients.

In addition to reviewing chronic heart failure treatment guidelines, pharmacotherapy of acute decompensation of chronic heart failure (ADHF), a condition where there is a paucity of evidence-based guidelines, will be briefly discussed. Treatment of the decompensated patient is often empiric with a greater reliance on specific hemodynamic goals. Significant heterogeneity exists concerning treatment approaches and is generally "tradition-based" rather than "evidence-based."

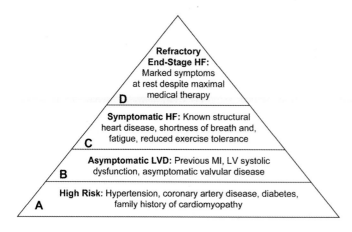

Figure 2.2 Disease progression of heart failure: ACC/AHA Heart Failure Stages. LVD, LV dysfunction. Adapted from Hunt SA, Baker DW, Chin MH *et al*. 2001 ACC/AHA Guidelines for the evaluation and management of chronic heart failure in the adult: executive summary. A report of the American College of Cardiology/American Heart Association Task Force on Practice Guidelines (Committee to Revise the 1995 Guidelines for the Evaluation and Management of Heart Failure). *Circulation* 2001; **104**: 2996–3007 with permission.

The pharmacotherapy of neurohormonal antagonism: the basis of chronic heart failure management

Angiotensin-converting enzyme inhibitors

The benefit of neurohormonal antagonism in patients with chronic heart failure secondary to LV systolic dysfunction is well accepted and has been supported by a large number of clinical trials over the past 20 years. This success supports the construct that inappropriate neurohormonal activation in patients with heart failure contributes to the pathologic process of LV remodeling. Strategies designed to inhibit the detrimental effect of angiotensin II on the cardiovascular system are utilized in all NYHA classes and ACC/AHA stages of heart failure. The effectiveness of inhibiting the renin–angiotensin–aldosterone system (RAAS) has been recognized since the publication of the landmark Cooperative North Scandinavian Enalapril Survival Study (CONSENSUS) in 1987 [6]. This trial demonstrated a profound reduction in mortality in severely ill NYHA class IV heart failure patients when the angiotensin-converting enzyme (ACE) inhibitor enalapril was added to digoxin and diuretics. These favorable results formed the basis for the neurohormonal interdiction hypothesis of heart failure management, which is now a universally accepted concept.

Studies following CONSENSUS reinforced this concept, reporting efficacy of ACE inhibition in the post-myocardial setting as well as in large cohorts of patients with asymptomatic to moderately symptomatic LV dysfunction [7–10]. The aggregate impact of ACE inhibitors on the survival of patients with symptomatic heart failure is a 15–20% improvement in the annual risk of death. ACE inhibitors have been studied in thousands of heart failure patients and have consistently improved symptoms, exercise tolerance, and quality of life measures. Therefore, strong evidence-based data exist for the benefit of ACE inhibition in patients presenting with LV dysfunction, regardless of functional class.

Although the benefit of ACE inhibitor therapy was initially thought to result primarily from attenuation of the harmful vasoconstrictive actions of angiotensin II (supporting the hemodynamic model of heart failure management), it is now recognized that

angiotensin II may cause deleterious effects on the cardiovascular system via multiple mechanisms, including atherogenic, profibrotic, and thrombogenic actions in addition to direct myocardial effects and augmentation of aldosterone activity [11] (Table 2.1). Indeed, a potential vasculoprotective effect of ACE inhibitors in addition to their known myocardial protective properties is supported by the results from the Heart Outcomes Prevention Evaluation (HOPE) trial, which identified a 17% relative risk reduction in new heart failure episodes when ACE inhibitor therapy (ramipril) was administered to patients with vascular disease or diabetes plus one additional risk factor in the absence of LV dysfunction [12].

The complete mechanism by which ACE inhibitors improve heart failure outcomes remains uncertain given the observation that angiotensin II levels, via ACE-independent conversion of angiotensin I to angiotensin II, gradually approach pretreatment levels weeks to months after initiation of ACE inhibition (ACE escape). It is speculated that potentiation of bradykinin activity, resulting from an ACE inhibitor-induced decrease in bradykinin metabolism, contributes to the therapeutic benefit of ACE inhibitors. Bradykinin promotes natriuresis and increases nitric oxide production by vascular endothelium resulting in vasodilation (Fig. 2.3). Additional mechanisms by which ACE inhibitors improve outcomes in heart failure, including anti-inflammatory actions and effects on oxidative stress, may also be operative [11].

Clinical use of ACE inhibitors

ACE inhibitors are recommended in heart failure stages B, C, and D (Fig. 2.4). Therefore, all patients

Table 2.1 Proposed actions of angiotensin II contributing to heart failure progression

Vasoconstriction
Sodium retention ($\uparrow$ Aldosterone)
Myocyte hypertrophy
Myocyte apoptosis
Vascular fibroproliferation
Endothelial dysfunction
$\uparrow$ Endothelin
Sympathetic activation
$\downarrow$ Thrombolysis
$\uparrow$ Oxygen free radicals

$\uparrow$ Increased; $\downarrow$ decreased.

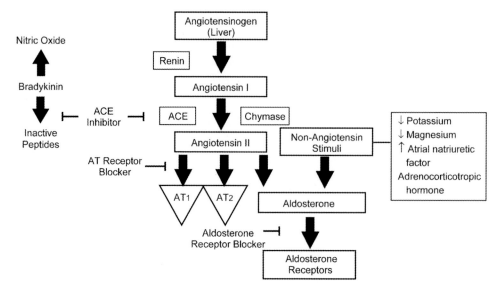

Figure 2.3 Activation of the renin–angiotensin–aldosterone system. Angiotensin II is converted from angiotensin I through angiotensin-converting enzyme (ACE) and chymase-dependent pathways. Angiotensin II produces its biologic effects by binding to angiotensin (AT) receptors. Aldosterone production is stimulated by angiotensin II as well as non-angiotensin mechanisms. ACE inhibitors block ACE-dependent conversion of angiotensin I to angiotensin II and prevent catabolism of bradykinin leading to increase nitric oxide production. Modified from Mann DL, Deswal A, Bozkurt B *et al*. New therapeutics for chronic heart failure. *Annu Rev Med* 2002; **53**: 59–74 with permission.

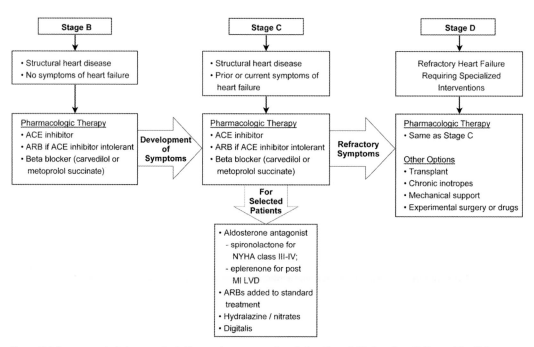

Figure 2.4 Recommended pharmacologic therapy for heart failure with left ventricular dysfunction; ACC/AHA Stages B, C and D. ACE, angiotensin-converting enzyme; ARB, angiotensin receptor blocker; NYHA, New York Heart Association Class; ACC, American College of Cardiology; AHA, American Heart Association; MI, myocardial infarction; LVD, left ventricular dysfunction. Adapted from Hunt SA, Abraham WT, Chin MH *et al*. [1] with permission.

with current or prior symptoms of heart failure and LV systolic dysfunction should be treated with an ACE inhibitor unless there is a major contraindication. Generally, the dose of ACE inhibitor shown to reduce cardiovascular events in the major clinical trials should be utilized, with the understanding that target dosing may not be achievable due to adverse effects (Table 2.2). Fortunately, there seem to be only small differences in clinical efficacy between low- and high-dose ACE inhibitors in most patients so it remains advantageous to administer intermediate or low-dose ACE inhibitor rather than stopping the drug completely [13].

The majority of symptomatic patients with stage C heart failure will be treated with multiple agents, including diuretics, which may limit the dose of ACE inhibitor tolerated because of hypotension or renal insufficiency. There is a reciprocal relationship that exists between ACE inhibitor dose and diuretic dose regarding tolerability. Typically, the higher the diuretic requirement, the more sensitive the blood pressure and renal function to ACE inhibitor treatment and the more carefully the drug should be initiated and titrated. Patients with hyponatremia secondary to symptomatic heart failure and volume retention are often exquisitely sensitive to ACE inhibitors. None the less, in the CONSENSUS trial, these patients derived significant benefit from ACE inhibitors and every effort should be made to maintain this treatment. During ACE inhibitor titration, renal function and serum potassium should be followed closely. The development of a cough should raise the question of worsening pulmonary congestion due to heart failure but may also be related to ACE inhibition in 5–10% of cases. The ACE inhibitor cough, which is typically non-productive and unpredictable, is probably related to increased kinin levels and therefore, switching to treatment with an angiotensin receptor blocker (see below) is often effective.

The question of whether concomitant aspirin therapy counteracts ACE inhibitor effects has been raised, but at the present time there are no definitive data concerning this issue. If aspirin therapy is indicated, most clinicians will administer low doses in patients requiring ACE inhibitors.

Angiotensin receptor blockers

The concept of enhanced blockade of the RAAS with the addition of a direct angiotensin II receptor (AT1) blocking agent is attractive and has been evaluated in multiple trials. Theoretically, blockade of the AT1 receptor would address the potentially detrimental effect of ACE escape and therefore result in significantly less angiotensin II activity at the receptor, less aldosterone production (the major stimulus being angiotensin II), and preservation of theoretical benefits from AT2 agonism (Fig. 2.3).

Table 2.2 Evidence-based therapies for inhibition of the renin–angiotensin–aldosterone system in heart failure

Drug	Initial daily dose(s)	Maximum dose(s)	Heart failure stage treated in clinical trials
ACE inhibitors			
Captopril	6.25 mg 3 times	50 mg 3 times	B, C
Enalapril	2.5 mg twice	10–20 mg twice	B, C
Fosinopril	5–10 mg once	40 mg once	C
Lisinopril	2.5–5 mg once	20–40 mg once	B, C
Quinapril	5 mg twice	20 mg twice	C
Ramipril	1.25–2.5 mg once	10 mg once	B, C
Trandolopril	1 mg once	4 mg once	B, C
ARBs			
Candesartan	4–8 mg once	32 mg once	C
Valsartan	20–40 mg twice	160 mg twice	B, C
Aldosterone antagonists			
Spironolactone	12.5–25 mg once	25 mg once or twice	C
Eplerenone	25 mg once	50 mg once	C

ACE, angiotensin-converting enzyme; ARB, angiotensin receptor blocker. Adapted from Hunt SA, Abraham WT, Chin MH *et al.* [1] with permission.

The Losartan Heart Failure Survival Study (ELITE II) was designed to compare the efficacy of an angiotensin receptor blocker (ARB) and ACE inhibitor, losartan and captoril respectively, in elderly patients with symptomatic heart failure due to LV systolic dysfunction (LV ejection fraction <40%) [14]. The investigators reported no difference between these agents regarding all-cause mortality. Since this trial was not statistically powered to determine equivalency of the two agents, ACE inhibitor therapy remains the treatment of choice for RAAS blockade in heart failure; however, differences regarding clinical efficacy between ACE inhibitors and ARBs seem to be narrowing as more investigations are completed. One criticism of ELITE II relates to the low dosing of losartan used in the study.

Recent studies utilizing ARBs as alternative treatment in ACE inhibitor-intolerant patients support the notion that ARBs are excellent substitutes for ACE inhibitors and are uniformly better tolerated. In addition, the utilization of ACE inhibitors and ARBs together has gained support for treating patients who remain symptomatic despite target dose ACE inhibitor treatment. The Valsartan Heart Failure Trial (Val-HeFT) enrolled 5010 patients to determine the benefit of valsartan (target dose 160 mg twice a day) added to ACE inhibitor in patients with symptomatic (NYHA class II–III; ACC/AHA stage C) heart failure [15]. The investigators reported a slight but statistically significant reduction in a clinical composite endpoint favoring the ARB, ACE inhibitor combination [15]. In addition, valsartan improved LV ejection fraction (LVEF) and reversed LV remodeling as measured by echocardiography [15]. A post-hoc subgroup analysis of 1610 patients on beta blocker and ACE inhibitor at baseline, however, identified increased mortality with the addition of valsartan (valsartan, 16.4% vs. placebo, 12.5%; $P = 0.018$), raising concerns about the combination of ARB, ACE inhibitor, and beta blocker.

The Candesartan in Heart Failure Assessment of Reduction in Mortality and Morbidity (CHARM) trial addressed this issue further by prospectively analyzing the effect of candesartan (target dose of 32 mg a day) in 4576 patients with low LVEF heart failure [16]. This study reported a statistically significant reduction in the combined endpoint of cardiovascular morbidity and mortality when candesartan was combined with an ACE inhibitor or an ACE inhibitor plus beta blocker [16]. The explanation for the disparity between Val-HeFT and CHARM regarding the so-called "triple therapy" group (ACE inhibitor, ARB and beta blocker-treated patients) is unclear but could be related to differences between the two ARBs, different dosing strategies, or merely chance [17]. One must consider that more validity may be given to the CHARM results since the assessment of triple therapy was a pre-specified endpoint.

Thus, results from Val-HeFT and CHARM support the concept of a clinical benefit to more complete antagonism of the RAAS. Furthermore, these studies allay concerns regarding the effectiveness of ARBs when employed in ACE inhibitor-intolerant patients. Both trials identified a highly significant survival advantage of ARB utilization in those patients intolerant to an ACE inhibitor and also identified a potential benefit to the addition of ARB to ACE inhibitor treatment in persistently symptomatic patients.

Clinical use of ARBs

The ARB is recommended for heart failure stages B, C, and D when ACE inhibitor cannot be used due to intolerable cough or the infrequent, but severe side effect of angioneurotic edema (Fig. 2.4). Substitution for the latter indication should be done with caution since angioneurotic edema has been reported rarely with ARBs. ARBs are not different from ACE inhibitors regarding the side effects of hypotension, renal insufficiency, and hyperkalemia. These problems are common with all inhibitors of the RAAS and must be closely monitored. Generally, all of the precautions taken during ACE inhibitor utilization must also be employed during ARB use.

As presented above, data from the CHARM and Val-HeFT trials indicate that ACE inhibitor and ARB may be more effective than either drug alone in symptomatic stage C patients (NYHA class II–IV); however, the adverse effects of angiotensin inhibition including hypotension, renal insufficiency, and hyperkalemia may be more pronounced. The use of an aldosterone antagonist in combination with an ACE inhibitor and ARB is discouraged due to the unacceptable risk of hyperkalemia. The evidence-based ARBs and recommended dosing guidelines are presented in Table 2.2.

Aldosterone antagonists

Elevated circulating levels of aldosterone play an integral role in the pathophysiology of heart failure. Aldosterone is an effector hormone of the RAAS and may produce detrimental effects via multiple mechanisms, including sodium and water retention, abnormal electrolyte homeostasis (magnesium and potassium), myocardial hypertrophy and fibrosis, vascular remodeling, and endothelial cell dysfunction [18]. In patients with heart failure, aldosterone levels increase primarily in response to angiotensin II; however, other factors (non-angiotensin stimuli) may also be important (Fig. 2.3).

Two major clinical trials currently direct the utilization of aldosterone antagonists in patients with heart failure and LV dysfunction. The Randomized Aldactone Evaluation Study (RALES) enrolled 1663 patients with moderate to severe heart failure (NYHA classes III–IV; LVEF <35%) to receive either spironolactone or placebo in combination with ACE inhibition and diuretics [19]. The study was stopped early because patients receiving spironolactone realized a remarkable 30% survival advantage including a reduction in the incidence of sudden cardiac death [19]. Benefit was also observed in the relatively small number of patients receiving beta blockers (approximately 10%). Not unexpectedly, a significant number of men on spironolactone experienced gynecomastia or breast pain ($P < 0.001$). Although significant hyperkalemia with spironolactone therapy was not observed in this rigorously performed and monitored trial, subsequent observations from a study done in Ontario, Canada identified a marked increase in hospitalization rates for hyperkalemia paralleling an increase in the number of spironolactone prescriptions for heart failure management [17].

More recently, the Eplerenone Post-acute Myocardial Infarction Heart Failure Efficacy and Survival Study (EPHESUS) enrolled 6632 patients and reported that the selective aldosterone antagonist eplerenone improves survival and reduces cardiovascular hospitalization in patients after myocardial infarction that have symptomatic LV dysfunction (average LVEF was 33%) [20]. Unlike the RALES trial, the majority of patients in EPHESUS also received beta blocker treatment (75%) in addition to ACE inhibitors and diuretics, thus supporting the safety of this combination. As expected, the trou-blesome side effect of gynecomastia and breast pain was not encountered in the eplerenone-treated patients given the selective mineralocorticoid receptor-blocking properties of eplerenone, which does not interfere with androgen or progesterone receptors.

Clinical use of aldosterone antagonists

Low-dose aldosterone antagonist therapy is recommended in stage C and D heart failure when symptoms are significant (NYHA classes III–IV) as well as in patients with symptomatic LV dysfunction following myocardial infarction. The decision to initiate this treatment in the heart failure patient must balance the potential of a reduction in heart failure death and hospitalization with the known risks of life-threatening hyperkalemia. The dose of aldosterone antagonist should be started low and, if tolerated, increased to target dosing which is 25 mg once a day of spironolactone and 50 mg once a day of eplerenone (Table 2.2). The risk of hyperkalemia may be substantial and recognition of the patient at risk is the key to the safe introduction and maintenance of this treatment. Although patients with creatinine levels as high as 2.4 mg/dL were allowed to be enrolled in RALES and EPHESUS, the risk of hyperkalemia increases substantially when the serum creatinine exceeds 1.6 mg/dL, particularly in elderly individuals, in whom creatinine may not reflect glomerular filtration rate. Extreme caution should be utilized if serum creatinine exceeds 2.0 mg/dL or if baseline serum potassium exceeds 5.0 mmol/L.

Frequent monitoring of renal function and serum potassium is necessary after introduction of therapy, particularly if moderate to high-dose ACE inhibitor or ARB are being utilized. Any changes in diuretic dose, ARB or ACE inhibitor dose should also prompt laboratory evaluation of electrolytes and renal function. Patients should be cautioned regarding potassium intake, and all medications, including non-prescription drugs, should be reviewed prior to initiating the aldosterone antagonist. As previously noted, the concomitant use of ACE inhibitor, ARB, and aldosterone antagonist should generally be avoided.

Beta-adrenergic receptor blockers

Although cardiac adrenergic drive supports cardiac performance early in the heart failure syndrome, chronic activation of the sympathetic nervous system has deleterious effects on the myocardium resulting in progressive LV remodeling and dysfunction. The degree of adrenergic activation correlates with mortality and in keeping with the neurohormonal interdiction hypothesis, current heart failure guidelines recommend blockade of the sympathetic nervous system in addition to the RAAS [1].

Beta blockers represent the most important therapy introduced for heart failure management over the past decade. The addition of an evidence-based beta blocker to an ACE inhibitor results in a 35% reduction in annual mortality related to heart failure (Fig. 2.5). Beta blockers have now been evaluated in over 20 000 heart failure patients and have been shown to possess a remarkable capacity for improving LV function and survival in patients with mild to severe symptoms, of both genders, and all age ranges. Following 4–6 months of treatment with an evidence-based beta blocker, one will expect an improvement in LVEF by at least 5–10% associated with an improvement in symptoms and functional capacity. Not infrequently, one may see a dramatic improvement in LV function and symptoms, particularly in those patients with hypertensive or dilated cardiomyopathy.

The primary action of beta blockers is to counteract the harmful effects of the sympathetic nervous system activated during heart failure. Several of the harmful effects of norepinephrine, the primary effector of sympathetic nervous system activation, include peripheral and coronary vasoconstriction, increased renin production, LV hypertrophy, myocardial ischemia, increased heart rate, programmed cell death (apoptosis), and arrhythmia [21]. The clinical benefits of beta blockers are mediated primarily

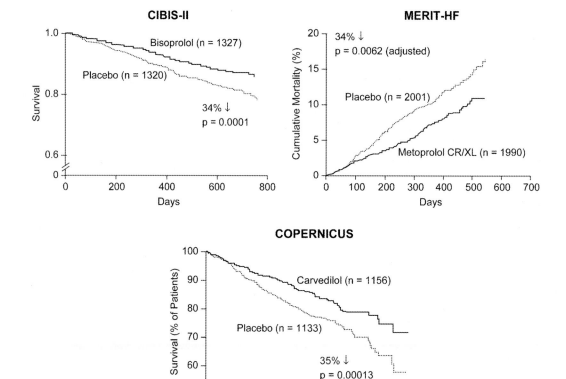

Figure 2.5 Major placebo-controlled mortality trials of beta blockade in heart failure. From CIBIS II, The Cardiac Insufficiency Bisoprolol Study II [26]; COPERNICUS, Effect of Carvedilol on Survival in Severe Chronic Heart Failure [27]; MERIT-HF, Metoprolol CR/XL Randomized Intervention Trial in Congestive Heart Failure [28] with permission.

by beta-1 adrenergic receptor blockade. However, more comprehensive adrenergic receptor blockade (alpha-1 and beta-2 adrenergic receptors) may result in added mortality benefit [22, 23]. Clearly, beta blockade in heart failure does not represent a "class effect" since studies have shown differences in efficacy between agents. In fact, one large trial utilizing the beta blocker bucindolol failed to show a significant reduction in mortality and was halted before completion of enrollment [24]. Similarly, beta blockers with partial agonist properties are contraindicated for heart failure management because of the risk of increased mortality [25]. The most commonly prescribed beta blocker in the United States, atenolol, has never been studied in a heart failure population and therefore its use for chronic heart failure management is not recommended.

Currently, there are three beta blockers that have been approved for heart failure management based upon results from large clinical trials. These drugs are the selective beta-1 antagonists metoprolol succinate and bisoprolol, and an agent with beta-1, beta-2, and alpha-1 blocking properties, carvedilol (Table 2.3). The Cardiac Insufficiency Bisoprolol Study II (CIBIS II) trial was the first randomized controlled trial of beta blocker therapy with sufficient statistical power to address all-cause mortality as a primary objective [26]. In CIBIS II, 2647 patients with LVEF <35% and moderate to severe heart failure (NYHA III–IV) on stable ACE inhibitor and diuretic therapy were randomized to receive either bisoprolol (target dose 10 mg per day) or placebo. The trial was stopped after 1.4 years, showing a significant survival advantage of 32% ($P = 0.002$) for those receiving bisoprolol. Bisoprolol also reduced sudden death by 45% ($P = 0.001$) and heart failure hospitalizations by 30% ($P < 0.001$).

The Metoprolol CR/XL Randomized Intervention Trial in Congestive Heart Failure (MERIT-HF) study enrolled 3991 patients, the majority with NYHA class II (41%) and class III (55%) heart failure with a mean LVEF of 28% [27]. Patients received standard background therapy with an ACE inhibitor or ARB, diuretics, and digoxin. Patients were randomized to receive either placebo or metoprolol succinate (metoprolol CR/XL) to a target dose of 200 mg a day. Similar to CIBIS II, this trial was also stopped after a mean follow-up of only one year because of a highly significant survival benefit in the metoprolol group (relative risk reduction for mortality was 34%, $P = 0.0062$). A beneficial response to metoprolol succinate was also observed regarding sudden death, heart failure hospitalizations, and functional classification.

The Carvedilol Prospective Randomized Cumulative Survival (COPERNICUS) study was designed to assess beta blockade in a more symptomatic group of patients than the previous trials [28]. In COPERNICUS, patients had symptoms at rest or with minimal activity despite treatment with standard heart failure therapies. Even in this very sick population, treatment with carvedilol improved survival at 10.4 months by 35% compared to placebo.

Results from the Carvedilol Post-Infarct Survival Controlled Evaluation (CAPRICORN) expand the efficacy of beta blockade to the patient with asymptomatic LV dysfunction (stage B) [29]. In the post-myocardial infarction cohort enrolled in this study, 1023 patients had asymptomatic LV dysfunction within one month post myocardial infarction and treatment with carvedilol, in addition to standard therapy including ACE inhibitor and antiplatelet therapy, was associated with a 31% relative mortality reduction compared with placebo.

Table 2.3 Evidence-based therapies for inhibition of the sympathetic nervous system in heart failure

Beta-adrenergic blockers	Initial daily dose(s)	Maximum dose(s)	Heart failure stage treated in clinical trials
Bisoprololol	1.25 mg once	10 mg once	C
Carvedilol	3.125 mg twice	25 mg twice (50 mg twice for patients >85 kg)	B, C
Metoprolol succinate	12.5–25 mg once	200 mg once	C

Adapted from Hunt SA, Abraham WT, Chin MH *et al.* [1] with permission.

The cumulative evidence base for the utilization of beta blocker therapy discussed above is robust and covers a broad spectrum of disease from asymptomatic LV dysfunction (NYHA class I; stage B) to severely symptomatic heart failure (NYHA class III–IV; stage C). As noted previously, there does not seem to be a class effect for beta blockade in treating heart failure. Currently the only two agents approved for heart failure management in the United States are metoprolol succinate and carvedilol, together with bisoprolol in Europe. Based on data from CAPRICORN and COPERNICUS, carvedilol is also approved for severe heart failure and asymptomatic LV dysfunction post myocardial infarction.

A controversy regarding possible clinical differences between beta-1 selective antagonists and comprehensive adrenergic blockade has been fueled by results from the Carvedilol or Metoprolol European Trial (COMET) [22, 23]. This study of over 3000 patients with moderate heart failure randomized patients to metoprolol tartrate (immediate-acting metoprolol) at a dose of 50 mg twice a day or carvedilol at a target dose of 25 mg twice a day plus standard heart failure therapy. The investigators reported a 17% survival advantage in those receiving carvedilol. The purpose of this trial was to compare the efficacy of selective beta-1 antagonism (metoprolol) with comprehensive adrenergic blockade (carvedilol). Controversy continues regarding the equivalency of the magnitude and duration of beta-1 blockade by the doses of the drugs used in COMET thus calling into question any firm conclusions drawn from the results. It is clear, however, that carvedilol significantly improves survival in patients with moderate heart failure compared to short-acting metoprolol. A direct comparison between carvedilol and metoprolol succinate, the agent used in MERIT-HF, has not been done and therefore results from COMET do not necessarily support a difference between these beta blockers.

Clinical use of beta-adrenergic receptor blockers

Institution of an evidence-based beta blocker is recommended in all stages and NYHA classes of heart failure (Fig. 2.4). Beta blocker therapy should be utilized as soon as LV dysfunction is identified. While the initiation and titration of beta blocker therapy was once delayed and proceeded with great trepida-tion due to concerns of worsening heart failure and hypotension in moderately ill and decompensated patients, it is now clear that these agents should be started early and perhaps even during hospitalization of decompensated heart failure, once adequate diuresis has been achieved. The clinician should understand that the acute pharmacologic effects of beta-1 receptor antagonism may result in acute hemodynamic compromise in the patient with symptomatic heart failure. Therefore, starting with very low doses and slow titration is recommended (see Table 2.3). Carvedilol should generally be started at 3.125 mg twice a day and titrated to a target dose of 25 mg twice a day. Metoprolol succinate is begun at 25 mg once a day and increased over several weeks to a target dose of 200 mg a day. The beneficial effects of beta blockade in heart failure are generally not evident until weeks to months after the initiation of therapy due to the time required for myocardial recovery from chronic catecholamine-induced injury. This beneficial "biologic effect" of beta blockade is thus differentiated from the acute "pharmacologic effect" of this therapy.

No longer are comorbid conditions such as chronic obstructive pulmonary disease (COPD), peripheral arterial disease, or diabetes mellitus contraindications to beta blocker use. While patients with a significant bronchospastic component to their COPD, or those with a remote history of asthma, may not tolerate beta-2 receptor blockade with carvedilol, selective beta-1 blockade with moderate dose metoprolol succinate may be successful. Patients with substantive metabolic derangement related to diabetes may better tolerate carvedilol because of its alpha antagonist and antioxidant properties [30].

The importance of initiating beta blockade is further emphasized by the recommendation that ACE inhibitor or ARB therapy should be reduced to lower doses if hypotension is preventing reasonable beta blocker dosing. Some have argued that beta blocker therapy should be the first agent started in those with a new diagnosis of heart failure [31]. An argument may also be made for insertion of a permanent pacemaker in those with chronotropic insufficiency who are not able to tolerate beta blockade. As conventional right ventricular-based pacing will induce left bundle branch block and therefore worsens cardiac function, a biventricular pacemaker is theoretically preferable. The authors have observed several instances where an improvement in systolic blood pressure following biventricular pacing in the appropriate candidate has allowed for optimization of beta blocker therapy.

Diuretic therapy in chronic heart failure

Treatment with a thiazide or loop diuretic is often necessary in patients with symptomatic (NYHA class II–IV, stages C and D) heart failure. The currently available diuretics and dose recommendations are listed in Table 2.4. Patients with stage B heart failure do not require diuretics for symptom relief or volume control. These patients may, however, require treatment with a thiazide diuretic for optimal blood pressure control. Rarely is a loop diuretic required in this heart failure subset unless used to control blood pressure when a thiazide diuretic may not be effective, as in the patient with significant renal insufficiency.

In stage C and D heart failure, diuretic therapy does not affect survival and is therefore utilized only for symptomatic benefit [1]. Given the fact that diuretic therapy may cause multiple deleterious effects in chronic heart failure including neurohormonal activation, a reduction in glomerular filtration rate, and metabolic and electrolyte disturbances, the lowest diuretic dose should be prescribed with a goal toward continued dose reduction whenever possible. Oftentimes, a flexible diuretic regimen is appropriate based upon daily weights or other signs

or symptoms of fluid retention. Patient compliance with sodium restriction will often aid in achieving the lowest possible diuretic dose while at the same time, allow for optimal dosing with the evidence-based ACE inhibitors and beta blockers. While spironolactone and eplerenone (discussed above) have mild diuretic properties, these agents are not typically effective alone when volume control is a problem.

Patients with advanced heart failure (NYHA class III–IV, stage C–D) often require high-dose diuretics for volume control and symptomatic benefit. In these patients, diuretic resistance may ensue necessitating combination therapy with loop and thiazide diuretics. A major effort should be given to reduce the frequency of this combination whenever possible due to the significant metabolic, electrolyte, and renal disturbances associated with this aggressive form of therapy. Prior to advancing to the combination of loop and thiazide diuretic, a trial of therapy with a loop diuretic and aldosterone antagonist is often warranted.

The major risk of diuretic therapy is hypokalemia and consequent ventricular arrhythmia. Therefore, careful monitoring of serum electrolytes is encouraged with aggressive potassium repletion when necessary. High-dose loop diuretic therapy, particularly if used in combination with thiazide diuretics, often leads to severe hypokalemia, even in the presence of potassium-sparing ACE inhibitor and aldosterone antagonist therapy.

Table 2.4 Oral diuretics recommended for the treatment of chronic heart failure

Drug	Initial daily dose(s)	Maximum daily dose	Duration of action
Loop diuretics			
Furosemide	20–40 mg once or twice	600 mg	6–8 h
Bumetanide	0.5–1.0 mg once or twice	10 mg	4–6 h
Torsemide	10–20 mg once	200 mg	12–16 h
Thiazide diuretics			
Chlorothiazide	250–500 mg once or twice	1000 mg	6–12 h
Chlorthalidone	12.5–25 mg once	100 mg	24–72 h
Hydrochlorothiazide	25 mg once or twice	200 mg	6–12 h
Indapamide	2.5 mg once	5 mg	36 h
Metolazone	2.5 mg once	20 mg	12–24 h
Potassium-sparing diuretics			
Amiloride	5 mg once	20 mg	24 h
Spironolactone	12.5–25 mg once	50 mg	2–3 days
Triamterene	50–75 mg twice	200 mg	7–9 h

Adapted from Hunt SA, Abraham WT, Chin MH *et al.* [1] with permission.

Pharmacologic therapy for selected patients

Isosorbide dinitrate/hydralazine

The concept of adding the vasodilators isosorbide dinitrate and hydralazine (ISDN/H) to standard evidence-based therapy in patients with persistent symptomatic heart failure has gained momentum recently following the publication of results from the African-American Heart Failure Trial (A-HeFT) [32]. While ISDN/H had previously shown some promise by eliciting a mild reduction in mortality in early heart failure trials, it was not subsequently proven to be advantageous when compared with ACE inhibitor therapy [33, 34]. A retrospective analysis of the early vasodilator trials, however, revealed a potential benefit of ISDN/H treatment in the subgroup of African Americans, suggesting that heart failure in blacks represents a different pathophysiologic state and may respond in a more favorable fashion to a nitric oxide donor (ISDN) and antioxidant (hydralazine). A-HeFT tested this hypothesis by randomizing 1050 African-American patients with heart failure (NYHA class III or IV; average LVEF 24%) receiving standard heart failure therapy (including ACE inhibitors, beta blockers, aldosterone antagonists) to a proprietary, fixed-dose combination of ISDN/H (Bidil; Nitromed, Bedford, MA, USA) [32, 35]. A 43% reduction in mortality was realized in the treatment group and the trial was terminated prematurely at a mean follow-up of only 10 months. Based on these results, ISDN/H has been approved for the treatment of heart failure in black patients. Whether this therapy is effective in other racial/ethnic groups or in patients with less severe heart failure remains to be determined [17, 35]. It should be emphasized that patients in A-HeFT received standard background heart failure therapy with ACE inhibitors and beta blockers. The ISDN/H combination is not recommended as first-line treatment for those that are ACE inhibitor naïve [1].

Nitrate therapy alone for heart failure management has not been extensively studied but may be effective for relief of symptoms such as exertional dyspnea or paroxysmal nocturnal dyspnea. ISDN is a potent venodilator but may also reduce afterload when systemic vascular resistance is severely elevated [1]. Targeted therapy based on specific symptoms in the individual patient may be effective.

Digoxin

While digoxin has been used to treat symptomatic heart failure for over 200 years, its utility in the current era of heart failure management is questionable. Typically, this agent is recommended in patients with NYHA class II to IV and stage C HF to improve symptoms and reduce the risk of decompensation and hospitalization. The Digitalis Investigation Group (DIG) trial, published in 1997, reported a significant reduction in heart failure hospitalizations when digoxin was added to standard heart failure therapy, but no mortality benefit was seen compared to placebo [36]. Very few patients in the DIG trial, however, received beta blocker and aldosterone antagonist therapy, thus raising questions as to the relevance of digoxin in present-day clinical practice.

It is important to realize that any clinical benefit from digoxin likely relates to its extracardiac actions, particularly its antagonism of the sympathetic nervous system, rather than its direct inotropic properties. Lower or sub-inotropic doses of digoxin (serum drug concentrations under 1.0 ng/mL) may be preferable, thus improving the risk-to-benefit ratio of this agent, particularly in the elderly who are at significant risk for toxicity [37].

Pharmacologic management of acutely decompensated heart failure

Acute decompensation of chronic heart failure (ADHF) comprises about 75% of all heart failure hospitalizations and is the most common reason for hospitalization in the elderly [38]. The pharmacologic approach to managing these patients focuses on the objectives presented in Table 2.5. To achieve these objectives, intravenous diuretic therapy is required in most situations, along with the rapid and appropriate selection and administration of intravenous vasoactive medications. Unlike the evidence-based therapies reviewed previously for chronic heart failure management, evidence-based guidelines for ADHF are not generally available. The recently released European Society of Cardiology Heart Failure Guidelines attempts to address

Table 2.5 Goals for patients hospitalized with heart failure

Relieve symptoms rapidly

Reverse hemodynamic abnormalities

Prevent end-organ dysfunction

Prevent death

Initiate patient education and evidence-based medications before discharge

Optimize evidence-based oral medications (ACE inhibitors, beta blockers, aldosterone antagonist)

Optimize patient education and heart failure disease management

ACE, angiotensin-converting enzyme.

the patient with ADHF but the recommendations are hampered by the absence of reliable clinical trial data [39]. Thus, the management of ADHF is less standardized and highly variable. The Acute Decompensated Heart Failure National Registry (ADHERE) has provided important observational data regarding therapy in over 100 000 patients and promises to significantly advance our understanding of ADHF [40].

Classification of hemodynamic profile

The specific therapeutic approach to the individual with ADHF can be targeted to their hemodynamic profile upon presentation. The use of a "four-square"

model can help identify specific hemodynamic profiles in the patient with ADHF based upon the history, physical examination, and initial laboratory assessment, thus aiding the clinician in the appropriate and expeditious selection of therapy (Fig. 2.6). The majority of patients admitted with ADHF fall into profile B – the wet and warm category, while a much smaller number are in profile C – wet and cold. In both instances, patients present with congestion requiring diuretic therapy. The profile B patient, however, is well perfused with a normal cardiac output whereas profile C represents the congested patient with peripheral hypoperfusion and near shock. Profile A patients (warm and dry) are not congested and have normal cardiac output, thus representing the "hemodynamic goal" for most patients presenting with ADHF. Profile L represents the least common presentation with low cardiac output in the absence of congestion. This specific profile may represent a profile C patient who has been diuresed too aggressively.

It should be emphasized that the majority of acute heart failure therapies, unlike the medications for chronic heart failure, are selected for their rapid favorable effects on the major determinants of LV function, including preload, afterload, and myocardial contractility. The medications commonly used to accomplish this goal are generally administered intravenously, exhibit pharmacokinetic properties that allow for rapid titration to hemodynamic

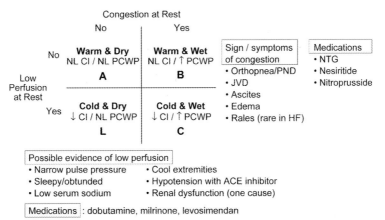

Figure 2.6 Four-square diagram of hemodynamic assessment of patients with heart failure. This diagram emphasizes the bedside presentation and vasoactive therapy of patients with acute decompensation of chronic heart failure. NTG, nitroglycerin; CI, cardiac index; PCWP, pulmonary capillary wedge pressure; JVD, jugular venous distention; PND, paroxysmal nocturnal dyspnea; NL, normal; ↑ elevated; ↓ decreased. Modified from Stevenson LA. Tailored therapy to hemodynamic goals for advanced heart failure. *Eur J Heart Failure* 1999; **1**: 251–257 with permission.

effect, and have a relatively short plasma half-life so that any untoward effect can be quickly terminated. Table 2.6 lists the specific hemodynamic responses generally observed during utilization of the common vasoactive therapies for ADHF.

Acute vasodilator therapy

Nitroglycerin

Nitroglycerin is often effective in the early management of patients presenting in profile B (congested with normal cardiac output) (Fig. 2.6). Nitroglycerin produces venous and arterial dilation through relaxation of vascular smooth muscle resulting primarily from *S*-nitrosothiol and nitric oxide production. The hemodynamic effect is one of preload and afterload reduction with an associated mild increase in stroke volume and cardiac output resulting in a reduction in ventricular filling pressure and pulmonary congestion. While nitroglycerin is generally considered a venodilator, its arterial vasodilating properties are unmasked in the setting of elevated systemic vascular resistance that commonly is present in ADHF of profile B. Nitroglycerin is usually started at an initial intravenous dose of 0.2–0.3 µg/kg per min and titrated to clinical effect. The occurrence of nitrate tolerance is universally recognized and necessitates continued dose titration during continuous infusion to maintain hemodynamic effect.

The only major randomized controlled trial to date assessing the efficacy of nitroglycerin in ADHF was the VMAC (Vasodilation in the Management of Acute Congestive Heart Failure) trial which showed that nitroglycerin was less effective than nesiritide and not different than placebo in improving a number of clinical and hemodynamic parameters (see below) [41].

Nitroprusside

Nitroprusside is a powerful venous and arterial vasodilator with potent preload- and afterload-reducing properties. This drug relaxes arterial and venous smooth muscle via the production of nitric oxide and nitrosothiols resulting in cyclic guanosine monophosphate (cGMP) production. Nitroprusside, by rapidly reducing ventricular filling pressures, is highly effective in improving symptoms of dyspnea and pulmonary congestion in profile B patients. Due to its potent afterload-reducing properties, this agent may also be effective in the profile C patient who is not hypotensive. These patients typically have a very high systemic vascular resistance and respond to afterload reduction with a marked improvement in stroke volume and cardiac output with minimal change in heart rate and blood pressure.

Nitroprusside is usually started at a dose of 0.03–0.1 µg/kg per min and its very short half-life (2 min) allows for rapid titration to hemodynamic effect. While this agent is quite effective in rapidly achieving hemodynamic goals in ADHF, it is used less frequently than other vasodilators because of the concern that its use requires an intensive care setting with invasive hemodynamic monitoring. In fact, data from the ADHERE Registry identifies nitroprusside use in only 1–2% of patients hospitalized with ADHF. Although cyanide and thiocyanate

Table 2.6 Intravenous agents for acute decompensation of chronic heart failure management

Therapy	CO	PCWP	BP	HR	Arrhythmia	Shorter onset	Longer offset
Dobutamine	↑↑↑	↓	↔	↑	↑↑	+++	0
Milrinone	↑↑	↓↓	↓	↑	↑↑	+	++
Nitroglycerin	↑	↓↓	↓↓	↔	↔	+++	0
Nesiritide	↑	↓↓	↓↓	↔	↔	++	++
Nitroprusside	↑↑	↓↓	↓↓	↔	↔	++++	0
Dopamine (µg/kg per min)							
Low (<3)	↔	↔	↔	↔	↔	+++	0
Moderate (3–7)	↑	↔	↑	↑	↑↑	+++	0
High (7–15)	↑↑	↔	↑↑	↑↑	↑↑↑	+++	0
Levosimendan[a]	↑↑	↓↓	↓	↑	↔	+++	+++ (metabolites)

[a]Investigational. CO, cardiac output; PCWP, pulmonary capillary wedge pressure; BP, blood pressure; HR, heart rate.

toxicity are the major side effects of nitroprusside administration, these problems are not common and occur only with prolonged administration in the setting of hepatic (cyanide toxicity) or renal (thiocyanate toxicity) dysfunction.

Nesiritide

Nesiritide is the recombinant form of B-type natriuretic peptide (BNP) and is the newest vasodilator approved for treatment of ADHF. This drug functions in a fashion similar to endogenous BNP which is produced by the cardiac ventricles when filling pressures and wall stress are elevated. Nesiritide produces arterial and venous vasodilation via the cGMP pathway by binding to vascular and endothelial receptors. In addition to its vasodilatory properties, nesiritide has a modest effect on renal excretion of salt and water [42]. This drug, similar to the other vasodilators, is effective primarily for the profile B patient who presents with dyspnea, congestion, and a systemic blood pressure above 90–100 mmHg. Nesiritide is administered intravenously, usually with a bolus of 2 µg/kg, followed by a continuous infusion of 0.01 µg/kg per min. The half-life of nesiritide is approximately 18 min, and its side effects are primarily related to its vasodilatory properties. Nesiritde is not proarrhythmic and has not been shown to cause tachyphylaxis. To avoid an unacceptable reduction in blood pressure, nesiritide should not be used if the systolic blood pressure is under 90 mmHg.

The Vasodilation in the Management of Acute Congestive Heart Failure (VMAC) trial evaluated the clinical effects of nesiritide compared with placebo or nitroglycerin in 498 patients with ADHF [41]. This is the largest randomized clinical trial to date evaluating vasodilator treatment of ADHF. The primary endpoints, change in pulmonary capillary wedge pressure (PCWP) and level of dyspnea, were assessed in both groups. Nesiritide decreased PCWP and improved dyspnea more rapidly and to a greater extent relative to both nitroglycerin and placebo. Nesiritide-treated patients had less adverse events when compared with those treated with nitroglycerin, the most common event being headache (8% in nesiritide vs. 20% in nitroglycerin). Importantly, the incidence of symptomatic hypotension was similar in both groups (4% in nesiritide and 5% in nitroglycerin).

Recent reports have raised questions concerning potential adverse effects of nesiritide on renal function and patient survival [43, 44]. Specifically, a meta-analysis of three select trials suggested a non-statistically significant increase in 30-day mortality when nesiritide therapy was compared with nitroglycerin and placebo [43]. While this finding merits further study, several methodological problems including the heterogeneity of the patient cohorts, nesiritide dosages, and background therapy with inotropes make the results inconclusive. When nesiritide was compared with nitroglycerin in an analysis of the ADHERE Registry, the in-hospital mortality odds ratio was 0.94 (95% CI 0.77–1.16; $P = 0.58$) in favor of nesiritide when adjusted for covariates and propensity score [45].

The risk of worsening renal function has also been identified in a recent report; however, this meta-analysis was not restricted to patients receiving nesiritide at the currently recommended dose [44]. Higher dosing of nesiritide has been associated with unacceptable hypotension that may certainly adversely affect renal perfusion. This finding is not unique to nesiritide, however, since most therapies for ADHF carry a substantial risk of temporarily adversely affecting renal perfusion, particularly during concomitant diuretic administration. The findings related to nesiritide are confounded by the observation that renal insufficiency was manageable and associated with a numerically lower mortality rate.

Positive inotropic therapy

The use of routine inotropic support to enhance myocardial contractility in ADHF should generally be discouraged. Basically, inotropic therapy is contraindicated for routine management of the patient with ADHF who has a hemodynamic profile of warm and wet (profile B) because of documented adverse effects on myocardial function, remodeling, and arrhythmia potential. There are, however, specific situations where positive inotropic support may be necessary, particularly in the profile C patient that exhibits only a mildly elevated systemic vascular resistance and is hypotensive. Dobutamine and milrinone are the positive inotropic medications that are currently available for clinical use. Levosimendan is a new inotrope that is currently under investigation.

Dobutamine enhances myocardial contractility via stimulation of myocardial beta-1 and possibly alpha-1 receptors, resulting in increased cyclic adenosine monophosphate (cAMP). In the profile C patient with pre-shock or shock syndrome, dobutamine is effective in improving cardiac output and renal perfusion while reducing ventricular filling pressures. The resulting potentiation of diuresis often further improves hemodynamics and reduces ventricular volumes and valvular insufficiency. The risk of dobutamine therapy, particularly at higher doses, is related primarily to atrial and ventricular arrhythmia as well as progression of the myopathic process and continued ventricular remodeling. When dobutamine therapy is considered warranted despite these risks, it should be administered in the lowest effective dose with careful attention to serum potassium levels and monitored rhythm.

Milrinone exhibits both direct inotropic and vasodilator properties by enhancing cAMP levels through inhibition of phosphodiesterase III. This compound evokes a marked reduction in vascular resistance but due to its long half-life, hypotension may be problematic. Milrinone should be considered only in profile C patients without significant hypotension. It may be used concurrently with dobutamine to increase inotropy since both drugs increase cAMP levels by complementary mechanisms. Due to the high arrhythmogenic risk of this therapy, the use of both agents together is not common practice and is typically reserved only as a pharmacologic bridge to device support. A 48-h infusion of milrinone in congested patients with ADHF (primarily profile B patients) identified an increased incidence of arrhythmia and hypotension related to milrinone treatment [46].

Levosimendan is an investigational agent that increases myocardial contractility by cAMP-independent mechanisms, thus potentially avoiding many of the adverse effects seen with dobutamine and milrinone. Levosimendan evokes a positive inotropic response primarily by increasing the sensitivity of myofilaments to intracellular calcium. This agent also exhibits mild vasodilator properties through its mild inhibition of phosphodiesterase III and by activation of potassium-dependent adenosine triphosphate channels [47]. Levosimendan produces the expected central hemodynamic effects of a drug that enhances inotropy and vasodilation. Direct comparison of this compound with dobutamine has been favorable thus far in clinical trials [48, 49]. Two seminal clinical studies with levosimendan assessing potential symptom and survival benefit will soon be completed (REVIVE and SURVIVE) and should provide definitive information regarding the role of this drug in the management of ADHF. Figure 2.7 provides a reasonable algorithm for the selection of pharmacologic therapy in ADHF.

Therapy for advanced heart failure and shock

When patients remain hemodynamically unstable despite utilization of the therapies discussed previously, then consideration for vasopressor support (dopamine, norepinephrine, vasopressin) should be considered. These patients have unfortunately advanced to stage D heart failure and it should be recognized that vasopressor medications provide only a temporary bridge to more definitive therapy. While the oral evidence-based therapies for chronic heart failure may be useful, hemodynamic instability may prevent their utilization at meaningful doses. The failure to identify a reversible disorder thus necessitating prolonged vasopressor support portends a poor outcome, particularly if the patient is not a candidate for mechanical support as a bridge to future definitive therapy such as cardiac transplantation [50].

Summary of pharmacologic strategies for heart failure

- ACE inhibitors (or ARB if ACE inhibitor intolerant) should be given to all patients with LV systolic dysfunction.
- One of the three evidence-based beta blockers should be used in all patients with LV systolic dysfunction.
- Aldosterone antagonists are recommended in patients with LV systolic dysfunction and persistent moderate to moderately severe symptoms.
- Diuretics are often necessary for volume control and symptomatic benefit in stages C and D heart failure.
- ISDN/H, digoxin, and ARBs may be added to ACE inhibitor, beta blocker, and diuretic therapy for those with persistent heart failure symptoms.

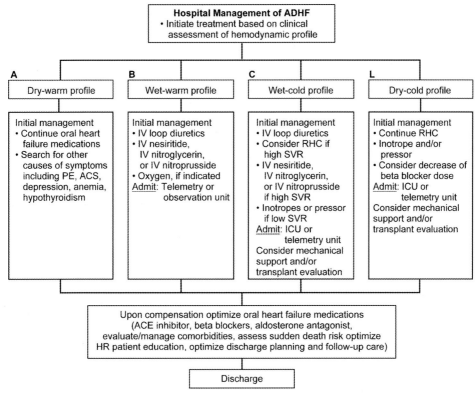

Figure 2.7 Assessment and treatment algorithm for acute decompensation of chronic heart failure (ADHF). This ladder diagram expands on the concept of the "four-square model" (see Fig. 2.6) with emphasis on treatment options for each type of clinical presentation of ADHF. ACS, acute coronary syndrome; IV, intravenous; PE, pulmonary embolism; RHC, right heart catheterization; SVR, systemic vascular resistance; ICU, intensive care unit. Modified from Fonarow GC, Weber JE. Rapid clinical assessment of hemodynamic profiles and targeted treatment of patients with acutely decompensated heart failure. *Clin Cardiol* 2004; 27 (suppl V): V1–V9 with permission from Clinical Cardiology Publishing Co., Inc., Mahwah, NJ 0743, USA.

- Use of an aldosterone antagonist with an ACE inhibitor and ARB is not recommended because of the risk of life-threatening hyperkalemia.
- Intravenous diuretics and vasoactive therapy (vasodilators, inotropes) are used for the management of ADHF. Table 2.6 presents the hemodynamic effects of intravenous vasoactive medications; Figs 2.6 and 2.7 outline a reasonable approach to the utilization of these therapies.

References

1 Hunt SA, Abraham WT, Chin MH *et al.* ACC/AHA 2005 guideline update for the diagnosis and management of chronic heart failure in the adult – summary article: a report of the American College of Cardiology/American Heart Association task force on the practice guidelines (writing committee to update the 2001 guidelines for the evaluation and management of heart failure). *Circulation* 2005; **112**: 1825–1852.

2 Fonarow GC for the Optimize-HF Steering Committee. Strategies to improve the use of evidence-based heart failure therapies: Optimize-HF. *Rev Cardiovasc Med* 2004; **5** (suppl 1): S45–S54.

3 Levy D, Kenchaiah S, Larson MG *et al.* Long-term trends in the incidence of and survival with heart failure. *N Engl J Med* 2002; **347**: 1397–1402.

4 Hunt SA, Baker DW, Chin MH *et al.* ACC/AHA guidelines for the evaluation and management of chronic heart failure in the adult: executive summary. A report of the American College of Cardiology/American Heart Association Task Force on Practice Guidelines (Committee to revise the 1995 Guidelines for the Evaluation and Management of Heart Failure). *J Am Coll Cardiol* 2001; **38**: 2101–2113.

5 Abraham WT (2005). New approaches in the prevention of heart failure. In: Topol ET, ed. *Updates, Textbook of Cardiovascular Medicine*, 2nd edn. Lippincott, Williams and Wilkins, New York, 2005; 8: 1–12.

6 The CONSENSUS Trial Study Group. Effects of enalapril on mortality in severe congestive heart failure. Results of the Cooperative North Scandinavian Enalapril Survival Study (CONSENSUS). *N Engl J Med* 1987; **316:** 1429–1435.

7 The SOLVD Investigators. Effect of enalapril on survival in patients with reduced left ventricular ejection fractions and congestive heart failure. *N Engl J Med* 1991; **325:** 293–302.

8 The SOLVD Investigators. Effect of enalapril on mortality and the development of heart failure in asymptomatic patients with reduced left ventricular ejection fractions. *N Engl J Med* 1992; **327:** 685–691.

9 Pfeffer MA, Braunwald E, Moye LA *et al.* Effect of captopril on mortality and morbidity in patients with left ventricular dysfunction after myocardial infarction. Results of the Survival and Ventricular Enlargement Trial. *N Engl J Med* 1992; **327:** 669–677.

10 The Acute Infarction Ramipril Efficacy (AIRE) Study Investigators. Effect of ramipril on mortality and morbidity of survivors of acute myocardial infarction with clinical evidence of heart failure. *Lancet* 1993; **342:** 821–828.

11 Unger T. The role of the renin-angiotensin system in the development of cardiovascular disease. *Am J Cardiol* 2002; 89 (suppl): 3A–10A.

12 The Heart Outcomes Prevention Evaluation Study Investigators. Effects of angiotensin-converting-enzyme inhibitor, ramipril, on cardiovascular events in high-risk patients. *N Engl J. Med* 2000; **342:** 145–153.

13 Packer M, Poole-Wilson PA, Armstrong PW *et al.* Comparative effects of low and high doses of the angiotensin-converting enzyme inhibitor, lisinopril, on morbidity and mortality in chronic heart failure. *Circulation* 1999; **100:** 2312–2318.

14 Pitt B, Poole-Wilson PA, Segal R *et al.* Effect of losartan compared with captopril on mortality in patients with symptomatic heart failure: randomized trial – the Losartan Heart Failure Survival study (ELITE II). *Lancet* 2000; **355:** 1582–1587.

15 Cohn JN, Tognoni G, for the Valsartan Heart Failure Investigators. A randomized trial of the angiotensin receptor blocker valsartan in chronic heart failure. *N Engl J Med* 2001; **345:** 1667–1675.

16 Young JB, Dunlap ME, Pfeffer MA *et al.* Mortality and morbidity reduction with candesartan in patients with chronic heart failure and left ventricular systolic dysfunction: results of the CHARM low-left ventricular ejection fraction trials. *Circulation* 2004; **110:** 2618–2626.

17 Young JB, Levine TB. Heart failure resulting from left ventricular systolic dysfunction. *Cardiol Rev* 2005; **22:** 7–16.

18 Weber KT. Efficacy of aldosterone receptor antagonism in heart failure: potential mechanisms. *Curr Heart Failure Rep* 2004; **I:** 51–56.

19 Pitt B, Zannad F, Remme WJ *et al.* The effect of spironolactone on morbidity and mortality in patients with severe heart failure. Randomized Aldactone Evaluation Study Investigators. *N Engl J Med* 1999; **341:** 709–717.

20 Pitt B, Remme W, Zannad F *et al.* Eplerenone, a selective aldosterone blocker, in patients with left ventricular dysfunction after myocardial infarction. *N Engl J Med* 2003; **348:** 1309–1321.

21 Joseph J, Gilbert EM. The sympathetic nervous system in chronic heart failure. *Prog Cardiovasc Dis* 1998; **41:** 9–16.

22 Poole-Wilson PA, Swedberg K, Cleland JG *et al.* Comparison of carvedilol and metoprolol on clinical outcomes in patients with chronic heart failure in the Carvedilol or Metoprolol European Trial (COMET): randomized controlled trial. *Lancet* 2003; **362:** 7–13.

23 Packer M. Do beta blockers prolong survival in heart failure only by inhibiting the beta 1-receptor? A perspective on the results of the COMET Trial. *J Cardiac Failure* 2003; **9:** 429–442.

24 Beta-Blocker Evaluation of Survival Trial (BEST) Investigators. A trial of the beta blocker bucindolol in patients with advanced chronic heart failure. *N Engl J Med* 2001; **344:** 1659–1667.

25 The Xamoterol in Severe Heart Failure Study Group. Xamoterol in severe heart failure. *Lancet* 1990; **336:** 1–6.

26 CIBIS II Investigators and Committees. The cardiac bisoprolol study II (CIBIS II): a randomized trial. *Lancet* 1999; **353:** 9–13.

27 MERIT-HF Study Group. Effect of metoprolol CR/XL in chronic heart failure: Metoprolol CR/XL Randomised Intervention Trial in Congestive Heart Failure (MERIT-HF). *Lancet* 1999; **353:** 2001–2007.

28 Packer M, Coats A, Fowler MB *et al.* Effect of carvedilol on survival in severe chronic heart failure. *N Engl J Med* 2001; **344:** 1651–1658.

29 The Capricorn Investigators. Effect of carvedilol on outcome after myocardial infarction in patients with left-ventricular dysfunction: the CAPRICORN randomized trial. *Lancet* 2001; **357:** 1385–1390.

30 Bakris GL, Fonseca V, Katholi RE *et al.* Metabolic effects of carvedilol vs metoprolol in patients with type 2 diabetes mellitus and hypertension: a randomized controlled trial. *JAMA* 2004; **292:** 2227–2236.

31 Sliwa K, Norton GR, Kone, N *et al.* Impact of initiating carvedilol before angiotensin-converting enzyme inhibitor therapy on cardiac function in newly diagnosed heart failure. *J Am Coll Cardiol* 2004; **44:** 1825–1830.

32 Taylor AL, Ziesche S, Yancy C *et al.* Combination of iso-

sorbide dinitrate and hydralazine in blacks with heart failure. *N Engl J Med* 2004; **351**: 2049–2057.

33 Cohn JN, Archibald DG, Ziesche S *et al.* Effect of vasodilator therapy on mortality in chronic congestive heart failure. *N Engl J Med* 1986; **314**: 1547–1552.

34 Cohn JN, Johnson G, Ziesche S *et al.* A comparison of enalapril with hydralazine – isosorbide dinitrate in the treatment of chronic congestive heart failure. *N Engl J Med* 1991; **325**: 303–310.

35 Yancy C. Comprehensive treatment of heart failure: state-of-the-art medical therapy. *Rev Cardiovasc Med* 2005; **6** (suppl 2): S43–S57.

36 The Digitalis Investigation Group. The effect of digoxin on mortality and morbidity in patients with heart failure. *N Engl J Med* 1997; **336**: 525–533.

37 Adams K, Gheorghiade M, Uretsky BF *et al.* Clinical benefits of low serum digoxin concentrations in heart failure. *J Am Coll Cardiol* 2002; **39**: 946–953.

38 American Heart Association: *Heart disease and stroke statistics – 2005 update.* American Heart Association, Dallas, TX, 2005.

39 Nieminen MS, Bohm M, Cowie MR *et al.* Executive summary of the guidelines on the diagnosis and treatment of acute heart failure: the Task Force on Acute Heart Failure of the European Society of Cardiology. *Eur Heart J* 2005; **26**: 384–416.

40 Adams KF, Fonarow GC, Emerman CL *et al.*, for the AD-HERE Scientific Advisory Committee and Investigators. Characteristics and outcomes of patients hospitalized for heart failure in the United States: rationale, design, and preliminary observations from the first 100,000 cases in the Acute Decompensated Heart Failure National Registry (ADHERE). *Am Heart J* 2005; **149**: 209–216.

41 Publication committee for the VMAC investigators: Intravenous nesiritide versus nitroglycerin for treatment of decompensated congestive heart failure. *JAMA* 2002; **287**: 1531–1540.

42 Marcus LS, Hart D, Packer M *et al.* Hemodynamic and renal excretory effects of human brain natriuretic peptide infusion in patients with congestive heart failure. *Circulation* 1996; **94**: 3184–3189.

43 Sackner-Bernstein JD, Kowalski M, Fox M *et al.* Short-term risk of death after treatment with nesiritide for decompensated heart failure: a pooled analysis of randomized controlled trials. *JAMA* 2005; **293**: 1900–1905.

44 Sackner-Bernstein JD, Skopicki HA, Aaronson KD. Risk of worsening renal function with nesiritide in patients with acutely decompensated heart failure. *Circulation* 2005; **111**: 1487–1491.

45 Abraham WT, Adams KF, Fonarow GC *et al.* ADHERE Scientific Advisory Committee and Investigators; AD-HERE Study Group. In-hospital mortality in patients with acute decompensated heart failure requiring intravenous vasoactive medications: an analysis from the Acute Decompensated Heart Failure National Registry (ADHERE). *J Am Coll Cardiol* 2005; **46**: 57–64.

46 Cuffe MS, Califf RM, Adams KF Jr. *et al.* Short-term intravenous milrinone for acute exacerbation of chronic heart failure: a randomized controlled trial. *JAMA* 2002; **287**: 1541–1547.

47 Yokoshiki H, Katsube Y, Sunagawa M *et al.* Levosimendan, a novel calcium sensitizer, activates the glibenclamide-sensitive potassium channel in rat arterial myocytes. *Eur J Pharmacol* 1997; **333**: 249–259.

48 Follath F, Cleland JG, Just H *et al.* Efficacy and safety of intravenous levosimendan compared with dobutamine in severe low-output heart failure (the LIDO study): a randomised double-blind trial. *Lancet* 2002; **360**: 196–202.

49 Moiseyev VS, Poder P, Andrejevs N *et al.* Safety and efficacy of a novel calcium sensitizer, levosimendan, in patients with left ventricular failure due to an acute myocardial infarction. A randomized, placebo-controlled, double-blind study (RUSSLAN). *Eur Heart J* 2002; **23**: 1422–1432.

50 Haas GJ, Young JB. (2002) Acute Heart Failure Management. In: Topol EJ, ed. *Textbook of Cardiovascular Medicine*, 2nd edn. Lippincott, Williams and Wilkins, New York, 2002: 1845–1865.

SECTION 2

Assessment of electrical and mechanical dyssynchrony

CHAPTER 3

Electrical activation sequence

Cecilia Fantoni, MD *& Angelo Auricchio,* MD, PhD

Electrical activation in the normal heart

The characterization and understanding of the cardiac electrical activation sequence *in vitro* and *in vivo* has been the first goal of cardiac physiology and clinical electrophysiology. It also constitutes the foundation for the interpretation of cardiac mechanical events. At present, a precise understanding of both electrical and mechanical events is particularly relevant in the context of non-pharmacological therapy for heart failure and more specifically, in patients with ventricular conduction disturbances.

Although characterization of cardiac electrical activation may be obtained non-invasively by different techniques, catheter-based mapping is still considered the "gold standard". Invasive evaluation of cardiac activation sequence can be obtained either by conventional catheter-based mapping technique or using more sophisticated, high-resolution, three-dimensional catheter-based mapping systems.

Conventional catheter-based mapping in dilated human hearts usually achieves only a gross estimate of the anatomy of the chambers. Moreover, given the limited number of recording sites that may be collected in a reasonable time and the lack of precision in marking specific anatomical locations, the characterization of the electrical activation is also not accurate [1, 2]. In contrast, the recently introduced catheter-based three-dimensional non-fluoroscopic contact and non-contact mapping techniques permit *in vivo* reconstruction of the cardiac anatomy and allow assessment of electrical activation sequence with high spatial and temporal resolution [3, 4]. Contact mapping usually uses bipolar signals

that represent local changes in electrical events with an associated higher sensitivity to rapidly changing events and a lower sensitivity to slowly changing events [5]. In contrast, unipolar signals (as recorded by non-contact mapping) retain at any given recording site electrical information across the whole transmural thickness with equal sensitivity to fast and slow conduction [6]. Given these different attributes, simultaneous unipolar and bipolar recordings may facilitate a more complete characterization and localization of electrical events, especially in severely diseased and dilated hearts.

Before discussing the pathological findings in patients with heart failure, it is important to review the normal atrial and ventricular activation sequence.

Atrial and atrioventricular conduction

In the normal heart, electrical activation originates from the sinus node, a 10–20-mm spindle-shaped structure located less than 1 mm from the epicardial surface in the high sulcus terminalis, at the junction of the superior vena cava and the right atrium. The sinus node is composed of a fibrous tissue matrix with closely packed cells of different types. Among these cells the most important ones are the nodal cells, also called "P cells," grouped in elongated clusters in the middle of the sinus node. These cells automatically and spontaneously depolarize and fire off action potentials at a regular rate, the most rapid within the normal heart, thus functioning as the dominant pacemaker. The firing rate of the nodal cells is dependent on various conditions, such as metabolic needs, atrial stretch, neural and humoral activation [7]; at rest it is usually between 60 and 100 beats per minute. Both adrenergic and cholinergic nerve terminations influence sinus node activity. Once the action potential has started in the sinus node, it spreads through both atria to reach the atrioventricular (AV) junction. The lack of insulation of the specialized nodal tissue, the sickle-shaped morphology with a long longitudinal axis and the caudal radiations facilitate communication between the sinus node and the right atrial myocardium [8].

The presence of specialized conduction pathways in the atria and their pathophysiological relevance are still disputed [9]. However physiological, but not anatomical, evidence indicates the presence of three intra-atrial pathways that conduct the impulse from the sinus to the AV node, running in the right atrium anteriorly, centrally and posteriorly respectively. Indeed, preferential and more rapid internodal conduction exists in some regions of the atria and may be due to isotropic conduction, size and geometry of the fibers, rather than to specialized tracts between the two nodes. The so-called "Bachmann bundle" [10], or anterior interatrial band, is a large muscle bundle that connects the right and the left atrium and conducts the electrical impulse from the right to the left side. In the normal human heart, propogation of the action potential from the sinus node through the atria takes approximately 100 ms.

The central fibrous body (annulus fibrosus) electrically isolates the atrial and ventricular myocardium, so that the AV node is the only physiologic electrical connection between atria and ventricles. The AV node consists of three different regions: the transitional cells zone also called nodal approaches, the compact portion or AV node itself, and the penetrating part or His bundle [11]. The AV nodal tissue conducts the electrical impulses very slowly; indeed, it takes approximately 80 ms to travel from the atrial to the ventricular side of the node. This delay between atrial and ventricular activation has functional importance, because it allows optimal ventricular filling. Like everywhere else in the heart, conduction in the AV node has no preferential direction; consequently, impulses can also be conducted retrogradely. Cells of the lower part of the AV node may exhibit spontaneous depolarization and consequent firing activity at an intrinsic lower rate compared with the sinus node. The AV node is richly innervated by both adrenergic and cholinergic fibers.

From the AV node the electrical impulse reaches the His bundle that continues to the distal part of the AV node, perforates the central fibrous body and penetrates the membranous septum. The proximal cells of the His bundle are very similar to the AV nodal cells, while the distal cells resemble those of the ventricular proximal branches (Purkinje cells). Within this distal system the electrical impulse is conducted approximately four times faster (3–4 m/s) than in the working myocardium (0.3–1 m/s) [12]. This difference is due to the fact that Purkinje cells are longer and have a higher content of gap junctions [13, 14]. Interestingly, neither sympathetic nor vagal stimulation affects normal conduction in the His bundle.

Ventricular conduction

The ventricular conduction system is usually described as a trifascicular structure consisting of a right bundle branch, and an anterior and posterior branch of the left bundle. These structures originate from the His bundle, at the superior margin of the muscular interventricular septum, immediately beneath the membranous septum. The right bundle branch proceeds intramyocardially as a thin, unbranched extension of the His bundle along the right side of the interventricular septum until it terminates in the Purkinje plexuses of the right ventricular (RV) apex, at the base of the anterior papillary muscle. Similarly, the left bundle branch also has a short intramyocardial route in the interventricular septum before giving rise to its two branches. The bifascicular vision of the left bundle branch is probably an oversimplification [15]; the left ventricular (LV) Purkinje network is made up of three main, widely interconnected portions, consisting of the anterior subdivision, the posterior subdivision and a centro-septal subdivision. This third medial subdivision supplies the mid-septal area of the LV and arises either from the main left bundle branch or from its anterior or posterior subdivision, or from both.

Three-dimensional electroanatomical mapping data collected in patients with heart failure support the trifascicular concept of the left bundle. The anterior subdivision is much longer and thinner than the posterior one and for this reason is more vulnerable to damage, so that conduction disturbances along this fascicle are much more common than the ones involving the posterior fascicle. The three subdivisions continue in a network of Purkinje fibers

[13, 16, 17], located subendocardially in the lower third of the septum and in the anterior free wall, and extending to the papillary muscles [13, 16].

The Purkinje fibers are large (10–30 μm diameter, 20–50 μm long), clear cells with many gap junctions that transform the individual cells into a widespread net, accounting for their very fast conduction velocity. During normal orthodromic excitation, fast propagation over these long fibers, together with the wide distribution of Purkinje–myocardial junctions, induces a high degree of electrical coordination between distant regions of the myocardium. The His bundle as well as the right and the left bundle branches are electrically isolated from the adjacent working myocardium. The only sites where the Purkinje system and the normal working cells are electrically coupled are the so-called Purkinje–myocardial junctions, located subendocardially both in the RV and in the LV. Consequently, these areas of conduction exit from the Purkinje fibers to

the working myocardium and result in the earliest activated and contracting regions of the ventricles [6, 12–14, 18, 19]. The distribution of the Purkinje–myocardial junctions is spatially inhomogeneous and the junctions themselves have variable degrees of electromechanical coupling [20]. The time between arrival of the impulse in the His bundle and the beginning of the ventricular electrical activation is approximately 20 ms [13].

In the normal heart, the first site of endocardial ventricular activation (endocardial breakthrough site) is usually in the LV, at the interventricular septum or in the anterior region (Fig. 3.1). Within approximately 10 ms the activation begins in the RV endocardium, near the insertion of the anterior papillary muscle, i.e. the exit of the right bundle branch (Fig. 3.1) [18]. After activation of these regions, depolarization wavefronts proceed simultaneously in the LV and RV, predominantly from apex to base and from septum to lateral wall in both

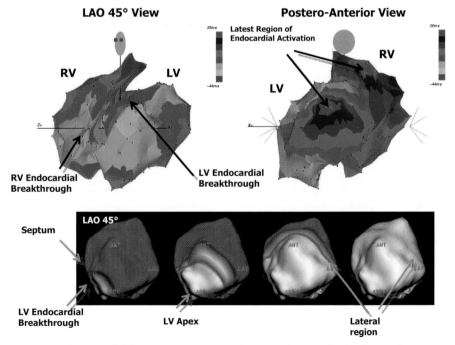

Figure 3.1 Upper panel: Color-coded (red indicating the earliest and purple the latest activation site) 10 ms isochronal maps, obtained with contact electroanatomical mapping system, of biventricular activation in a normal heart. The earliest endocardial ventricular activation site (breakthrough site) is recorded in the LV anterior septal region (red spot). The latest activated regions are the posterolateral walls of both RV and LV. Lower panel: Unipolar isopotential maps, recorded with non-contact mapping system of LV activation sequence in a normal heart. The LV endocardial breakthrough is recorded in the septum. The activation wavefront (white spot) proceeds fast toward the anterior, then to the lateral region and finally to the posterior region.

ventricles (Fig. 3.1). The latest activated endocardial region of the RV is the basal area near the AV sulcus and the pulmonary conus. Overall, the postero-lateral/basal area of the LV is the last part of the heart to be depolarized [18] (Fig. 3.1).

Simultaneous depolarization wavefront occurs centrifugally from the endocardium to the epicardium [18, 19]. However, the earliest ventricular epicardial activation site (epicardial breakthrough site) occurs usually at the pretrabecular area of the RV from where there is a radial spread towards the apex and the base, within the subepicardial layers.

In a normal heart, the duration of total ventricular electrical activation is 50–80 ms [18]. The short ventricular activation time stresses the important role of the Purkinje fibers system in the synchronization of electrical myocardial activity.

Electrical activation in heart failure patients

Abnormal impulse generation and propagation is frequently observed in patients with heart failure. Both functional and structural alterations (cardiac remodeling) are responsible for such abnormalities. Cardiac remodeling commonly refers to persistent changes in the properties of myocardium in response to abnormal external stresses. Although most notably, cardiac remodeling occurs in the setting of structural heart diseases such as myocardial infarction, hypertrophy, and heart failure, it may occur also in the absence of anatomic dysfunction, as is the case during abrupt changes in heart rate and/or activation sequence. Indeed, remodeling is a prominent feature of atrial fibrillation and flutter, ventricular pacing or intrinsic conduction delays and sustained tachycardia.

In this regard, remodeling constitutes a fundamental response of the heart to stress caused by abnormal activation of the cardiac chambers. It is mediated by changes in gene expression, which in turn, alter the type and amounts of myocyte proteins, the distribution and function of subcellular organelles, the size and morphology of individual cells, the properties of the extracellular matrix, and ultimately those of the entire organ. Although electrical and structural remodeling are important adaptive mechanisms, allowing the heart to main-

tain its primary blood pumping function in face of abnormal external stresses, maladaptive consequences of remodeling likely and significantly contribute to disease progression and bad prognosis in patients with heart disease, particularly those with congestive heart failure.

Sinus node incompetence and atrial arrhythmias are frequently observed in patients with heart failure. Pathologic AV conduction occurs in more than half of these patients; moreover, approximately one-third of heart failure patients present with ventricular conduction disturbances, left bundle branch block being the most common.

When the normal, physiological and synchronous sequence of electrical activation is lost, the electrical impulse is conducted primarily through the working myocardium with slow conduction properties, rather than through the rapid specialized conduction system. As a consequence, during abnormal electrical conduction the time required for complete activation of the atrial and ventricular muscle is much longer than during physiological conduction and furthermore a pathologic and asynchronous activation pattern occurs.

Regardless of specific activation pattern, it should be considered that the conduction delay and the degree of asynchrony during abnormal conduction are determined by specific myocardial properties. First of all, conduction velocity through the normal working myocardium is up to four times slower than conduction velocity through the specialized conduction system. Moreover, conduction velocity is approximately two times faster in the direction parallel to muscle fibers length (isotropic conduction) than in the direction perpendicular to them (anisotropic conduction) [21]. It has been demonstrated that, despite the presence of an intact specialized conduction system, ectopically generated impulses rarely penetrate the rapid conduction system and probably only at the Purkinje–myocardial junctions [13, 19, 22]. In this way, the ectopic impulses often propagate through the working myocardium before reaching a Purkinje–myocardial junction and entering the specialized fast conducting system. Consequently, during ectopic impulse generation, the activation sequence is primarily determined by the slow conduction through the working myocardium [22]. Also, the fibers that are closest to the endocardial surface, even though not part of the Purkinje system, conduct impulses faster than the intramyocardial and epicardial fibers [23]. This fact, together with the smaller endocardial circumference compared with its epicardial counterpart, explains the reason why total time required for electrical activation is shorter in the endocardial layers than in the epicardial ones.

Electrical atrial remodeling

In patients with heart failure, a pathological and diffuse involvement of the atrial myocardium has frequently been described [24, 25]. Both atria are usually enlarged with widespread substitution of functioning myocardial cells by regions of fibrosis and scars. Apoptotic processes, repeated ischemic events and chronic inflammation, induced by increased mechanical stress and consequent metabolic changes, can partially explain such histological alterations [26]. At a subcellular level, atrial stretch leads to alteration in gene expression which may result in pathologic ion channel function, with consequent abnormal transmembrane currents and action potentials that constitute the pathophysiological base for so-called "electrical atrial remodeling" [27], and are responsible for abnormal and slow conduction.

Since the sinus node extends over a variably large area of the right atrium, it is often involved by these pathologic alterations [28]. Patients with heart failure usually present with an abnormally caudal localization of the sinus node complex, due to loss of functioning myocardial cells in the upper regions of the right atrium. Structural alterations, abnormal loading conditions, and imbalanced neurohumoral influences account for the sinus node function impairment. Increase of intrinsic sinus cycle length, prolongation of the sinus node recovery time and slowing of the sinoatrial conduction velocity have all been observed in heart failure patients [29]. All together these phenomena may lead to important derangement of sinus node function with consequent bradycardia and chronotropic incompetence, which may favor the onset and persistence of focal or reentrant atrial arrhythmias [29].

Mapping data in heart failure patients have depicted the "electrical atrial remodeling" process as being governed by the presence of low atrial voltages, areas of electrical silence (scars) and widespread fractionated signals and double potentials [30]. In this subset atrial electrophysiology is characterized by slow conduction throughout both the atria and the Bachmann's bundle, increase of effective atrial refractory period and demonstration of functional conduction delays at the crista terminalis [31]. All together, these phenomena lead to prolongation of total intra-atrial activation time and internodal conduction time, with consequent severe impairment of atrial mechanical contraction capacity and overall function.

Left bundle branch block

Left bundle branch block (LBBB) results from block or conduction delays in any of several sites of the left-sided intraventricular conduction system, including the main left bundle branch or its subdivisions or, less commonly, within the fibers of the distal His bundle. The result is an abnormal and slow pattern of electrical activation within the LV due to conduction through the working myocardium. LBBB usually appears in patients with underlying heart diseases, typically in patients with dilated cardiomyopathy of any etiology.

Recent electrophysiological findings have demonstrated that LBBB is a rather complex and heterogeneous electrical disease [32–34]. There is increasing evidence that disarray of myocardial layers may partly account for this heterogeneity [33]. Endocardial activation maps have demonstrated the similarity in the sequence of electrical activation during LBBB and RV pacing [35]; this similarity has led to the use of AV sequential RV apical pacing as a model for "experimental LBBB" [36]. Alternatively, an animal model of LBBB can be easily created by ablation of the proximal part of the left bundle branch [37, 38].

Early informations on electrical activation pattern in patients with LBBB came from data of Wyndham *et al.* [39] and Vassallo *et al.* [40], who respectively mapped the LV epicardial and endocardial activation in patients with LBBB, as well as during RV apical pacing [2]. More recently, detailed information on the spread of activation in patients with LBBB has been provided using catheter-based high-resolution three-dimensional mapping data [33, 34].

In patients with a LBBB-QRS morphology, the first endocardial ventricular activation occurs in the RV, usually in a single or double breakthrough located in the anterolateral region, within milliseconds after the beginning of the earliest QRS complex (Fig. 3.2). In the RV, the activation proceeds rapidly from the breakthrough site to the apex, to the septum, to the outflow tract and to the basal region around the tricuspidal annulus through the intact right-sided Pukinje system. Simultaneously, the activation wavefront spreads slowly to the left side of the septum (trans-septal conduction). Usually, the earliest LV endocardial activation (LV breakthrough site) occurs at a single septal site or at the anterior region, usually 40–70 ms later than the earliest RV activation. Nevertheless, it has been demonstrated that in patients with LBBB trans-septal conduction time has a binary distribution with a clear division below 20 ms and above 40 ms [33]. About one-third of heart failure patients with LBBB show a near-normal trans-septal time (i.e. less than 20 ms). The abrupt prolongation in trans-septal time is always correlated to a change in the breakthrough site; indeed, patients with a near-normal trans-septal time (≤20 ms) present with a septo-basal or anterior endocardial LV breakthrough site. In contrast, patients with an abnormal, prolonged trans-septal time (≥40 ms) usually present with a mid-septal or apical-septal LV breakthrough site. This observation strongly suggests that LV breakthrough occurring at anterior or basal septal location is probably related to conduction which still proceeds through one or more septal branches of the His-Purkinje system.

On the other hand, the mid-septal or septo-apical LV breakthrough site may indicate a slow cell-to-cell activation sequence from RV to LV through the working septal myocardium.

Detailed analysis of the ventricular activation process using contact and non-contact mapping techniques (i.e. unipolar and bipolar signals) simultaneously [33] demonstrated that in patients with LBBB activation is significantly different in the subendocardial layers compared with the intramyocardial ones. Both techniques revealed that the activation wavefront spreads from the septal or anterior LV breakthrough site both superiorly and inferiorly, toward the anterolateral wall. Nevertheless, three-dimensional contact mapping demonstrated that the activation front slowly proceeds from the anterior to the lateral and posterolateral region of LV with a continuous activation pattern, similar to one observed in normal hearts, but significantly slower (Fig. 3.2). In contrast, non-contact three-dimensional mapping technique showed that the activation front cannot cross directly from the anterior and superior region to the lateral wall due to a block to the conduction (Fig. 3.3); this wavefront reaches the lateral or posterolateral regions of the LV by propagating inferiorly around the apex, giving rise to a very characteristic and unique "U-shaped" discontinuous activation pattern. According to data of both mapping systems, LV activation ultimately ends at the basal region of the lateral or posterolateral wall, near the mitral valve annulus (Figs 3.2

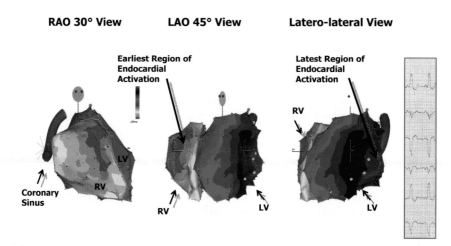

Figure 3.2 Color-coded electroanatomical 10 ms isochronal maps, acquired with contact mapping system, of RV and LV activation in a patient with left bundle branch block, and depressed LV ejection fraction. The earliest ventricular activation site is recorded at the RV anterolateral region (red spot). After about 45 ms, a single LV septal breakthrough site is noted. The latest activated region is the posterolateral wall of the LV (blue to purple isochronal lines).

**LV Endocardial
Breakthrough**

**LV latest activated
region**

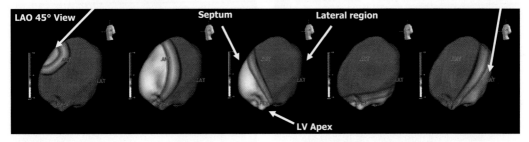

Figure 3.3 Upper panel: Unipolar isopotential maps, recorded with non-contact mapping system of LV activation sequence in a heart failure patient with left bundle branch block and dilated cardiomyopathy. The LV endocardial breakthrough is recorded in the mid septum, from where the activation wavefront (white spot) proceeds in a U-shaped activation pattern rotating around the apex, due to the presence of a functional block at the

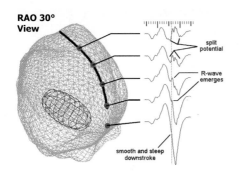

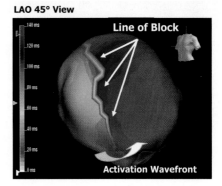

anterior region. Lower panel: Intracardiac non-contact electrograms showing fragmented, multiphasic signals possibly indicating a reduction of conduction velocity and inability to propogate throughout anterior region (left side). Unipolar isochronal map, acquired with non-contact mapping system, of the LV showing the anterior location of functional line of block (right side).

and 3.3). Total LV endocardial activation time in patients with LBBB is much longer (80–150 ms) than in patients without conduction delays (50–80 ms).

Local unipolar electrograms confirm the presence of fragmented, double, or multiphasic components (Fig. 3.3) in the anterior region where the wavefront is not able to cross according to non-contact mapping data [33, 34, 41]. The conduction block is best represented by a line (line of block) that generally parallels the septum, directed from the base toward the apex, in the anterior or anterolateral region of the LV [33] (Fig. 3.3). Functional behavior of this line of block is demonstrated by a change in its location during ventricular pacing at different sites, with different cycle lengths and AV delays (Fig. 3.4). Interestingly, this functional conduction block can be easily recognized by unipolar signals used by non-contact mapping and is not identified by bi-

polar electrograms used by contact mapping. This may suggest that the largest conduction delay is located more intramurally than subendocardially; therefore it is conceivable that a functional block to the conduction emerges from anisotropic conduction due to disarray of intramyocardial layers of tissue, each with potentially different characteristics of conduction.

These findings substantiate and may explain the remarkable heterogeneity of LBBB. Indeed, QRS morphology does not correlate to specific activation patterns whereas duration of the QRS complex does. Almost all patients with LBBB and QRS duration longer than 150 ms have a prolonged trans-septal time and an anterior location of the line of block (Fig. 3.5); in contrast, patients who present with LBBB but a QRS shorter than 150 ms show a short trans-septal time and a lateral location of the line of block (Fig.

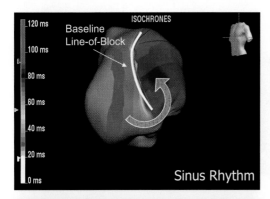

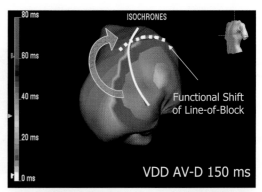

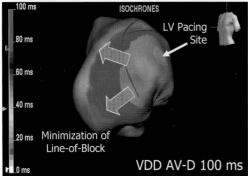

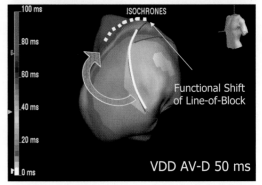

Figure 3.4 Unipolar isochronal LV map in a heart failure patient with left bundle branch block (upper left panel). During intrinsic activation the conduction block (line of block) is located in the anterior region. During atrial-synchronous LV pacing (LV lateral wall) at different AV delays (AV-D), a shift of the line of block is recorded, which demonstrates the functional behavior of the block. At AV delays of 150 ms and 50 ms, the line of block was shorter and more superiorly located than during intrinsic activation. At an atrioventricular delay of 100 ms (lower left panel), minimization of the line of block is observed.

3.5). This observation may suggest that these latter patients present with lesser degree of electrical inter- and LV-intraventricular dyssynchrony and in general a more homogeneous electrical activation process. Early evidence exists that those patients with a shorter QRS duration may require a different delivery of cardiac resynchronization therapy [33, 34].

Recently, electrical activation processes in heart failure patients with LBBB have been further characterized in their transmural events. By combining conventional catheter mapping technique and three-dimensional non-contact mapping system, the epi-endocardial ventricular activation sequence (i.e. the transmural activation sequence limited to the regions adjacent to the epicardial anterior and lateral coronary veins) has been evaluated [42] (Fig. 3.6). By comparing the timing of the earliest detectable ventricular epicardial activation, recorded at the anterior vein, with the time of the earliest LV endocardial activation by non-contact mapping, it was possible to show that in patients with a short endocardial breakthrough time or trans-septal time, the transmural activation sequence at the anteroseptal region showed an endo- to epicardium sequential activation timing (Fig. 3.6). In contrast, in patients with a prolonged trans-septal time, the transmural activation timing was reverted, as the epicardium was activated earlier than the endocardium (Fig. 3.6). Notably, total LV endocardial activation time was significantly longer in patients with a short trans-septal time and an endo- to epicardium sequential activation timing than in those with a prolonged trans-septal time and a reversed epi- to endocardium timing (Fig. 3.6). This can probably be explained by the fact that patients with a short trans-septal time present with more pronounced disease of the working myocardial tissue and better preserved conduction capacities through the proximal specialized conduction system. Indeed, many patients with an ischemic cardiomyopathy demonstrate this

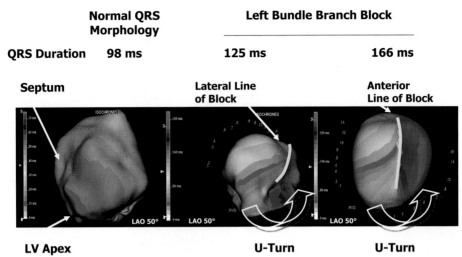

Normal QRS Morphology	Left Bundle Branch Block	
QRS Duration 98 ms	125 ms	166 ms
Septum	Lateral Line of Block	Anterior Line of Block
LV Apex	U-Turn	U-Turn

Figure 3.5 Relation between QRS duration and LV activation sequence as assessed by unipolar isochronal maps. In patients with normal QRS duration (left panel) a homogeneous and continuous activation pattern occurs within the LV. In patients with LBBB, a functional conduction block determines a discontinuous, U-shaped LV activation pattern. In patients with LBBB and QRS duration below 150 ms the conduction block is usually located in a more lateral position (middle panel). In contrast, patients with LBBB and QRS longer than 150 ms consistently display an anterior location of the line of block (right panel).

type of conduction abnormality. Whether these two groups of patients have a different outcome and response to both pharmacological and non-pharmacological therapies remains to be determined. This observation, however, indicates that at least two, and probably multiple, independent activation wavefronts occur as a result of different conduction capabilities of the epicardium and endocardium in patients with LBBB. Thus, different merging patterns can take place, according to variable degrees of injury and disarray and consequent conducting velocities in the different layers and regions.

Right bundle branch block

Right bundle branch block (RBBB) is the result of conduction block or delay in any portion of the right-sided intraventricular conduction system. The delay may occur in the distal His bundle, in the main right bundle branch or in the distal portions of the RV conduction system. The result is an abnormal and slow pattern of electrical activation within the RV due to conduction through the working myocardium.

The relative fragility and mechanical structure of the right-sided conduction system may explain the high prevalence of this conduction delay in the general population without evidence of structural heart disease. Nevertheless, new onset of RBBB in a patient carries a significant risk of underlying coronary heart disease and represents the substrate for developing congestive heart failure. Furthermore, in the presence of structural heart disease, the coexistence of RBBB suggests a more advanced disease, such as an involvement of the proximal anterior descending coronary artery or three-vessel disease. RBBB has been proven to be as important as LBBB as a predictor of mortality in heart failure patients [43]. Up to 15% of heart failure patients that are candidates for cardiac resynchronization therapy present with RBBB.

Both conventional catheter mapping and three-dimensional high-resolution electroanatomical catheter mapping techniques [44] have shown that in patients with RBBB, the earliest ventricular activation site is located in the LV, usually at the septum (Fig. 3.7). The septal activation coincides with the beginning of the QRS complex. After a considerable delay (50–70 ms), the activation starts at the RV septum, due to a slow left-to-right trans-septal conduction. The electrical activation of the entire RV occurs slowly, most likely as a result of cell-to-cell conduction: from the septal breakthrough site, the activation front proceeds toward the RV anterior wall, and then to the right lateral wall and to the outflow tract, both of which are the latest activated regions. Due to this activation pattern, RV anterior

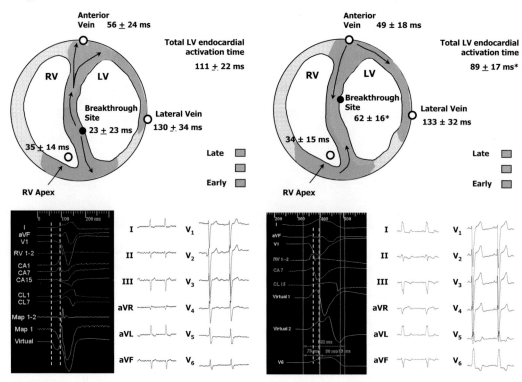

Figure 3.6 Transmural electrical activation sequence as assessed by combining conventional catheter mapping and non-contact mapping techniques. In the lower panel, along with surface ECG, intracardiac bipolar recordings of RV (RV1–2), unipolar LV non-contact (virtual) electrograms, as well as epicardial unipolar recordings acquired through microcatheters inserted into the anterior (CA) and lateral (CL) epicardial veins are shown. In patients with a relatively short time to LV endocardial breakthrough (left side), an endo- to epicardial activation timing in the anteroseptal region of the LV occurs. In contrast, in patients with prolonged time to LV endocardial breakthrough, an epi- to endocardium activation timing is recorded (right side) (see text).

and lateral regions are delayed with respect to onset of the QRS, thus mirroring on the right side of the heart a pattern of delayed activation that is similar to that usually observed in the LV of patients with LBBB (Fig. 3.7). As a result, total RV endocardial activation time in patients with RBBB is much longer (80–120 ms) than in patients without a conduction delay (50–80 ms).

In an otherwise structurally healthy heart with RBBB, LV activation propagates rapidly through the intact left-sided conduction system, from the septum toward the anterior and then to the lateral wall, accounting for the earliest part of the QRS complex. For this reason, much or all of the RV undergoes depolarization after activation of the LV has been completed. Consequently during RBBB, the electrical forces generated by the RV are not masked by the predominant and largest LV electrical forces, but now appear as a delayed component in the QRS

complex, resulting in the characteristic RBBB morphology on the surface ECG.

In patients with an electrocardiographic RBBB pattern and underlying cardiomyopathy, the QRS morphology is significantly different from the characteristic RBBB appearing in otherwise structurally normal hearts. Indeed, most of these heart failure patients demonstrate a specific electrocardiographic pattern defined by Rosenbaum *et al.* as "RBBB masking LBBB" [45], characterized by a broad, slurred, sometimes notched R wave on leads I and aVL, together with a leftward axis deviation, as most frequently noted in LBBB QRS morphology (Fig. 3.7). Recent electroanatomical mapping data [44] have demonstrated that in patients presenting with RBBB and underlying cardiomyopathy, not only is RV activation abnormally delayed, but LV activation is also delayed as much as in patients presenting with LBBB. Furthermore, the LV activation pattern

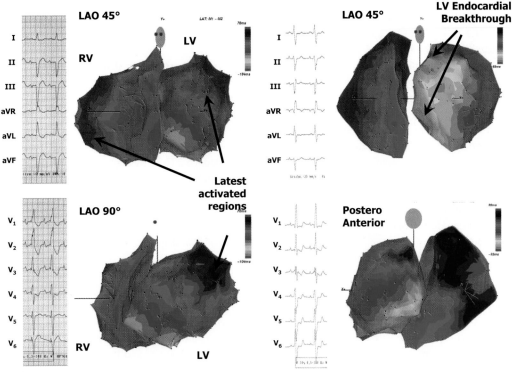

Figure 3.7 Left panels: ECG and color-coded electroanatomical 10 ms isochronal maps of biventricular activation in a patient with heart failure and "RBBB masking LBBB" QRS morphology. The earliest ventricular endocardial activation site (red spot) is located in the inferior LV septum and, after approximately 60 ms, the activation starts also in the RV septum. Then, the activation proceeds in both ventricles very slowly, from the septal breakthrough sites toward the anterior regions . The lateral regions of both ventricles are activated very late. Right panels: ECG and color-coded electroanatomical 10 ms isochronal maps of biventricular activation in a patient with heart failure and pure RBBB pattern. Two LV endocardial breakthrough sites, one in the septum and one in the anterior region, are noted.

observed in these patients resembles that observed in patients with LBBB, which explains the characteristic ECG pattern. These patients usually present clinically with a severe biventricular ischemic cardiomyopathy, with large areas of myocardial injury, due to a significant lesion of the left anterior descendent coronary artery. Notably, the few heart failure patients presenting with pure RBBB differed from the ones with "RBBB masking LBBB" by presenting an additional LV anterobasal breakthrough site in addition to the septal site, thus suggesting preserved conduction capacities throughout the anterior fascicle of the left bundle (Fig. 3.7).

Electrical activation during cardiac resynchronization therapy

The understanding of the detrimental mechani-cal consequences related to asynchronous electrical activation has stimulated attempts to alter AV and inter- and intraventricular timing to provide a more synchronous activation pattern in patients with heart failure. Cardiac resynchronization therapy (CRT), the aim of which is to provide hemodynamic benefit by correcting an electrical disturbance, can be delivered either by pacing the LV alone or pacing both ventricles, synchronized with the atrial electrical activation. The mechano-energetic effects induced by this novel non-pharmacological therapy have been extensively discussed in Chapter 4.

While the mechanical effects elicited by CRT have been well characterized, the electrical spread of activation during atrial-synchronous LV pacing only or biventricular pacing has not been investigated in great detail. Moreover, the relationship between changes in electrical synchrony and the resulting changes in the contractile or mechanical synchrony with CRT is poorly understood.

Regardless of how CRT is delivered, it is important to stress that patients with heart failure frequently present with pathological interatrial and/or intra-atrial conduction times [30]. Thus, atrial pacing may further prolong these delays [31], significantly contributing to loss of the atrial mechanical function and consequently worsening of biventricular mechanics. Furthermore, AV timing modulates the degree of pre-excitation of RV, and more importantly of the LV, so that it is always important to take the AV delay into account when discussing spread of activation and fusion of the wavefronts generated at different sites.

Inter- and intraventricular electrical delays are almost always accompanied by a wide QRS complex, but clinical studies have shown a poor correlation between shortening of the QRS duration with CRT and hemodynamic improvement. Because the QRS complex is mostly derived from epicardial potentials, this would indicate that epicardial electrical synchrony cannot predict mechanical improvement with CRT. Indeed, it has been shown in a canine model of heart failure with LBBB that improvements in hemodynamic function and mechanical synchrony with CRT are not correlated to correction of epicardial electrical asynchrony [46]. Similarly, another animal study of LBBB in the non-failing heart demonstrated that hemodynamic function was optimized with LV pacing only if endocardial electrical synchrony was also present [47]. This was accomplished by selecting an AV delay that allowed fusion between LV stimulus and intrinsic conduction through the right bundle branch. These findings raise the hypothesis that endocardial and epicardial surfaces may exhibit different degrees of electrical fusion and thus synchrony during LV pacing, such that hemodynamic improvement might be observed with increased endocardial electrical synchrony, without a clear correlation to epicardial electrical synchrony or QRS duration.

Although in animal models more data about the ventricular activation sequence during CRT have been collected, different methodologies do not permit full comparison of the findings among the studies. Moreover, the ventricular activation sequence obtained in the canine model may not entirely correspond to human pathological findings, and extrapolation of such observations may not entirely apply to humans.

Electrical activation during single site left ventricular pacing

Detailed epicardial and endocardial characterization of the electrical activation during atrial synchronous LV epicardial single site pacing in an animal model with normal ventricular function has been recently provided [48]. This gives us very useful insights into how synchrony may arise during CRT delivered by LV pacing alone. Faris *et al.* evaluated the transition from dyssynchronous to synchronous LV activation pattern by constructing activation time maps for both endo- and epicardial surfaces, as a function of lengthening the AV delay [48]. They showed that, at short AV delays during epicardial LV pacing, LV activation pattern was asynchronous in both the endocardial and the epicardial surfaces without possibility of merging with the intrinsic conduction which was traveling through the right bundle branch. In this situation, both inter- and LV intraventricular electrical asynchrony were usually increased. In contrast, at longer AV delays, the electrical activation pattern became more synchronous in both the epicardial and the endocardial surfaces, due to increasing degree of fusion between the wavefront propagating from the LV epicardial pacing site and the intrinsic wavefront originating from the right bundle branch. This activation pattern led to a significant reduction of both inter- and LV intraventricular electrical asynchrony. Finally, at very long AV delays, electrical asynchrony increased again, indicating that the heart was primarily activated from the intrinsic conduction system through the right bundle branch, rather than from the LV stimulus. In this last example, activation of both ventricles resembled what is usually observed during intrinsic LBBB, with consequent significant inter- as well as LV intraventricular electrical asynchrony. Interestingly, the transition from dyssynchronous to synchronous activation occurred at similar AV delays in the epicardial and endocardial surfaces [49].

Characterization of the ventricular activation sequence during single site LV pacing in humans is considerably limited. In the normal heart, the spread of ventricular electrical activation occurs within 50–80 ms via conduction through the Purkinje network, and contraction occurs with similar synchrony. In heart failure patients with ventricular conduction delay of LBBB pattern, the electrical activation sequence is significantly altered (U-shaped pattern), creating regions of early and late activation/contraction, delayed by as much as 100–150 ms (Fig. 3.8). Regions of latest activation, usually the LV lateral or posterolateral walls, are considered the target pacing site of the LV (Figs 3.9 and 3.10). Thus, pre-excitation of the LV lateral or posterolateral wall is the usual way for providing CRT.

When CRT is delivered with LV pacing alone and at a short AV delay, i.e. before the spontaneous impulse coming from the RV can break through into the LV, a single LV endocardial breakthrough site is noted (Figs 3.4 and 3.9). This endocardial breakthrough site is located not far from the epicardial pacing site and it usually occurs 30–60 ms from delivery of the stimulus, after transmural propagation from epicardium to endocardium. From the endocardial breakthrough site, LV activation spreads radially toward both the posterior wall and the septum, through the working myocardial cells. Once the anterior region of the LV is reached, activation is usually no more able to proceed and reflects inferiorly around the apex, giving rise to a discontinuous activation sequence (Figs 3.4 and 3.9). Due to the fact that LV activation by pacing is always conducted via working myocardium, this leads to a reversed "U-shaped" activation pattern, which is directionally reversed (lateral wall–septum) as compared to intrinsic LBBB (septum–lateral wall). A slight change in the location of the functional block may occur compared to intrinsic LBBB (Figs 3.8 and 3.9). As a consequence, during epicardial LV pacing alone without fusion with the intrinsic wavefront coming from the right side, no reduction or even an increase of both inter- and LV intraventricular electrical asynchrony may occur. This phenomenon is also confirmed by an increase of total biventricular and LV endocardial activation times and QRS duration. Despite that, a significant hemodynamic benefit has been consistently reported, probably related to the fact that all regions of the LV are homogeneously electrically and mechanically delayed. Thus, this results in a reduction of the relative mechanical dispersion within the LV and increase of pump efficiency.

The line-of-block usually changes in location and in length as the AV delay changes (i.e. with different degrees of fusion between the activation wavefronts coming from the left and the right side). A minimization of the line-of-block may be noted at a particular AV-delay (Fig. 3.4). The AV delay at which this phenomenon occurs may or may not be coincident with the most optimal "hemodynamic" AV delay. Indeed, the "hemodynamic" optimal AV delay is the result of three independent components: (1) preload maximization, (2) mechanical retiming of lateral and septal walls which is dependent on the spread of activation front(s) within epicardium/endocardium, and (3) the region of collision of different wavefronts within the LV.

At an optimal AV delay a significant degree of fusion may occur between the wavefront initiated by the epicardial LV lead and the intrinsic one originating from the right bundle branch. In this situation, LV electrical activation may resemble that occurring during simultaneous biventricular pacing, depending very much on the selected AV delay. Two different endocardial LV breakthrough sites, one in the septum and one in the lateral region, may be noted, leading to two opposite propagating wavefronts merging in the anterior or middle portion of the LV. In this way, both inter- and LV intraventricular electrical asynchrony are reduced, with consequent reduction of total biventricular and LV activation times.

There has been confirmation that pacing from the epicardium as delivered during CRT does not enter into the Purkinje system. When the pacing site coincides with the intrinsically latest activated region, spread of the activation can be predicted: indeed, the latest activated site is located 180° apart from LV pacing site (Fig. 3.9), being now very close to the intrinsic LV endocardial breakthrough site occurring during LBBB. Moreover, recent mapping data showed that during LV only pacing from the epicardial surface (i.e. from a lateral epicardial vein), a slow activation front spreads at the epicardium both homogeneously and radially (Fig. 3.9). Simultaneous with the spreading of this wavefront at the epicardial layer, the activation front dives into the most inner myocardial layers, thus breaking through at the endocardium 30–60 ms after the LV epicardial pacing. Once the wavefront has reached

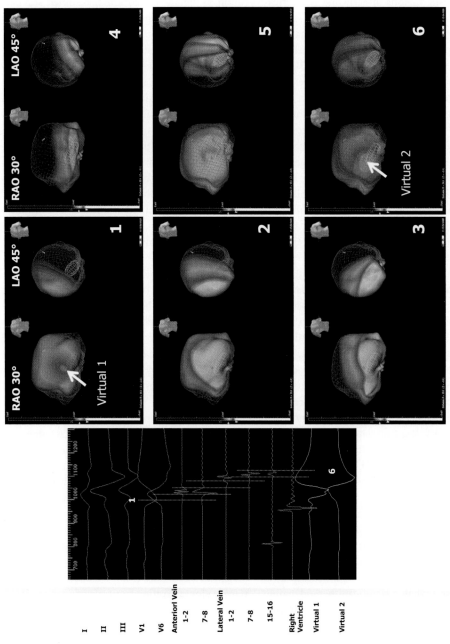

Figure 3.8 Non-contact mapping LV activation sequence during intrinsic left bundle branch block. The different timings of the activation sequence are drawn on the ECG. The left panel shows surface ECG (light blue), intracardiac bipolar RV recordings (red), unipolar LV non-contact (white) electrograms, as well as epicardial bipolar recordings acquired through microcatheters inserted into the anterior and lateral epicardial veins (green). Each panel is taken at a corresponding point, as noted by the white lines. The activation starts in the LV septum and proceeds toward the anterior wall, but once this region is reached the activation front is no longer able to proceed and reflects around the apex, giving rise to a characteristic U-shaped activation pattern (see text).

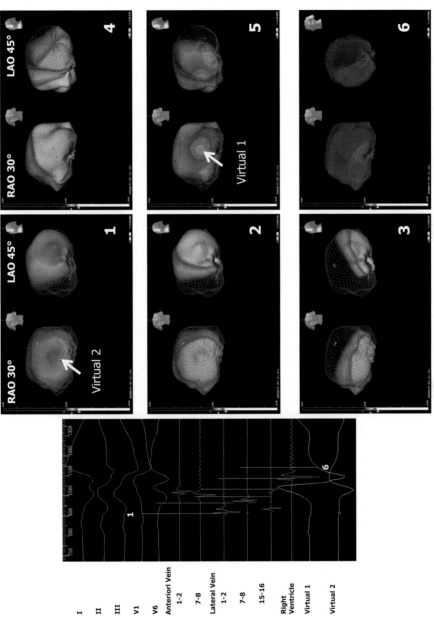

Figure 3.9 Non-contact mapping LV activation sequence in the same patient of Fig. 3.8, during single site LV pacing (lateral epicardial vein). The left panel shows along with the surface ECG (light blue), intracardiac bipolar RV recordings (red), unipolar LV non-contact (white) electrograms, as well as epicardial bipolar signals recorded through microcatheters inserted into the anterior and lateral epicardial veins (green). Each panel is taken at a corresponding point, as noted by the white lines. The endocardial activation starts in the lateral wall, very close to the epicardial pacing site. From this spot activation proceeds to epicardial layers, which are activated before transmural activation occurs. Pacing from LV epicardium gives rise to a reversed U-shaped laterosseptal activation pattern. In this particular example, because LV single site pacing is delivered at a short AV delay, no fusion occurs between the activation wavefront generated by the pacing lead and the intrinsic wavefront through the AV node and the right bundle branch (see text).

the endocardium, it proceeds through the working subendocardial cells. Therefore, LV transmural activation is variable and determined predominantly by the time needed for the paced stimulus to break through into the endocardium, as well as by the propagation velocity within the myocardial and subendocardial layers.

Electrical activation during biventricular pacing

During biventricular pacing, LV and RV may be stimulated simultaneously or sequentially (RV-LV or LV-RV). Biventricular pacing is most commonly delivered from the RV endocardial surface, usually at the RV apex, and from the LV epicardial surface, most commonly from a lateral or posterolateral vein.

Precise assessment of electrical activation sequence during biventricular pacing is very limited both in animals and human beings. The study by Lambiase et al. [41] is the only one that has been conducted in patients with this specific goal; however, this study included a small, highly selected cohort of patients with heart failure undergoing CRT. Their observations are, however, intriguing. In agreement with other authors [33, 34], Lambiase et al. showed that patients with heart failure and ventricular conduction delays had a slow conduction zone within the LV. Pacing the LV from an area without slow conduction increased the hemodynamic gain and was accompanied by a reduction in both LV activation time and QRS width.

Mapping data obtained in our laboratory by combining conventional and three-dimensional mapping techniques in heart failure patients with LBBB [33], have shown that during simultaneous biventricular pacing from RV apex and an epicardial lateral vein, delivered with a short AV delay that preempts intrinsic conduction through the AV node, an initial LV endocardial breakthrough site occurs in the mid or apical LV septum. This breakthrough site originates from right-to-left impulse propagation from the RV pacing site. Interestingly, the time needed by the right activation wavefront to cross the septum and to reach the LV is usually close to the time needed by the wavefront originating from the LV pacing site to break from the epicardium into the endocardium (30–60 ms). This results in two near simultaneous LV endocardial

breakthrough sites, one in the septum and one in the lateral region (Fig. 3.10). The spread of these two wavefronts is consistently different, since the wavefront generated by RV pacing is primarily located at the endocardium, whereas the wavefront generated by LV pacing spreads mostly at the epicardium and myocardium. Once the activation wavefront originating from RV stimulus has reached LV endocardium after trans-septal conduction, it propagates from the septum toward the anterior and then the lateral LV region (Fig. 3.10). At the same time, it crosses the intramyocardial layers, reaching the epicardium after a variable delay and propagates in the same direction of the endocardial front, but much more slowly, within the subepicardial layers. In this way an endo- to epicardium activation gradient is noted in the septoanterior LV region. From the LV pacing site, activation soon spreads over the epicardium, radially toward both the anterior and the posterior regions. At the same time, the wavefront breaks into the endocardium and propagates in the same directions within the inner layers. In this way an epi- to endocardium activation gradient is created in the lateral and posterolateral LV regions. The two activation wavefronts originating from the two pacing sites collide most frequently at the level of the anterosuperior region of the LV, where an area of slow conduction is often located (Fig. 3.10). In this way, biventricular pacing is able to abolish the typical "U-shaped" activation pattern that characterizes LV activation in heart failure patients with LBBB (Fig. 3.10).

Furthermore, given the coexistence of epicardial and endocardial activation wavefronts coming from opposite directions, it can also be postulated that transmural activation sequence is more synchronized (Fig. 3.11). Simultaneous with LV depolarization, RV activation spreads circumferentially from the RV pacing site toward the base (i.e. the posterior region and the outflow tract, being the latest activated regions of the RV). Therefore, biventricular pacing is able to reduce and in some cases to abolish inter- and LV intraventricular electrical asynchrony, with a significant reduction of both biventricular and LV activation times as reflected by a reduction of QRS duration.

Recent data from Lambiase et al. [41] indicate that simultaneous pacing from the LV endocardium and endocardial RV apex elicited the largest

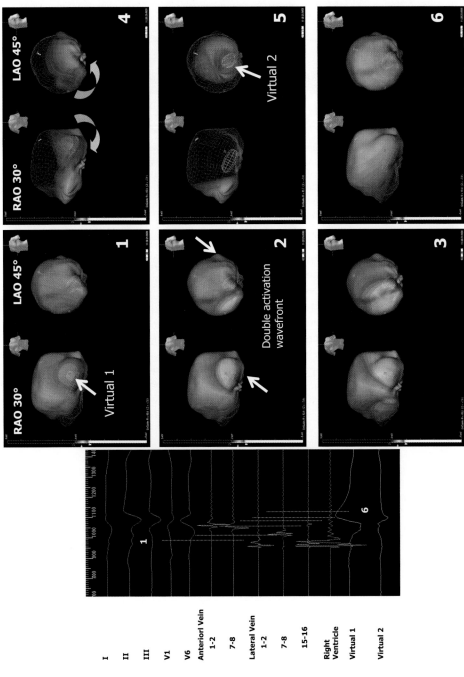

Figure 3.10 Non-contact mapping LV activation sequence in the same patient as Fig. 3.8 during biventricular pacing, delivered at the RV apex and a lateral epicardial vein. The left panel shows along with the surface ECG (light blue), intracardiac bipolar RV recordings (red), unipolar LV non-contact (white) electrograms, as well as epicardial bipolar signals recorded through microcatheters inserted into the anterior and lateral epicardial veins (green). Each panel is taken at a corresponding point, as noted by the white lines. Two wavefronts have been generated by the two pacing sites. A fusion occurs at the anterior region and then proceeds to the inferior wall of the LV. The QRS duration is much shorter than during intrinsic activation (Fig. 3.8) or LV only pacing (Fig. 3.9).

| RAO 30° | LAO 45° | RAO 30° | LAO 45° | RAO 30° | LAO 45° |

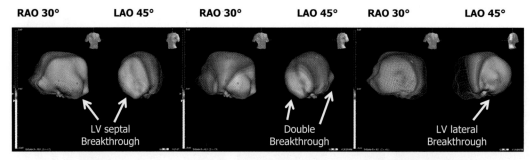

| **Right Ventricular Apical Pacing** | **Biventricular Pacing** | **Left Ventricular Epicardial Pacing** |

Figure 3.11 Non-contact mapping LV activation sequence in the same patient as Fig. 3.8, during RV apical pacing, biventricular pacing (RV apex and LV lateral epicardial vein) and during LV single site pacing (lateral vein). During RV apical pacing, LV activation starts at the apex, after right-to-left trans-septal conduction. During biventricular pacing a fusion between two activation wavefronts coming from the septum and LV lateral wall takes place. During LV pacing from a lateral vein, LV activation starts in the lateral wall and then proceeds with a reversed lateral-septum "U-shaped" pattern.

increase in hemodynamic function, the shortest LV endocardial activation time, and the narrowest QRS complex. This observation is consistent with data by Garrigue *et al.* [49] who demonstrated that LV endocardial pacing led to a significantly greater hemodynamic improvement and narrower QRS complex compared with LV epicardial pacing. The exact three-dimensional electrical and mechanical characterization during this novel approach still needs to be defined.

Conclusions

Characterization of the spread of electrical activation in both RV and LV has enabled a much better understanding of how CRT may potentially be applied in different patient populations presenting with different activation patterns. Understanding of the transmural activation sequence may be of great interest for further improving the mechanical benefits achieved by CRT.

References

1 Cannom DS, Wyman MG, Goldreyer BN. Initial ventricular activation in left-sided intraventricular conduction defects. *Circulation* 1980; **62**: 621–631.

2 Vassallo JA, Cassidy DM, Miller JM *et al.* Left ventricular endocardial activation during right ventricular pacing: effect of underlying heart disease. *J Am Coll Cardiol* 1986; **7**: 1228–1233.

3 Gepstein L, Hayan G, Ben-Haim SA. A novel method for nonfluoroscopic catheter-based electroanatomical mapping of the heart. In vitro and in vivo accuracy results. *Circulation* 1997; **95**: 1611–1622.

4 Schilling RJ, Peters NS, Davies DW. Simultaneous endocardial mapping in the human left ventricle using a noncontact catheter: comparison of contact and reconstructed electrograms during sinus rhythm. *Circulation* 1998; **98**: 887–898.

5 De Bakker JMT, Hauer RNW, Simmens TA. Activation mapping: Unipolar versus bipolar recording. In: Zipes DP, Jalife J, eds. *Cardiac Electrophysiology – From Cell to Bedside*, 3rd edn. WB Saunders, Philadelphia, 2000: 1068–1078.

6 Scher AM, Young AC, Malmgreen AL *et al.* Spread of electrical activity through the wall of the ventricle. *Circ Res* 1953; **1**: 539–547.

7 Cao J, Chen LS, KenKnight BH *et al.* Nerve sprouting and sudden cardiac death. *Circ Res* 2000; **86**: 816–821.

8 Sanchez-Quintana D, Cabrera JA, Farré J *et al.* Sinus node revisited in the era of elctroanatomical mapping and catheter ablation. *Heart* 2005; **91**: 189–194.

9 Sherf L, James TN. Fine structure of cells and their histologic organization within internodal pathways of the heart: clinical and electrocardiographic implications. *Am J Cardiol* 1979; **44**: 345–369.

10 Khaja A, Flaker G. Bachmann's bundle: does it play a role in atrial fibrillation? *Pacing Clin Electrophysiol* 2005; **28**: 855–863.

11 Ho SY, McComb JM, Scott CD *et al.* Morphology of the

cardiac conduction system in patients with electrophysiologically proven dual atrioventricular nodal pathways. *J Cardiovasc Electrophysiol* 1993; **4**: 504.

12 Scher AM, Young AC, Malmgreen AL *et al*. Activation of the interventricular septum. *Circ Res* 1955; **3**: 56–64.

13 Myerburg RJ, Nilsson K, Gelband H. Physiology of canine intraventricular conduction and endocardial excitation. *Circ Res* 1972; **30**: 217–243.

14 Hoffman BF, Cranefield PF, Stuckley JH *et al*. Direct measurement of conduction velocity in *in situ* specialized conduction system of mammalian heart. *Proc Soc Exp Biol Med* 1959; **102**: 55–57.

15 Kulbertus HE, Demoulin J-C. The left hemiblocks: significance, prognosis and treatment. *Schweiz Med Wochenschr* 1982; **112**: 1579–1584.

16 Uhley HN, Rivkin L. Peripheral distribution of the canine A-V conduction system. *Am J Cardiol* 1960; **5**: 688–691.

17 Truex RC, Copenhaver WM. Histology of the moderator band in man and other mammals with special reference to the conduction system. *Am J Anat* 1947; **80**: 173–200.

18 Durrer D, Dam v. RT, Freud GE *et al*. Total excitation of the isolated human heart. *Circulation* 1970; **41**: 899–912.

19 Spach MS, Barr RC. Analysis of ventricular activation and repolarization from intramular and epicardial potential distributions for ectopic beats in the intact dog. *Circ Res* 1975; **37**: 830–843.

20 Rawling DA, Joyner RW, Overholt ED. Variations in the functional electrical coupling between the subendocardial Purkinje and ventricular layers of the canine left ventricle. *Circ Res* 1985; **57**: 252–261.

21 Spach MS, Miller WT, Geselowitz DB *et al*. The discontinuous nature of propagation in normal canine cardiac muscle. Evidence for recurrent discontinuities of intracellular resistance that affect the membrane currents. *Circ Res* 1981; **48**: 39–54.

22 Prinzen FW, Augustijn CH, Arts T *et al*. Redistribution of myocardial fiber strain and blood flow by asynchronous activation. *Am J Physiol* 1990; **259**: H300–H308.

23 Myerburg RJ, Gelband H, Nilsson K *et al*. The role of canine superficial ventricular fibers in endocardial impulse conduction. *Circ Res* 1978; **42**: 27–35.

24 Li D, Fareh S, Leung TK *et al*. Promotion of atrial fibrillation by heart failure in dogs: atrial remodelling of a different sort. *Circulation* 1999; **100**: 87–95.

25 Ohtani K, Yutani C, Nagata S *et al*. High prevalence of atrial fibrosis in patients with dilated cardiomyopathy. *J Am Coll Cardiol* 1995; **25**: 1162–1169.

26 Verheule S, Wilson E, Everett T *et al*. Alteration in atrial electrophysiology and tissue structure in a canine model of chronic atrial dilatation. *Circulation* 2003; **107**: 2615–2622.

27 Morton JB, Sanders P, Vohra JK *et al*. The effect of chronic atrial stretch on atrial electrical remodeling in patients

with an atrial septal defect. *Circulation* 2003; **107**: 1775–1782.

28 Sanders P, Kistler PM, Morton JB *et al*. Remodeling of sinus node function in patients with congestive heart failure. Reduction of sinus node reserve. *Circulation* 2004; **110**: 897–903.

29 Olgin JE, Kalman JM, Fitzpatrick AP *et al*. Role of right atrial endocardial structures as barriers to conduction during human type I atrial flutter: activation and entrainment mapping guided by intracardiac echocardiography. *Circulation* 1995; **92**: 1839–1848.

30 Sanders P, Morton JB, Davidson NC *et al*. Electrical remodeling of the atria in congestive heart failure. Electrophysiological and electroanatomic mapping in humans. *Circulation* 2003; **108**: 1461–1468.

31 Bernheim A, Ammann P, Sticherling C *et al*. Right atrial pacing impairs cardiac function during resynchronization therapy. *J Am Coll Cardiol* 2005; **45**: 1482–1487.

32 Rodriguez L-M, Timmermans C, Nabar A *et al*. Variable patterns of septal activation in patients with left bundle branch block and heart failure. *J Cardiovasc Electrophysiol* 2003; **14**: 135–141.

33 Auricchio A, Fantoni C, Regoli F *et al*. Characterization of left ventricular activation in patients with heart failure and left bundle branch block. *Circulation* 2004; **109**: 1133–1139.

34 Fung JWH, Yu CM, Yip G *et al*. Variable left ventricular activation pattern in patients with heart failure and left bundle branch block. *Heart* 2004; **90**: 17–19.

35 Verbeek X, Vernooy K, Peschar M *et al*. Intraventricular resynchronization for optimal left ventricular function during pacing in experimental left bundle branch block. *J Am Coll Cardiol* 2003; **42**: 558–567.

36 Ono S, Nohara R, Kambara H *et al*. Regional myocardial perfusion and glucose metabolism in experimental left bundle branch block. *Circulation* 1992; **85**: 1125–1131.

37 Verbeek X, Vernooy K, Peschar M *et al*. Quantification of interventricular asynchrony during left bundle branch block and ventricular pacing. *Am J Physiol* 2002; **283**: H1370–H1378.

38 Liu L, Tockman B, Girouard S *et al*. Left ventricular resynchronization therapy in a canine model of left bundle branch block. *Am J Physiol* 2002; **282**: H2238–H2244.

39 Wyndham CRC, Smith T, Meeran MK *et al*. Epicardial activation in patients with left bundle branch block. *Circulation* 1980; **61**: 696–703.

40 Vassallo JA, Cassidy DM, Marchlinski FE *et al*. Endocardial activation of left bundle branch block. *Circulation* 1984; **69**: 914–923.

41 Lambiase PD, Rinaldi A, Hauck J *et al*. Non-contact left ventricular endocardial mapping in cardiac resynchronization therapy. *Heart* 2004; **90**: 44–51.

42 Fantoni C, Regoli F, Kawabata M, Klein HU, Auricchio

A. Reversed transmural activation timing in patients with heart failure and left bundle branch block. *Eur Heart J* 2004: (suppl): 2320.

43 Hesse B, Diaz LA, Snader CE *et al.* Complete bundle branch block as an independent predictor of all-cause mortality: report of 7,073 patients referred for nuclear exercise testing. *Am J Med* 2001; **110**: 253–259.

44 Fantoni C, Kawabara M, Massaro R *et al.* Right and left ventricular activation sequence in patients with heart failure and right bundle branch block. A detailed analysis using 3D non-fluoroscopic electroanatomic mapping system. *J Cardiovasc Electrophysiol* 2005; **16**: 112–119.

45 Rosenbaum MB. Types of right bundle branch block and their clinical significance. *J Electrocardiol* 1968; **1**: 221–229.

46 Leclercq C, Faris O, Tunin R *et al.* Systolic improvement and mechanical resynchronization does not require electrical synchrony in the dilated failing heart with left bundle-branch-block. *Circulation* 2002; **106**: 1760–1763.

47 Prinzen FW, van Ooosterhout MFM, Vanagt WYR *et al.* Optimization of ventricular function by improving the activation sequence during ventricular pacing. *Pacing Clin Electrophysiol* 1998; **21**: 2256–2560.

48 Faris OP, Evans FJ, Dick AJ *et al.* Endocardial versus epicardial electrical synchrony during LV free-wall pacing. *Am J Physiol Heart Circ Physiol* 2003; **285**: H1864–H1870.

49 Garrigue S, Jais P, Espil G *et al.* Comparison of chronic biventricular pacing between epicardial and endocardial left ventricular stimulation using Doppler tissue imaging in patients with heart failure. *Am J Cardiol* 2001; **88**: 858–862.

CHAPTER 4

Myocardial mechano-energetics

Tammo Delhaas, MD, PhD *& Frits W. Prinzen,* PhD

Introduction

Until approximately a decade ago the mechanical effects of asynchronous electrical activation were almost completely neglected, despite the first evidence for detrimental mechanical effects being published 80 years ago by Wiggers. Nowadays, interest in this issue is rapidly growing, related to the increasing numbers of reports on the beneficial effects of cardiac resynchronization therapy (CRT) [1, 2] and adverse effects of conventional right ventricular (RV) pacing [3–5]. It is also becoming increasingly clear that duration of the QRS complex has little predictive value with respect to short-term hemodynamic and long-term clinical outcome under these circumstances.

Fortunately, information on cardiac mechanics is also rapidly increasing due to the development of dedicated non-invasive imaging techniques for assessment of regional myocardial function. Insights into regional myocardial mechanics during asynchronous activation is not only helpful in assessing the cause of disturbed pump function, it also gives clues to long-term structural, contractile, and electrophysiological adaptations in the heart. In this chapter we will discuss cardiac mechanics and energetics during asynchronous and resynchronized activation. To this purpose information from studies in animal experimental models and from patients will be used as well as that from mathematical models of cardiac mechanics.

Electromechanical coupling

As in any muscle, cardiac contraction is evoked by an action potential. The action potential triggers calcium influx through L-type calcium channels, initiating calcium-induced calcium release by the sarcoplasmic reticulum (SR). Transport and binding of calcium, released from the SR, takes some time, which gives rise to a time delay between the depolarization and onset of force development. The entire electromechanical delay amounts to approximately 30 ms [6]. On a global basis this delay can be observed as the delay between the R wave of the ECG and the rise in left ventricular (LV) pressure.

In the healthy heart ventricular activation occurs through impulse conduction through the rapid conduction system. Endings of this system are located in the subendocardium. From there, the impulses are conducted through the slower conducting working myocardium. Accordingly, during normal sinus rhythm in hearts without conduction abnormalities the electrical activation is relatively synchronous (activation of the ventricles occurring within 70 ms). Earliest activation occurs in the LV septal endocardium and latest in the epicardium of the LV lateral wall [7].

The consequences of this sequence of electrical activation for the sequence of contraction have been studied only recently, partly due to technical limitations of studying transmural differences in contraction in high detail. These differences could be investigated in a mathematical model of LV mechanics. Surprisingly, the model showed that a mechanical activation sequence similar to the well-described electrical activation sequence during sinus rhythm would result in considerably more asynchronous contraction than actually measured *in vivo* [8]. The more synchronous contraction patterns, as observed *in vivo*, could only be achieved when activating the contraction system synchronously (Fig.

4.1). Therefore, this evidence suggests that onset of contraction might even be more synchronous than electrical activation and that this would require differences in electromechanical delay between endo- and epicardium, compensating for the ~40 ms delay between endo- and epicardial electrical activation [8]. This idea is supported by transmural differences in excitation–contraction coupling processes at the cellular level [9]. The presence of a regionally different electromechanical delay may also explain why modern non-invasive techniques show quite synchronous ventricular contraction patterns [10], one study even showing an earlier onset in the LV free wall than in the septum [11].

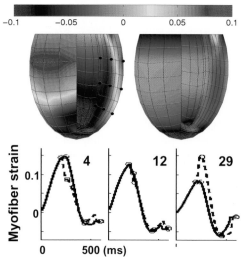

Figure 4.1 Distribution of myofiber strain during the isovolumic contraction phase in a mathematical model of LV mechanics [8]. The left panel depicts the strain distribution calculated from a simulation, assuming mechanical activation with a sequence equal to that of electrical activation during normal sinus rhythm, the right panel that simulating absolutely synchronous mechanical activation. Notice that in this figure early shortening and pre-stretch occur as negative and positive strains, respectively. Myofiber strain tracings in the lower part of the figure are derived from the endocardium, mid myocardium, and epicardium, indicated by the middle row of dots indicated in the upper left panel. Note that during sinus rhythm simulation significant differences exist in the distribution of early systolic strain, as apparent from the different colors and the regional difference in strain tracing (broken lines). The figures in the lower panel indicate the time of mechanical activation during sinus rhythm simulation. Modified after Kerckhoffs *et al.* [8].

To date, it is not known whether the electromechanical coupling is influenced by altered sequences of activation, hypertrophy, or heart failure. Because, for the heart as a pump, the synchrony of contraction is more important than that of impulse conduction, studies on electromechanical coupling in dyssynchronous hearts appear to be important in increasing our knowledge of the mechanisms of action of CRT and other therapies.

Contraction patterns in asynchronous hearts

During ventricular pacing [12, 13] and in diseases affecting the ventricular conduction system, such as left bundle branch block (LBBB) [14], the normal physiological sequence of electrical activation is disturbed. Under these circumstances the impulse is conducted through the slowly conducting working myocardium, rather than through the rapidly conducting specialized conduction system. As a consequence, the time required for activation of the entire ventricular muscle, for example expressed as QRS duration, is at least twice as long as that during normal sinus rhythm. QRS prolongation by abnormal activation is even greater in patients with ischemic heart disease [13].

Asynchronous electrical activation also leads to asynchronous and dyscoordinate contraction. During the 1980s and 1990s, this was studied in detail in animal experiments by using ventricular pacing [15–19]. As expected from the fairly tight electromechanical coupling, regions with earliest electrical activation (black in bulls-eye plot in lower left panel of Fig. 4.2) also start to contract first (lower blue tracing, Fig. 4.2). Because all other muscle fibers are still in a relaxed state, the early activated fibers can shorten rapidly by up to 10% before the onset of the ejection phase. This rapid early systolic shortening is followed by minimal systolic shortening, sometimes even holo-systolic stretch, and premature relaxation. In contrast, in late-activated regions (yellow in bulls-eye plot of Fig. 4.2) the fibers are stretched by up to 15% during early systole (lower red tracing in Fig. 4.2). This stretch is followed by doubling of net systolic shortening and by delayed relaxation [16, 19]. Therefore, during asynchronous activation local contraction patterns differ not only in the onset of contraction,

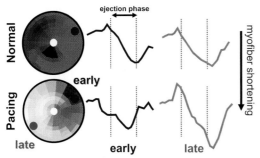

Figure 4.2 Bulls-eye plots of electrical activation of the LV endocardium (left panels) and strain tracings during normal activation (upper row) and ventricular pacing (lower row). Asynchronous activation (endocardial time differences of ~30 ms, dark color indicating earliest activation) leads to early onset of shortening (lower blue tracing) while late activated regions are stretched during early systole, followed by pronounced shortening during the ejection phase. Derived from data presented by Prinzen *et al.* [16] and Verbeek *et al.* [60].

but also, and more importantly, in the pattern of contraction. These contraction patterns imply that opposing regions of the ventricular wall are out of phase and that energy generated by one region is dissipated in opposite regions. Therefore, not only does pump output decrease, but also the efficiency to do so (see below).

In various studies in normal canine heart the onset of segment shortening was found to be closely related to the timing of electrical activation [6, 10, 15]. The cause of the complicated regional differences in contraction pattern is most likely related to local differences in myocardial fiber length during the early systolic phase. Fiber length is presumably closely related to sarcomere length, an important determinant of contractile force [20]. In studies using two isolated papillary muscles in series asynchronous stimulation caused a downward shift in the force–velocity relation in the earlier activated muscle and an upward shift in the later activated one [21]. Therefore, the regional differences in contraction pattern during ventricular pacing are most likely caused by regional differences in effective preload. Accordingly, during ventricular pacing regional systolic fiber shortening increases with increasing isovolumic stretch [22]. Similarly, a close correlation exists between the time of local electrical activation and the degree of systolic fiber shortening. This relation was found to be independent of

the region investigated and for multiple sites of pacing, suggesting a universal property [17] (Fig. 4.3).

Consequences for local energetics

Global LV pump work, generated by the summed action of the myocardial fibers, can be derived from LV pressure–volume loops. Total mechanical work (e.g. external mechanical work and the so-called potential mechanical work) is defined as the pressure–volume area (PVA), which is the area bounded by the pressure–volume trajectory during systole and both the end-systolic and end-diastolic pressure–volume relationship curves [23]. Local mechanical work can be derived from local fiber stress–fiber strain loops (Fig. 4.4). It is therefore conceivable that local differences in wall motion and deformation during asynchronous electrical activation will be reflected in local differences in myocardial work. This was demonstrated in dogs with epicardial pacing at different sites by construction of local fiber stress–fiber strain diagrams and calculation of local external and total mechanical work analogous to the PVA concept used for the entire left ventricle [18, 19]. Regions close to the pacing site showed early systolic shortening at low pressure, followed by minimal systolic shortening, sometimes even holo-systolic stretch at higher ventricular pressures. As a consequence the area of the fiber stress–fiber strain loops is small or even negative, indicating

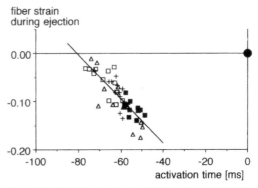

Figure 4.3 Plot of local subepicardial fiber strain during the ejection phase versus local electrical activation time during right atrial (normal activation, filled squares), LV free wall (open squares), LV apex (+) and RV outflow tract pacing (triangles). The activation time was normalized to the moment of maximum rate of rise of LV pressure. A strain value of –0.10 represents 10% shortening. Modified after Delhaas *et al.* [17].

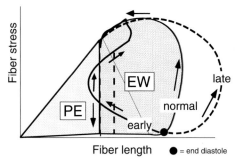

Figure 4.4 Schematic of the calculation of local work during normal and abnormal activation. Simplified fiber stress–fiber length (s–L) relations in regions with early, normal, and late activation are presented. PE, potential energy; EW, external work. External work is determined as the area of the s–L loop, and potential work is the area of the triangle delineated by the origin, the end-systolic fiber length–stress point and the end-systolic fiber length point. Fiber length was defined as L/L_0, the ratio of fiber length at time t and at zero cavity volume. Total work is the sum of PE and EW [18, 19].

low external work or work being performed on that particular region. In regions remote from the pacing site the loops are wide and external work can be up to twice that during synchronous ventricular activation. Total myocardial work (sum of external work and potential energy) is reduced by 50% in early activated regions and is increased by 50% in late activated regions, as compared with the situation during atrial pacing [18, 19].

A limitation to these studies is that for calculation of local fiber stress several assumptions had to be made. Fiber stress cannot be measured reliably since the measuring devices used can easily damage the local myocardial structure in the direct environment of the measuring site. Another approach is to simulate fiber stress–strain relations during asynchronous electrical activation in a finite element computational model of LV cardiac electromechanics [24]. This model has been validated [25, 26] and includes fiber orientation as well as physiological active and passive material properties. Depolarization times during simulated pacing were determined assuming that pulses are exclusively conducted through the working myocardium with a higher wave velocity parallel (0.75 m/s) than perpendicular (0.3 m/s) to the myofiber [25]. Wall mechanics were determined by solving the equations of force equilibrium. Active myofiber stress development depended on time, sarcomere length and sarcomere shortening velocity and was initiated at the time of depolarization.

Figure 4.5 presents data on electrical activation times, sarcomere length at the start of ejection and stroke work, as calculated throughout the RV and LV walls. The spread of electrical activation occurs gradually, as has been shown by various experimental [10, 16, 18, 27] and clinical measurements [13, 28]. Regional differences in sarcomere length at the beginning of the ejection phase were calculated due to early onset of contraction in early activated region and stretch of the not yet activated regions. Calculations of stress–strain diagrams show that the stress–strain loop in the early depolarized region progressed in a clockwise direction, indicating negative stroke work. The model also calculates that maximum active fiber stress decreases by ~35% in early activated regions and increases by ~10% in late activated ones (Fig. 4.6). This observation was never made for calculated fiber stress in animal experiments, where differences in maximum active fiber stress between early and late activated regions were estimated to be in the order of 10% maximally [18]. While measurements are limited to a transmural average or one single layer, the model shows that behavior is similar in all layers.

The area of the myofiber stress–strain loops, representing stroke work, gradually increased from negative values in early depolarized to supranormal values in late depolarized regions (Fig. 4.5). This finite element model of LV electromechanics, in which known principles of propagation of depolarization, time-dependent contraction of myofibers, and equilibria of forces were applied, realistically simulates LV mechanics during RV apex pacing by only changing the sequence of depolarization. It therefore shows that the apparently complex events observed during pacing are caused by well-known basic physiological processes.

In the light of the considerable mechanical differences between regions, it is not surprising that during asynchronous activation myocardial blood flow [16, 18, 29, 30], oxygen consumption [18, 31], and glucose uptake also differ between regions [29]. Compared with sinus rhythm, myocardial blood flow and oxygen consumption are 30% lower in early activated regions and 30% higher in late activated regions [16, 18].

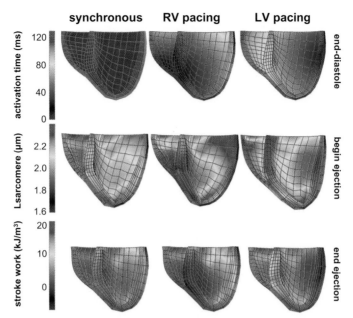

Figure 4.5 Anterior views of the heart, showing cross-sections of the walls, and LV and RV endocardium. Top panel: Electrical activation times as calculated from simulated synchronous activation and for simulated RV and LV pacing, represented on the mesh at end-diastole. Mid panel: Sarcomere length for the three simulations, represented on the deformed mesh at the beginning of LV ejection. Bottom panel: Stroke work per unit volume of tissue (kJ/m³) for the three simulations. Stroke work is represented on the mesh at end-systole. During synchronous activation sarcomere length and stroke work are distributed fairly uniform throughout the LV and RV wall. During asynchronous activation sarcomere length at begin ejection and stroke work are reduced in early activated regions and increased in late activated regions, irrespective of whether the regions are in the RV or LV wall. Modified after Kerckhoffs *et al.* [24].

Figure 4.6 Myofiber stress–sarcomere length loops in the LV midwall for an early (left), mid (middle), and late (right) activated region, as calculated from a mathematical model of LV mechanics. Black dashed loops denote loops for normal sinus rhythm, while red loops indicate loops during RV apex pacing. The triangles and circles indicate the opening and closing of valves for the SR and RVA simulation respectively. The arrows indicate the direction of the loop progression through time. Note that in the early depolarized region the red loop progresses in a clockwise direction (negative external work), while all other loops progress in a counter-clockwise direction (positive external work). Modified after Kerckhoffs *et al.* [26].

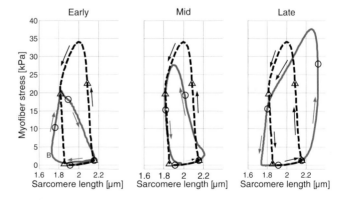

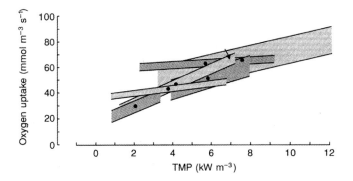

Figure 4.7 Correlation between oxygen uptake and total myocardial work (TMP), as obtained from measurements in open-chest anesthetized dogs during pacing at the right atrium, LV apex, and RV outflow tract in 16 sub-epicardial regions. Each gray area represents the 95% confidence intervals of data from one experiment. The dots denote the centers of the estimated relations. Modified after Delhaas et al. [18].

A good correlation was found between local mechanical work and oxygen consumption during ventricular pacing (Figs 4.7 and 4.8) [18]. This indicates that regional differences in blood flow are a physiological adaptation to the differences in mechanical work. This idea is supported by the finding that regional differences in blood flow during pacing disappear during total coronary vasodilation by adenosine [32] and, hence, that coronary perfusion is not hampered by abnormal contraction and relaxation patterns. Another argument in favor of matching demand and supply during asynchronous activation is the fact that septal blood flow after chronic experimental LBBB was reduced without signs of hibernation [30]. Only at higher heart rates, when myocardial perfusion becomes more critical, does impairment of blood flow due to the abnormal conduction play a possible role [33].

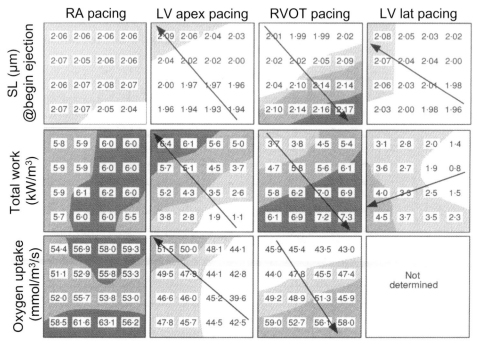

Figure 4.8 Mean maps of sub-epicardial sarcomere length (SL), total work, and oxygen uptake during RA, LV apex, RV outflow tract, and LV lateral (lat) wall pacing in the canine heart. Depicted is a region of approximately 4 × 4 cm on the anterior and lateral LV wall. Gradients are indicated by arrows. Modified after Delhaas et al. [18].

Effect of asynchronous activation on systolic and diastolic pump function

The dyscoordinate contraction patterns caused by abnormal ventricular activation, especially during RV apex pacing and LBBB, induce a wealth of systolic and diastolic hemodynamic perturbations, which are summarized in Fig. 4.9. An abnormality usually limited to ventricular pacing is uncoupling between atrial and ventricular contraction, leading to impaired filling and mitral regurgitation. The asynchronous activation of the ventricles usually leads to inter- and intraventricular asynchrony. During RV pacing and LBBB interventricular asynchrony leads to delayed LV activation and consequently an altered trans-septal pressure gradient that in its turn leads to abrupt pre-ejection posterior interventricular wall motion [34]. This may result in displacement of the posterior papillary muscle towards the mitral annulus, causing early systolic regurgitation. The increased intraventricular asynchrony gives rise

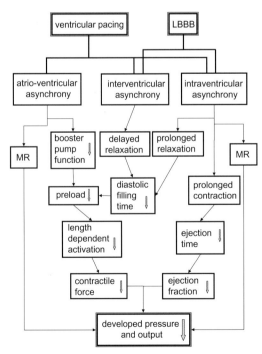

Figure 4.9 Possible relationship between the various consequences of asynchronous activation of the ventricles, due to ventricular pacing or conduction disturbances, and the deterioration of pump function over time. For details see text. LBBB, left bundle branch block; MR, mitral regurgitation.

to prolonged isovolumic contraction and relaxation phases without an increase in total duration of systole. Consequently, duration and extent of ejection are reduced [35–37]. Zhou and colleagues used this property in proposing the Z-ratio, being the ratio of the sum of LV ejection and filling times to the total RR interval. This Z-ratio dissociates the effects of abnormal ventricular activation and systolic disease [36].

Dyscoordination between the two LV papillary muscles can also create mitral valve regurgitation. This combination of factors may lead to LV dilation and increased pulmonary wedge pressure [38]. During RV pacing and LBBB, the increased interventricular asynchrony may also lead to an increased interval between left atrial and LV contraction, potentially leading to suboptimal LV filling and reduction in preload [13, 38–41].

The effects of asynchronous electrical activation on LV pump function are independent of changes in pre- and afterload [35, 42–44]. The pump function-reducing effect of dyssynchronous activation has been observed not only under resting conditions, but also during various loading conditions [45] and exercise [38]. Ventricular pacing also reduces exercise capacity when compared with atrial pacing [46]. Impairments in regional and global cardiac pump function have been observed in patients and animals with LBBB, even if LBBB was not accompanied by other cardiovascular diseases [30, 37]. Ventricular pacing also deteriorates pump function in patients with coronary artery disease [47]. Therefore, it appears that dyssynchrony is an important independent determinant of cardiac pump function.

In invasive hemodynamic studies in animals as well as in patients the maximal rate of rise of LV pressure (LV dP/dt_{max}) is a sensitive marker of reduced systolic function due to dyssynchrony [48–50]. LV dP/dt_{max} is dependent on preload, but since this parameter hardly changes with changing pacing site or mode, LV dP/dt_{max} appears an appropriate marker of dyssynchrony-induced changes in LV contractility. The sensitivity of this isovolumic measure of contractility may be due to the large differences in muscle fiber length changes during this phase (see above). It is probable that forces generated by the already activated fibers are dissipated by the internal resistance of fibers that have not yet been activated.

The negative inotropic effect of pacing has also been characterized using the LV function curve (i.e. output at a range of different preloads) [51] and the end-systolic pressure–volume relation. Concerning the latter, most studies report a rightward shift of this pressure–volume relation (i.e. an increased pressure–volume intercept) [43, 44]. This implies that for each end-systolic pressure the LV has to operate at a larger LV volume, thus leading to ventricular dilatation. This effect comes on top of the LV dilatation caused by mitral valve regurgitation.

Also the rate of ventricular relaxation is slower during ventricular pacing. Isovolumic relaxation parameters, like LV dP/dt_{min} and Tau, are strongly influenced by pacing [48, 50, 52]. Parameters of auxotonic relaxation (rate of segment lengthening or LV volume increase) are also lower during ventricular pacing than during sinus rhythm, but the difference is less pronounced than for the isovolumic relaxation parameters [45, 50].

All these changes following asynchronous activation combined may lead to a lower cardiac output and systolic arterial and LV pressure (Fig. 4.9). In general, stroke volume is affected more than systolic LV pressure [44, 48, 49], presumably because baroreflex regulation partly compensates for decreases in blood pressure. This idea is supported by increased catecholamine levels [53] and increased systemic vascular resistance [38] during ventricular pacing.

Some experimental studies report a correlation between QRS duration and systolic LV function [42, 44, 54], while other studies could not find such a correlation [48, 55, 56]. A possible explanation for the inconsistent correlation between QRS duration and LV function is that QRS duration is a measure of the duration of activation of both RV and LV and that it is not related to the sequence of activation. This idea is supported by the finding that LV function correlates better with the duration of LV endocardial activation than with QRS duration [44]. It is also important to keep in mind that QRS width is not related to the amount of early or late activated myocardium. For example, in Wolff–Parkinson–White syndrome the QRS can be very wide, whereas only a small part of the LV is activated early. Various studies also indicate that the pathway of activation may be a determinant of ventricular function. A ventricular pacing site with relatively good hemodynamic performance is, for example, the LV apex [12, 55, 57], an

observation even made in human hearts [58]. Electrical mapping during LV apex pacing indicates an electrical activation proceeding from apex to base simultaneously in septum and LV lateral wall. Even though LV activation is somewhat dyssynchronous, there is no dyssynchrony between opposite walls. Apex to base conduction in combination with a lack of septal–lateral dyssynchrony may be a good approximation of the activation during normal sinus rhythm. When more pacing sites are added during LV apex pacing, this does not improve LV function, and sometimes even reduces it [48, 55], despite reduction in QRS duration. This finding further emphasizes the importance of a good sequence of ventricular activation.

Beside intraventricular asynchrony, interventricular asynchrony may also be a determinant of ventricular pump function. In an extensive overview of studies on RV and LV pacing it appears that RV pacing consistently leads to more severe reduction in LV function than does LV pacing (reviewed in [59]). Even at similar intraventricular asynchrony, LV dP/dt_{max} is lower during RV than during LV pacing [60]. Also in the mathematical model of the RV and LV, mentioned above, where all elements have the same mechanical properties, hemodynamic deterioration was more pronounced during RV than during LV pacing [24]. This suggests an important role for interventricular asynchrony and, related to that, interventricular mechanical coupling (or interaction). In the section below, evidence will be presented that interventricular coupling may be even more important in failing hearts than it is in normal hearts.

Ventricular efficiency

Another important consequence of ventricular dyssynchrony is its effect on ventricular oxygen consumption. In isolated, isovolumically beating hearts ventricular pacing reduces oxygen consumption and developed LV pressure to the same amount, so that efficiency is not influenced [42]. In a similar preparation Boerth and Covell reported a smaller reduction in oxygen consumption than in pressure development, resulting in a decrease in efficiency [35]. In anesthetized open-chest dogs [61] (Fig. 4.10) and in conscious dogs [62] RV apex pacing decreased mechanical output, whereas myocar-

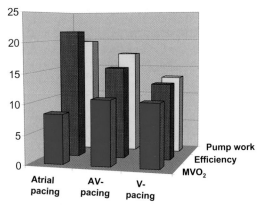

Figure 4.10 External pump work (yellow bars, product of systolic aortic pressure, cardiac output and oxygen equivalent of mechanical cardiac work, × 10⁻² mmHg L/min), myocardial oxygen consumption (red bars, MVo₂, μmol/min per g) and efficiency (green bars, 100 × external work/MVo₂, %) during atrial pacing, AV-sequential pacing and single-chamber pacing in anesthetized dogs. Data derived from Baller *et al.* [61].

dial oxygen consumption was unchanged or even increased, compared with atrial pacing. As a consequence, efficiency decreased by 20–30% in these studies. Efficiency of conversion of metabolic to pumping energy is of particular interest in patients with compromised coronary circulation, since increased oxygen consumption over longer periods of time (as during milrinone therapy) leads to increased mortality [63].

Structural and electrical remodeling due to asynchronous activation and contraction

Early electrical and contractile remodeling due to asynchrony

Like many mechanical disturbances to the heart muscle, the mechanical effects of asynchronous electrical activation lead to changes in cardiac structure and function. For long-term clinical outcome these "remodeling" effects may be at least as important as the acute hemodynamic effects.

A particular adaptation of the heart to ventricular pacing is that after stopping this abnormal activation, repolarization remains abnormal, a phenomenon called T wave, or cardiac, memory. Rosen [64] compared cardiac memory with memory processes in nervous systems throughout nature. Indeed, his

group has found evidence that short-term (<1 h) cardiac memory involves changes in ion channels and phosphorylation of target proteins [65] and that long-term memory (~3 weeks of pacing) involves altered gene programming and protein expression [64, 66]. While the T waves during cardiac memory may appear similar to some that predict arrhythmias during ischemia, the exact clinical relevance of cardiac memory is unclear. Costard-Jäckle *et al.* have demonstrated opposite changes in repolarization in regions remote from and close to a pacing site, starting within the first hour of ventricular pacing [67]. These investigators showed that these electrophysiological changes restored synchrony of repolarization, after being asynchronous immediately upon ventricular pacing.

The repolarization abnormalities related to cardiac memory also have a mechanical counterpart. After a period of ventricular pacing relaxation is disturbed immediately after restoring sinus rhythm [68]. Furthermore, following an acute decrease of ejection fraction upon initiating ventricular pacing, ejection fraction decreases further over the period of a week. Also, after returning to atrial pacing, ejection fraction only slowly recovers its pre-pacing value [69] (Fig. 4.11). It seems likely that changes in ion channel function underlie the reduction in ejection fraction during the first week of changed electrical activation, both from normal to asynchronous activation and vice versa [65]. Therefore, electrical and contractile remodeling occurs soon after changes in activation, and it takes some time to restore these ion channel functions.

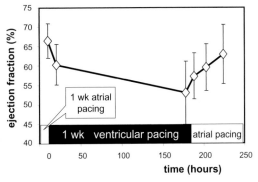

Figure 4.11 Time course of ejection fraction, as determined in patients before and 2 h and one week after onset of RV apex pacing as well as after 2, 24 and 32 h of returning to atrial pacing. Data derived from Nahlawi *et al.* [69].

Long-term adaptations

Longer lasting (>1 month) ventricular pacing and LBBB lead to major structural changes, such as ventricular dilatation and asymmetric hypertrophy [30, 43, 70, 71]. The ventricular dilatation appears to be related to the fact that the left ventricle operates at a larger volume (see above). Global hypertrophy may be induced by this global dilatation as well as by the increased sympathetic stimulation [53].

The asymmetry of hypertrophy appears to be more prominent during LV lateral wall pacing than during RV pacing and LBBB [30, 43, 71]. Nevertheless, during LV and RV pacing as well as LBBB the asymmetry of hypertrophy is characterized by more pronounced growth of late activated myocardium, the same tissue that shows enhanced contractile performance due to early systolic pre-stretch (Fig. 4.12). Because in all regions of the heart circulating hormones have the same concentration, the asymmetry of hypertrophy most likely illustrates the important influence of local stretch on local growth. In LBBB patients LV dilatation and asymmetric hypertrophy have also been observed [70].

In juvenile canine hearts it has been observed that ventricular pacing leads to fiber disarray [72], which potentially is also the result of the regionally different, and abnormal distribution of mechanical work [16, 18, 73]. In chronically paced ventricles myocyte diameter is increased in late activated regions [43]

(Fig. 4.12), but the number of capillaries per myocyte did not change (van Oosterhout, unpublished data). Therefore, the diffusion distance for oxygen increases, potentially leading to compromised oxygenation. The latter is known to render hypertrophic myocardium susceptible to ischemia.

In diseases like infarction and hypertension ventricular remodeling appears, at least initially, to have the function of compensating for the loss of function and the increased load, respectively. However, dilatation and hypertrophy do not reduce the asynchronous activation induced by pacing or LBBB, but rather increase it [30, 43]. This is due to the longer path length of impulse conduction (dilatation) and the larger muscle mass to be activated (hypertrophy). Moreover, chronic asynchronous activation also reduces expression of gap-junction channels [74], which is associated with a slower conduction velocity, especially in the later activated regions [75]. In the latter study it was also shown that action potential duration and refractory period decrease in the late activated myocardium. In canine hearts with non-ischemic dilated cardiomyopathy, induced by rapid RV pacing, similar electrophysiological changes were found [76]. Molecular and cellular mechanisms of slower conduction turned out to be complicated. Slowing of conduction velocity was not directly related to reduced Connexin 43 (Cx43) expression, but rather to changes in phos-

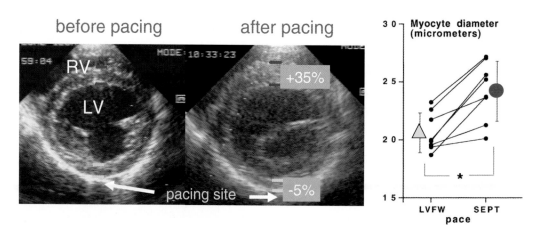

Figure 4.12 Left panel: Cross-sectional LV short-axis echocardiographic images from a dog before and six months after onset of LV free wall pacing. Note the decreased LV free wall thickness (yellow lines), increased septal wall thickness (red lines), and increased LV cavity in the image after six months of pacing compared with baseline image. Right panel: Myocyte diameter in LV free wall (LVFW) and septum (SEPT) of chronically paced hearts. Lines connect data from the same animal. Yellow triangle and red circle indicate the mean value in the corresponding region. Modified after Van Oosterhout *et al.* [43].

phorylation and localization of Cx43. It has to be investigated whether this electrical remodeling can also lead to cardiac arrhythmias.

In contrast to the regionally different electrical remodeling in asynchronous hearts, other remodeling processes turn out to be uniform. In the model of chronic LV pacing the activity of various metabolic enzymes was reduced equally in early and late activated regions (Fig. 4.13). Interestingly, when compared with samples from hearts subjected to volume (atrioventricular block) [77] or pressure overload hypertrophy [71], the same enzyme activities were reduced in pressure overload but not in increased in volume overload. Therefore, these data indicate that metabolic remodeling is not dependent on the degree of local hypertrophy, but rather on systemic factors. The functional importance of the reduced activity of metabolic enzymes in paced hearts in unclear, but it is not impossible that exhaustion at the metabolic level can contribute to the development of heart failure [78].

All these processes may lead to a vicious circle, where dilatation and hypertrophy further reduce LV pump function, directly or by increasing asynchrony of activation (Fig. 4.14). As is the case after myocardial infarction, initial compensatory hypertrophy may result in heart failure many years later. Trials in patients with RV apex pacing, where onset of asynchronous activation is exactly known, indicate that it may take more than five years before initially healthy hearts start to show signs of failure [3]. However, if hearts are already compromised when ventricular pacing is started, heart failure may develop within a year [5]. LBBB is also known to be an independent risk factor for cardiac morbidity and mortality [79, 80].

Mechanical resynchronization

LBBB is the most predominant intraventricular conduction abnormality, with a prevalence of about 30% in patients with heart failure. As discussed in more detail elsewhere in this book (Chapter 3), in LBBB activation spreads from the right bundle branch (RBB) to the RV wall and, after trans-septal conduction, it spreads within the left ventricle from septum to LV lateral wall. Resynchronization can, at least theoretically, be achieved in two ways. First of all, by stimulating the RV and LV wall (almost) simultaneously. This gives rise to two activation wavefronts, merging approximately in the middle. Alternatively, resynchronization is obtained by pacing at the LV lateral wall using an atrioventricular interval that allows merging of the intrinsic activation originating from the RBB with the wavefront derived from the LV pacing lead. Due to the tight excitation–contraction coupling in the heart, CRT also improves coordination of contraction between

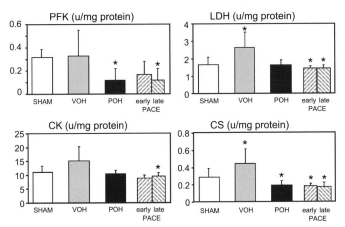

Figure 4.13 Enzyme activity of fructose-6-phosphate kinase (PFK, glycolytic enzyme), lactate dehydrogenase (LDH, glycolytic enzyme), creatine kinase (CK, transfer of P_i from ATP to creatine phosphate and vice versa) and citrate synthase (CS, Krebs cycle enzyme) in LV free wall in control (white bar), volume overload hypertrophy (chronic AV block [77], gray bar), pressure overload hypertrophy (aortic stenosis [71], black bar) and chronically paced hearts [43]. For the latter group samples were taken from early and late activated regions (denoted by opposite hatching). *$P < 0.05$ vs. SHAM.

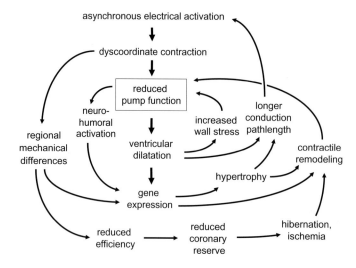

Figure 4.14 Possible relation between asynchronous electrical activation, abnormal contraction, LV pump function, ventricular remodeling and the progression towards heart failure. For details see text.

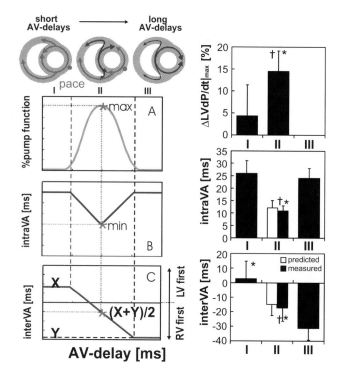

Figure 4.15 Left panels: Schematic representation of a path length model of ventricular impulse conduction (upper) and predicted results for LV pump function (A), intraventricular (intraVA, B) and interventricular asynchrony (interVA, C) as a function of the AV delay during single site LV pacing. Situations I, II, and III denote the situations during short (complete capture), intermediate and (very) long AV delay (~ baseline LBBB). X = interVA during LV pacing at short AV delay and Y = interVA during baseline; (X+Y/2) predicts optimal resynchronization. Right panels: Data for a group of canine LBBB hearts on LV dP/dt$_{max}$, intraVA, and interVA in situations I, II, and III. Changes in LV dP/dt$_{max}$ are relative to LBBB (III) values. The open bars in II denote the values predicted by the model, the closed ones denote the measured values. •$P < 0.05$ vs. III, †$P < 0.05$ vs. I. Modified after Verbeek *et al.* [107].

the cardiac chambers and within the LV wall as shown using different imaging techniques.

In LBBB activation spreads from the right bundle branch (RBB) to the right ventricular wall and, after transseptal conduction, within the left ventricle from septum to LV lateral wall. Conceptually, resynchronization occurs when two activation wave-fronts, originating from opposite walls, merge in the middle (upper left panel of Fig. 4.15). This can be achieved by stimulating the RV and LV wall (almost) simultaneously or by pacing the LV lateral wall at an AV interval that allows the activation wave from that pacing site to merge with the wave originating from the RBB. With the tight excitation-contraction coupling in the heart, such stimulation is also expected to improve the coordination of contraction.

Figure 4.15 shows that, according to these simple assumptions, maximal hemodynamic effect is expected when intraventricular asynchrony is minimal. Under these conditions interventricular asynchrony is predicted to have a value equal to the average of interventricular asynchrony during LBBB and during LV pacing at short AV-delay (the (X+Y/2) value, lower left panel of figure 4.15) [107]. The right panels of figure 15 depict data from canine LBBB hearts, indicating that predictions from this concept on resynchronization closely match experimental observations. Also in patients during LV and biventricular pacing interventricular asynchrony accurately predicted the AV-delay at which optimal LV pump function occurred [81].

The principle of merging wavefronts of contraction by biventricular pacing is illustrated by data obtained in normal canine hearts using MRI tagging, a technique considered to be the current gold standard of tissue deformation (Fig. 4.16). During normal ventricular activation (right atrial pacing) the myocardial fibers shorten regularly and uniformly, as depicted by the appearance of the blue color as systole proceeds (upper row). During single site RV and LV pacing (third and fourth row) the contraction wave starts from the site of pacing and proceeds to the opposite wall in a quite regular fashion. Note the stretching of the opposite wall during early and mid-systole, as indicated by the yellow color. Also note that the situation during RV apex pacing is similar to that during LBBB. During simultaneous RV and LV (biventricular) pacing two contraction waves start from opposite sites, merging approximately in the middle [27]. So when compared with single site ventricular pacing, biventricular pacing clearly creates a pattern of contraction that approaches the normal situation better. However, it can also be observed that in these hearts without conduction disturbances the pattern of contraction during right atrial pacing is more uniform than during biventricular pacing. This is also associated with slightly depressed hemodynamics during biventricular pacing [27, 55]. These data are in agreement with observations in the Pacing Therapies in Congestive Heart Failure (PATH-CHF) trial, which showed that in patients without ventricular dyssynchrony LV pump function did not improve by biventricular pacing, but rather worsened upon starting biventricular pacing [107].

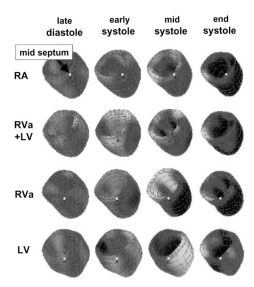

Figure 4.16 Strain renderings of the LV created by mapping myocardial circumferential strain (Ecc) as color on a volume reconstruction of the LV. Blue indicates contraction (negative Ecc), red indicates the reference state (Ecc = 0), and yellow indicates stretch (positive Ecc). Data are shown for late diastole, early systole, mid-systole, and end-systole (sequential columns from left to right). Data obtained using MRI tagging during RA, biventricular RV apex (RVa), and LV lateral wall (LV) pacing, from top to bottom. Black dot next to each heart indicates the location of the midseptum. Modified after Wyman *et al.* [27].

While biventricular pacing clearly resynchronizes asynchronous hearts, it may worsen the synchrony and sequence of activation in hearts without conduction block. Therefore, in the era of ever-increasing enthusiasm about CRT, it should be realized that starting biventricular pacing therapy in some patients may have adverse effects. In this respect even the recognition of CRT "non-responders" may be a euphemism, because, as discussed above, inducing dyssynchrony may actually worsen a patient's condition in the short or long term.

That biventricular pacing improves contraction patterns in patients with abnormal ventricular conduction has been shown several times, especially using ultrasound techniques [82, 83], as discussed in more detail elsewhere in this book (Chapters 5 and 6). These studies showed more simultaneous myocardial velocity patterns within the left ventricle and between right and left ventricles.

Breithardt *et al.* used strain rate imaging in order to quantify tissue deformation more accurately in patients before and during CRT [84]. They found that deformation (strain) describes resynchronization better than the velocity of tissue displacement (TDI). However, strain imaging is, as of yet, a considerably more complex technique. The value of this study is that it shows normalization of myocardial strains in patients similar to those shown by MRI tagging in animal studies [10, 19, 30, 85] and that after improvement the strain rate imaging technique may be a valuable tool in optimizing CRT.

Because abnormal systolic strains, like those present during asynchronous activation, also have consequences for local energetics (see above), it is reconfirming that positron emission tomography (PET) studies show more uniform distribution of blood flow and glucose uptake upon resynchronization [29, 31, 86, 87]. The finding that this recovery of blood flow occurs within two weeks after onset of CRT [29] and disappears within 15 min after stopping CRT [87] shows that the septal underperfusion during LBBB is merely due to abnormal load distribution, as had already been supposed on the basis of basic physiologic observations (see above).

The more uniform distribution of cardiac contraction during CRT also leads to a higher efficiency of the entire LV chamber. Nelson *et al.* showed elegantly that resynchronization increases LV dP/dt_{max} while even slightly decreasing myocardial oxygen consumption, as measured using coronary sinus blood flow and arteriocoronary sinus oxygen content differences [88]. A similar increase in LV dP/dt_{max} in these patients, evoked by dobutamine infusion, significantly increased myocardial oxygen consumption. Therefore, restoration of coordination of contraction by CRT improves cardiac function through a mechanism different from that of inotropic stimulation. The observation that CRT improves ventricular efficiency is important for two reasons. First, there is evidence that, in general, failing hearts have a reduced ratio between work performed and oxygen consumed (mechanical efficiency) [89]. Also, these hearts often have compromised energy metabolism, as evidenced by a reduced ratio of phosphocreatine to total ATP [90]. So any relief of the compromised energy metabolism can be expected to have a relevant benefit.

As far as is known, no other therapies in heart failure improve cardiac efficiency. While inotropic drugs increase myocardial oxygen consumption in parallel with contractility, vasodilators decrease both parameters. The effect of phosphodiesterase III inhibitors depends on the vasodilative and inotropic effects as well [91]. The potentially harmful effect of longer lasting increase of myocardial energy expenditure through inotropic therapy has, for example, been shown for enoximone [63].

The improved efficiency from CRT is unlikely to be due to alterations in intrinsic myocyte function. Rather, the net effect is observed at the chamber level because of the more coordinate contraction in different regions of the LV wall. This process is analogous to that of a poorly timed automotive engine; each piston continues to burn fuel, but when timing is suboptimal, there is reduced effective compression and engine power, wasted work, and lower fuel economy [88].

Many studies have shown improvements in the parameters of cardiac pump function, such as LV dP/dt_{max}, pulse pressure, cardiac output, and ejection fraction [83, 92–96]. Such improved systolic pump function is achieved at unchanged or even decreased filling pressures, denoting a true improvement of ventricular contractility through improved coordination of contraction. This is also indicated by a leftward shift of the end-systolic pressure–volume point during CRT [94, 95]. Further improvement in pump function is possibly mediated by reduction of mitral regurgitation [97] and prolongation of diastolic filling time. These beneficial effects occur almost immediately after starting resynchronization [93].

The mysterious benefits of LV pacing

While in clinical practice CRT usually implies biventricular pacing, all acute hemodynamic studies show that single site LV pacing improves hemodynamic as least as well, if not better, than biventricular pacing [92–94]. Also long-term results are equally good for LV and biventricular pacing [98]. When using single site LV pacing in patients with LBBB-like conduction disturbances one presumably achieves resynchronzation by fusion of the LV pacing wavefront with that derived from the RBB [60, 99]. The better cardiac pump function shown during LV pacing than during biventricular pacing could even be attributed to using the RBB as "infinite electrode" as opposed to the RV pacing lead.

After all, by using the RV pacing site in biventricular pacing, one renders the RV asynchronous.

However, improvements by LV pacing are also reported in patients with atrial fibrillation [100] and even in patients with narrow QRS complex [101]. LV pacing at very short atrioventricular delay in patients with LBBB in sinus rhythm also improves LV function more than is anticipated from the degree of electrical resynchronization (Fig. 4.17) [93, 107]. This is further emphasized by findings in a canine model of dyssynchrony and heart failure, in which LV pacing was associated with electrical asynchrony and mechanical synchrony and hemodynamic improvement [85]. A possible explanation for the relatively good performance of LV pacing is that during LV pacing in failing hearts, septal pre-stretch is less, either due to altered material properties or elevated RV pressure. Since early systolic pre-stretch determines the degree of subsequent systolic shortening, reduced pre-stretching could just create alteration

of mechanical activity, as compared to the LBBB situation, to the extent that mechanical contraction becomes virtually uniform.

Another possible explanation is provided by work of Bleasdale *et al.* [101]. These investigators measured LV pressure–volume diagrams in patients with both narrow and wide QRS complex and varying levels of venous pressures. In patients with central venous pressure of more than 15 mmHg LV pacing at a short atrioventricular interval increased LV filling through a mechanism called interventricular coupling or diastolic ventricular interaction. The idea is that in hearts with high central venous pressures the RV occupies much of the pericardial space. Therefore, early LV activation may allow the left ventricle to fill first at the expense of the right ventricle, thereby increasing its Frank–Starling effect.

One aspect of the good performance of LV pacing in heart failure patients may be that CRT could be applied with a simpler (i.e. classical DDD) pacemaker. However, its greatest value may be in the fact that pacing therapy may be applied to patient populations other than just those with conduction disturbances. To do so, however, we will first need to improve our understanding of the acute and long-term effects of any potentially new indication.

Long-term effects of cardiac resynchronization therapy

A variety of cardiac and extracardiac processes triggered by CRT are responsible for the long-term beneficial effect of CRT. These effects can be understood when considering the reversal of all effects of asynchronous activation, as depicted in Fig. 4.14. The improved pump function reduces neurohumoral activation, which is evidenced by an increase in heart rate variability and a reduction in plasma brain natriuretic peptide (BNP) levels [102]. Furthermore, the improved contractility and pump efficiency at a smaller end-diastolic volume reduces mechanical ventricular stretch. These two effects may well explain the decrease of end-diastolic and end-systolic LV volume over time, referred to as reverse remodeling (Fig. 4.18) [1, 83]. As it was elegantly demonstrated by Yu *et al.* [83], such reverse remodeling points to structural improvement in the myocardium. These authors showed the increasing reverse remodeling effect of resynchronization over

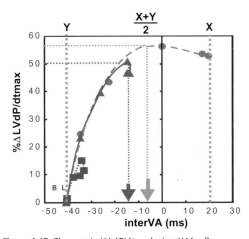

Figure 4.17 Changes in LV dP/dt_{max} during LV (red), biventricular (green), and RV pacing (blue) in a patient, plotted versus intraventricular asynchrony (interVA). The various interVA values were obtained by pacing at various AV delays, with shorter AV delays leading to less negative, during LV pacing even positive, interVA values. In this patient biventricular pacing reduced interVA from a baseline value of –43 ms to –15 ms (green arrow), which is below the optimal (X + Y)/2 value (orange arrow). This impaired interventricular resynchronization was accompanied by a smaller increase in LV dP/dt_{max} during biventricular than during LV pacing. This difference was observed in 11 out of 22 patients [107]. X = interVA during LV pacing at short AV delay and Y = interVA during baseline.

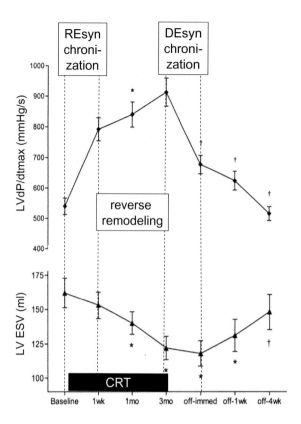

Figure 4.18 Changes in LV dP/dt_{max} (upper panel) and end-systolic volume (lower panel) before and after biventricular pacing (CRT) as well as when pacing was suspended for four weeks. *Significant difference vs. baseline. †Significant difference vs. biventricular pacing for three months. Data indicate the effects of acute resynchronization (upon CRT on) and desynchronization (upon CRT off) as well as reverse remodeling (reduction in LV end-systolic volume. Modified after Yu et al. [83].

time by measuring the time course of LV cavity volume and LV dP/dt_{max} during the first three months after onset of CRT and during a month after temporarily stopping CRT. After stopping CRT, still some beneficial effect of CRT was noticeable, pointing to adaptation in the tissue (Fig. 4.18).

Preliminary data from a study in canine LBBB hearts showed that isolated LBBB induces LV dilatation as well as hypertrophy and that these derangements are almost completely reversed by biventricular pacing. Interestingly, biventricular pacing reversed the hypertrophy in the LV wall, especially in the late activated LV lateral wall [103]. This observation may be important, because after initiation of LBBB the development of asymmetric hypertrophy [30] is associated with molecular changes, especially in the most hypertrophied LV lateral wall [74–76]. Recently, unequal distribution of wall thickness at anterior, inferior, septal, and lateral wall has been observed in patients with dilated cardiomyopathy undergoing CRT (A Auricchio and CM Yu, personal communication), thus confirming the animal observation. At three-month follow-up after CRT

initiation, reduction of LV mass and regional wall thickness was demonstrated in a significant number of patients, which represents structural reverse remodeling. However, such benefit was only observed in volumetric responders, but was worsened in nonresponders (A Auricchio and CM Yu, personal communication).

Another potentially important consequence of the reverse remodeling process upon CRT is the improvement in myocardial perfusion reserve [87]. These investigators showed that three months of CRT improved myocardial perfusion reserve (Fig. 4.19) [87]. The exact cause of this beneficial effect is not yet clear. These investigators show a correlation between reduction of an indicator of wall stress and the increase of hyperemic blood flow, suggesting a role for reverse remodeling. On the other hand, the almost complete disappearance of the beneficial effect on hyperemic blood flow upon temporarily stopping CRT suggests that the (mechanical) resynchronization may be another factor involved. Because perfusion reserve indicates the safety margin against myocardial ischemia, this may certainly be

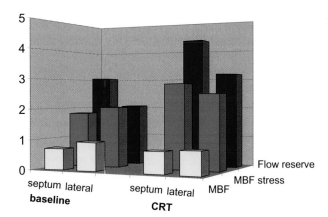

Figure 4.19 Myocardial blood flow during rest (MBF) and hyperemia (MBF stress, both mL/min per mL of myocardium) and the flow reserve, as measured with PET and $H_2^{15}O$ in patients before (baseline) and after three months of biventricular pacing. Data derived from table 3 of Knaapen *et al.* [87].

additive to all other mechanisms in increasing life expectancy of patients.

Most recently, the importance of reverse remodeling has been emphasized by a study showing that reverse remodeling is a strong predictor of decreased total mortality and even more accurate for cardiac mortality [104]. These fascinating data indicate how important the long-term changes in cardiac tissue are for clinical outcome.

While CRT is usually applied to adult, often elderly patients, there may also be a role for resynchronization in children. Experience in this field is, however, small [105]. Janousek *et al.* presented two cases where either stopping RV apex pacing and allowing junctional narrow QRS rhythm or upgrading an RV apex pacemaker to a biventricular one resulted in clear reverse remodeling and clinical improvement [106].

References

1 St. John Sutton MG, Plappert T, Abraham WT *et al.* Effect of cardiac resynchronization therapy on left ventricular size and function in chronic heart failure. *Circulation* 2003; **107**: 1985–1990.

2 Cleland JG, Daubert JC, Erdmann E *et al.* The effect of cardiac resynchronization on morbidity and mortality in heart failure. *N Engl J Med* 2005; **352**: 1539–1549.

3 Andersen HR, Nielsen JC, Thomsen PEB *et al.* Long-term follow-up of patients from a randomised trial of atrial versus ventricular pacing for sick-sinus syndrome. *Lancet* 1997; **350**: 1210–1216.

4 Sweeney MO, Hellkamp AS, Ellenbogen KA *et al.* Adverse effect of ventricular pacing on heart failure and atrial fibrillation among patients with normal baseline QRS duration in a clinical trial of pacemaker therapy for sinus node dysfunction. *Circulation* 2003; **107**: 2932–2937.

5 Wilkoff BL, Cook JR, Epstein AE *et al.* Dual-chamber pacing or ventricular back-up pacing in patients with an implantable defibrillator. *JAMA* 2002; **288**: 3115–3123.

6 Prinzen FW, Augustijn CH, Allessie MA *et al.* The time sequence of electrical and mechanical activation during spontaneous beating and ectopic stimulation. *Eur Heart J* 1992; **13**: 535–543.

7 Durrer D, Dam v. RT, Freud GE *et al.* Total excitation of the isolated human heart. *Circulation* 1970; **41**: 899–912.

8 Kerckhoffs RCP, Bovendeerd PHM, Kotte JCS *et al.* Homogeneity of cardiac contraction despite physiological asynchrony of depolarization: a model study. *Ann Biomed Eng* 2003; **31**: 536–547.

9 Cordeiro JM, Greene L, Heilmann C *et al.* Transmural heterogeneity of calcium activity and mechanical function in the canine left ventricle. *Am J Physiol* 2004; **286**: H1471–1479.

10 Wyman BT, Hunter WC, Prinzen FW *et al.* Mapping propagation of mechanical activation in the paced heart with MRI tagging. *Am J Physiol* 1999; **276**: H881–H891.

11 Zwanenburg JJ, Gotte MJ, Kuijer JP *et al.* Timing of cardiac contraction in humans mapped by high-temporal-resolution MRI tagging: early onset and late peak of shortening in lateral wall. *Am J Physiol* 2004; **286**: H1872–1880.

12 Lister JW, Klotz DH, Jomain SL *et al.* Effect of pacemaker site on cardiac output and ventricular activation in dogs with complete heart block. *Am J Cardiol* 1964; **14**: 494–503.

13 Vassallo JA, Cassidy DM, Miller JM *et al.* Left ventricular endocardial activation during right ventricular pacing: effect of underlying heart disease. *J Am Coll Cardiol* 1986; **7**: 1228–1233.

14 Vassallo JA, Cassidy DM, Marchlinski FE *et al.* Endocardial activation of left bundle branch block. *Circulation* 1984; **69**: 914–923.

15 Badke FR, Boinay P, Covell JW. Effect of ventricular pacing on regional left ventricular performance in the dog. *Am J Physiol* 1980; **238**: H858–H867.

16 Prinzen FW, Augustijn CH, Arts T *et al.* Redistribution of myocardial fiber strain and blood flow by asynchronous activation. *Am J Physiol* 1990; **259**: H300–H308.

17 Delhaas T, Arts T, Prinzen FW *et al.* Relation between regional electrical activation time and subepicardial fiber strain in the canine left ventricle. *Eur J Physiol (Pflugers Arch)* 1993; **423**: 78–87.

18 Delhaas T, Arts T, Prinzen FW *et al.* Regional fibre stress-fibre strain area as estimate of regional oxygen demand in the canine heart. *J Physiol (Lond)* 1994; **477**: 481–496.

19 Prinzen FW, Hunter WC, Wyman BT *et al.* Mapping of regional myocardial strain and work during ventricular pacing: experimental study using magnetic resonance imaging tagging. *J Am Coll Cardiol* 1999; **33**: 1735–1742.

20 Ter Keurs HEDJ, Rijnsburger WH, Van Heuningen R *et al.* Tension development and sarcomere length in rat cardiac trabeculae. Evidence of length-dependent activation. *Circ Res* 1980; **46**: 703–714.

21 Tyberg JV, Parmley WW, Sonnenblick EH. In-vitro studies of myocardial asynchrony and regional hypoxia. *Circ Res* 1969; **25**: 569–579.

22 Prinzen FW, Delhaas T, Arts T *et al.* Regional electromechanical coupling during ventricular pacing. Paper presented at: Cardiac arrhythmias, pacing and electrophysiology, 1998, Athens.

23 Suga H, Hayashi T, Suehiro S *et al.* Equal oxygen consumption rates of isovolumic and ejecting contractions with equal systolic pressure-volume areas in canine left ventricle. *Circ Res* 1981; **49**: 1082–1091.

24 Kerckhoffs RCP, Faris OP, Bovendeerd PHM *et al.* Intra- and interventricular asynchrony of electromechanics in the ventricularly paced heart. *J Engin Math* 2003; **47**: 201–216.

25 Kerckhoffs RCP, Faris OP, Bovendeerd PHM *et al.* Timing of depolarization and contraction in the paced canine ventricle: model and experiment. *J Cardiovasc Electrophysiol* 2003; **14**: S188–S195.

26 Kerckhoffs RCP, Faris OP, Bovendeerd PHM *et al.* Electromechanics of the paced left ventricle simulated by a straightforward mathematical model: comparison with experiments. *Am J Physiol* 2005; **289**: H1889–1897.

27 Wyman BT, Hunter WC, Prinzen FW *et al.* Effects of single- and biventricular pacing on temporal and spatial dynamics of ventricular contraction. *Am J Physiol* 2002; **282**: H372–H379.

28 Auricchio A, Fantoni C, Regoli F *et al.* Characterization of left ventricular activation in patients with heart failure and left bundle-branch block. *Circulation* 2004; **109**: 1133–1139.

29 Nowak B, Sinha AM, Schaefer WM *et al.* Cardiac resynchronization therapy homogenizes myocardial glucose metabolism and perfusion in dilated cardiomyopathy and left bundle branch block. *J Am Coll Cardiol* 2003; **41**: 1523–1528.

30 Vernooy K, Verbeek XAAM, Peschar M *et al.* Left bundle branch block induces ventricular remodeling and functional septal hypoperfusion. *Eur Heart J* 2005; **26**: 91–98.

31 Lindner O, Vogt J, Kammeier A *et al.* Effect of cardiac resynchronization therapy on global and regional oxygen consumption and myocardial blood flow in patients with non-ischaemic and ischaemic cardiomyopathy. *Eur Heart J* 2005; **26**: 70–76.

32 Amitzur G, Manor D, Pressman A *et al.* Modulation of the arterial coronary blood flow by asynchronous activation with ventricular pacing. *Pacing Clin Electrophysiol* 1995; **18**: 697–710.

33 Beppu S, Matsuda H, Shishido T *et al.* Functional myocardial perfusion abnormality induced by left ventricular asynchronous contraction: experimental study using myocardial contrast echocardiography. *J Am Coll Cardiol* 1997; **29**: 1632–1638.

34 Little WC, Reeves RC, Arciniegas J *et al.* Mechanism of abnormal interventricular septal motion during delayed left ventricular activation. *Circ Res* 1982; **65**: 1486–1490.

35 Boerth RC, Covell JW. Mechanical performance and efficiency of the left ventricle during ventricular stimulation. *Am J Physiol* 1971; **221**: 1686–1691.

36 Zhou Q, Henein M, Coats A *et al.* Different effects of abnormal activation and myocardial disease on left ventricular ejection and filling times. *Heart* 2000; **84**: 272–276.

37 Grines CL, Bashore TM, Boudoulas H *et al.* Functional abnormalities in isolated left bundle branch block. *Circulation* 1989; **79**: 845–853.

38 Leclercq C, Gras D, Le Helloco A *et al.* Hemodynamic importance of preserving the normal sequence of ventricular activation in permanent cardiac pacing. *Am Heart J* 1995; **129**: 1133–1141.

39 Rosenqvist M, Isaaz K, Botvinick EH *et al.* Relative importance of activation sequence compared to atrioventricular synchrony in left ventricular function. *Am J Cardiol* 1991; **67**: 148–156.

40 Mark JB, Chetham PM. Ventricular pacing can induce hemodynamically significant mitral valve regurgitation. *Anesthesiology* 1991; **74**: 375–377.

41 Twidale N, Manda V, Holliday R *et al.* Mitral regurgi-

tation after atrioventricular node catheter ablation for atrial fibrillation and heart failure: acute hemodynamic features. *Am Heart J* 1999; **138**: 1166–1175.

42 Burkhoff D, Oikawa RY, Sagawa K. Influence of pacing site on left ventricular contraction. *Am J Physiol* 1986; **251**: H428–H435.

43 Van Oosterhout MFM, Prinzen FW, Arts T *et al.* Asynchronous electrical activation induces inhomogeneous hypertrophy of the left ventricular wall. *Circulation* 1998; **98**: 588–595.

44 Park RC, Little WC, O'Rourke RA. Effect of alteration of left ventricular activation sequence on the left ventricular end-systolic pressure-volume relation in closed-chest dogs. *Circ Res* 1985; **57**: 706–717.

45 Bahler RC, Martin P. Effects of loading conditions and inotropic state on rapid filling phase of left ventricle. *Am J Physiol* 1985; **248**: H523–H533.

46 Harper GR, Pina IL, Kutalek SP. Intrinsic conduction maximizes cardiopulmonary performance in patients with dual chamber pacemakers. *Pacing Clin Electrophysiol* 1991; **14**: 1787–1791.

47 Betocchi S, Piscione F, Villari B *et al.* Effects of induced asynchrony on left ventricular diastolic function in patients with coronary artery disease. *J Am Coll Cardiol* 1993; **21**: 1124–1131.

48 Prinzen FW, van Oosterhout MFM, Vanagt WYR *et al.* Optimization of ventricular function by improving the activation sequence during ventricular pacing. *Pacing Clin Electrophysiol* 1998; **21**: 2256–2260.

49 Rosenqvist M, Bergfeldt L, Haga Y *et al.* The effect of ventricular activation sequence on cardiac performance during pacing. *Pacing Clin Electrophysiol* 1996; **19**: 1279–1287.

50 Zile MR, Blaustein AS, Shimizu G *et al.* Right ventricular pacing reduces the rate of left ventricular relaxation and filling. *J Am Coll Cardiol* 1987; **10**: 702–709.

51 Gilmore JP, Sarnoff SJ, Mitchell JH *et al.* Synchronicity of ventricular contraction: observations comparing hæmodynamic effects of atrial and ventricular pacing. *Br Heart J* 1963; **25**: 299–307.

52 Heyndrickx GR, Vantrimpont PJ, Rousseau MF *et al.* Effects of asynchrony on myocardial relaxation at rest and during exercise in conscious dogs. *Am J Physiol* 1988; **254**: H817–H822.

53 Lee MA, Dae MW, Langberg JJ *et al.* Effects of long-term right ventricular apical pacing on left ventricular perfusion, innervation, function and histology. *J Am Coll Cardiol* 1994; **24**: 225–232.

54 Karpawich PP, Justice CD, Chang C-H *et al.* Septal ventricular pacing in the immature canine heart: A new perspective. *Am Heart J* 1991; **121**: 827–833.

55 Peschar M, de Swart H, Michels KJ *et al.* Left ventricular septal and apex pacing for optimal pump function in canine hearts. *J Am Coll Cardiol* 2003; **41**: 1218–1226.

56 Buckingham TA, Candinas R, Schlapfer J *et al.* Acute hemodynamic effects of atrioventricular pacing at different sites in the right ventricle individually and simultaneously. *Pacing Clin Electrophysiol* 1997; **20**: 909–915.

57 Klotz DH, Lister JW, Jomain SL *et al.* Implantation sites of pacemakers after right ventriculotomy and complete heart block. *JAMA* 1963; **186**: 929–931.

58 Vanagt WY, Verbeek XA, Delhaas T *et al.* The left ventricular apex is the optimal site for pediatric pacing: correlation with animal experience. *Pacing Clin Electrophysiol* 2004; **27**: 837–843.

59 Prinzen FW, Peschar M. Relation between the pacing induced sequence of activation and left ventricular pump function in animals. *Pacing Clin Electrophysiol* 2002; **25**: 484–498.

60 Verbeek X, Vernooy K, Peschar M *et al.* Intra-ventricular resynchronization for optimal left ventricular function during pacing in experimental left bundle branch block. *J Am Coll Cardiol* 2003; **42**: 558–567.

61 Baller D, Wolpers H-G, Zipfel J *et al.* Comparison of the effects of right atrial, right ventricular apex and atrioventricular sequential pacing on myocardial oxygen consumption and cardiac efficiency: a laboratory investigation. *Pacing Clin Electrophysiol* 1988; **11**: 394–403.

62 Owen CH, Esposito DJ, Davis JW *et al.* The effects of ventricular pacing on left ventricular geometry, function, myocardial oxygen consumption and efficiency of contraction in conscious dogs. *Pacing Clin Electrophysiol* 1998; **21**: 1417–1429.

63 Packer M, Carver JR, Rodeheffer RJ *et al.* Effect of oral milrinone on mortality in severe chronic heart failure. *N Engl J Med* 1991; **325**: 1468–1475.

64 Rosen MR. The heart remembers: clinical implications. *Lancet* 2001; **357**: 468–471.

65 Plotnikov AN, Yu H, Geller JC *et al.* Role of L-type calcium channels in pacing-induced short-term and long-term cardiac memory in canine heart. *Circulation* 2003; **107**: 2844–2849.

66 Patberg KW, Plotnikov AN, Quamina A *et al.* Cardiac memory is associated with decreased levels of the transcriptional factor CREB modulated by angiotensin II and Calcium. *Circ Res* 2003; **93**: 472–478.

67 Costard-Jäckle A, Franz MR. Slow and long-lasting modulation of myocardial repolarization produced by ectopic activation in isolated rabbit hearts: Evidence for cardiac 'memory'. *Circulation* 1989; **80**: 1412–1420.

68 Alessandrini RS, McPherson DD, Kadish AH *et al.* Cardiac memory: a mechanical and electrical phenomenon. *Am J Physiol* 1997; **272**: H1952–H1959.

69 Nahlawi M, Waligora M, Spies SM *et al.* Left ventricular function during and after right ventricular pacing. *J Am Coll Cardiol* 2004; **44**: 1883–1888.

70 Prinzen FW, Cheriex EM, Delhaas T *et al.* Asymmetric thickness of the left ventricular wall resulting from asynchronous electrical activation. A study in patients with left bundle branch block and in dogs with ventricular pacing. *Am Heart J* 1995; **130**: 1045–1053.

71 Van Oosterhout MFM, Arts T, Muijtjens AMM *et al.* Remodeling by ventricular pacing in hypertrophying dog hearts. *Cardiovasc Res* 2001; **49**: 771–778.

72 Karpawich PP, Justice CD, Cavitt DL *et al.* Developmental sequelae of fixed-rate ventricular pacing in the immature canine heart: An electrophysiologic, hemodynamic and histopathologic evaluation. *Am Heart J* 1990; **119**: 1077–1083.

73 Waldman LK, Covell JW. Effects of ventricular pacing on finite deformation in canine left ventricles. *Am J Physiol* 1987; **252**: H1023–H1030.

74 Spragg DD, Leclercq C, Loghmani M *et al.* Regional alterations in protein expression in the dyssynchronous failing heart. *Circulation* 2003; **108**: 929–932.

75 Spragg DD, Akar FG, Helm RH *et al.* Abnormal conduction and repolarization in late-activated myocardium of dyssynchronously contracting hearts. *Cardiovasc Res* 2005; **67**: 77–86.

76 Akar FG, Spragg DD, Tunin RS *et al.* Mechanisms underlying conduction slowing and arrhythmogenesis in nonischemic dilated cardiomyopathy. *Circ Res* 2004; **95**: 717–725.

77 Peschar M, Vernooy K, Vanagt WYR *et al.* Absence of reverse electrical remodeling during regression of volume overload hypertrophy in canine ventricles. *Cardiovasc Res* 2003; **58**: 510–517.

78 van Bilsen M, Smeets PJ, Gilde AJ *et al.* Metabolic remodelling of the failing heart: the cardiac burn-out syndrome? *Cardiovasc Res* 2004; **61**: 218–226.

79 Schneider JF, Thomas Jr HE, Kreger BE *et al.* Newly acquired left bundle branch block: the Framingham study. *Ann Intern Med* 1979; **90**: 303–310.

80 Casiglia E, Spolaore P, Ginocchio G *et al.* Mortality in relation to Minnesota code items in elderly subjects. *Jpn Heart J* 1993; **34**: 567–577.

81 Yu Y, Kramer A, Spinelli J *et al.* Biventricular mechanical asynchrony predicts hemodynamic effect of uni- and biventricular pacing. *Am J Physiol* 2003; **285**: H2788–2796.

82 Sogaard P, Egeblad H, Kim WY *et al.* Tissue Doppler imaging predicts improved systolic performance and reversed left ventricular remodeling during long-term cardiac resynchronization therapy. *J Am Coll Cardiol* 2002; **40**: 723–730.

83 Yu CM, Chau E, Sanderson JE *et al.* Tissue Doppler echocardiographic evidence of reverse remodeling and improved synchronicity by simultaneously delaying regional contraction after biventricular pacing therapy in heart failure. *Circulation* 2002; **105**: 438–445.

84 Breithardt OA, Stellbrink C, Herbots L *et al.* Cardiac resynchronization therapy can reverse abnormal myocardial strain distribution in patients with heart failure and left bundle branch block. *J Am Coll Cardiol* 2003; **42**: 486–494.

85 Leclercq C, Faris O, Tunin R *et al.* Systolic improvement and mechanical resynchronization does not require electrical synchrony in the dilated failing heart with left bundle-branch block. *Circulation* 2002; **106**: 1760–1763.

86 Neri G, Zanco P, Zanon F *et al.* Effect of biventricular pacing on metabolism and perfusion in patients affected by dilated cardiomyopathy and left bundle branch block: evaluation by positron emission tomography. *Europace* 2003; **5**: 111–115.

87 Knaapen P, van Campen LM, de Cock CC *et al.* Effects of cardiac resynchronization therapy on myocardial perfusion reserve. *Circulation* 2004; **110**: 646–651.

88 Nelson GS, Berger RD, Fetics BJ *et al.* Left ventricular or biventricular pacing improves cardiac function at diminished energy cost in patients with dilated cardiomyopathy and left bundle-branch block. *Circulation* 2000; **102**: 3053–3059.

89 Suga H, Igarashi Y, Yamada O *et al.* Mechanical efficiency of the left ventricle as a function of preload, afterload, and contractility. *Heart Vessels* 1985; **1**: 3–8.

90 De Sousa E, Veksler V, Minajeva A *et al.* Subcellular creatine kinase alterations: implications in heart failure. *Circ Res* 1999; **85**: 68–76.

91 Hasenfuss G, Holubarsch C, Heiss HW *et al.* Myocardial energetics in patients with dilated cardiomyopathy: influence of nitroprusside and enoximone. *Circulation* 1989; **80**: 51–64.

92 Blanc JJ, Etienne Y, Gilard M *et al.* Evaluation of different ventricular pacing sites in patients with severe heart failure: results of an acute hemodynamic study. *Circulation* 1997; **96**: 3273–3277.

93 Auricchio A, Stellbrink C, Block M *et al.* Effect of pacing chamber and atrioventricular delay on acute systolic function of paced patients with congestive heart failure. The Pacing Therapies for Congestive Heart Failure Study Group. The Guidant Congestive Heart Failure Research Group. *Circulation* 1999; **99**: 2993–3001.

94 Kass DA, Chen C-H, Curry C *et al.* Improved left ventricular mechanics from acute VDD pacing in patients with dilated cardiomyopathy and ventricular conduction delay. *Circulation* 1999; **99**: 1567–1573.

95 Dekker AL, Phelps B, Dijkman B *et al.* Epicardial left ventricular lead placement for cardiac resynchronization therapy: optimal pace site selection with pressure-volume loops. *J Thorac Cardiovasc Surg* 2004; **127**: 1641–1647.

96 Leclercq C, Cazeau S, Le Breton H *et al.* Acute hemody-

namic effects of biventricular DDD pacing in patients with end-stage heart failure. *J Am Coll Cardiol* 1998; **32**: 1825–1831.

97 Yu C-M, Fung W-H, Lin H *et al.* Predictors of left ventricular reverse remodeling after cardiac resynchronization therapy for heart failure secondary to idiopathic dilated or ischemic cardiomyopathy. *Am J Cardiol* 2002; **91**: 684–688.

98 Touiza A, Etienne Y, Gilard M *et al.* Long-term left ventricular pacing: assessment and comparison with biventricular pacing in patients with severe congestive heart failure. *J Am Coll Cardiol* 2001; **38**: 1966–1970.

99 Turner MS, Bleasdale RA, Vinereanu D *et al.* Electrical and mechanical components of dyssynchrony in heart failure patients with normal QRS duration and left bundle-branch block, inpact of left and biventricular pacing. *Circulation* 2004; **109**: 2544–2549.

100 Etienne Y, Mansourati J, Gilard M *et al.* Evaluation of left ventricular based pacing in patients with congestive heart failure and atrial fibrillation. *Am J Cardiol* 1999; **83**: 1138–1140.

101 Bleasdale RA, Turner MS, Mumford CE *et al.* Left ventricular pacing minimizes diastolic ventricular interaction, allowing improved preload-dependent systolic performance. *Circulation* 2004; **110**: 2395–2400.

102 Adamson PB, Kleckner K, Van Hout WL *et al.* Cardiac resynchronization therapy improves heart rate variability in patients with symptomatic heart failure. *J Am Coll Cardiol* 2003; **108**: 266–269.

103 Vernooy K, Verbeek XAAM, Crijns HJGM *et al.* Nonuniform workload and remodeling of the left ventricle, induced by left bundle branch block, is reversed by biventricular pacing. *Circulation* 2004; **110**: III-481 (abstract).

104 Yu CM, Bleeker GB, Fung JW *et al.* Left ventricular reverse remodeling but not clinical improvement predicts long-term survival after cardiac resynchronization therapy. *Circulation* 2005; **108**: 266–269.

105 Strieper M, Karpawich P, Frias P *et al.* Initial experience with cardiac resynchronization therapy for ventricular dysfunction in young patients with surgically operated congenital heart disease. *Am J Cardiol* 2004; **94**: 1352–1354.

106 Janousek J, Tomek V, Chaloupecky V *et al.* Dilated cardiomyopathy associated with dual-chamber pacing in infants: improvement through either left ventricular cardiac resynchronization or programming the pacemaker off allowing intrinsic normal conduction. *J Cardiovasc Electrophysiol* 2004; **15**: 470–474.

107 Verbeek XAAM, Auricchio A, Yu Y *et al.* Tailoring cardiac resynchronization therapy using interventricular asynchrony. Validation of a simple model. *Am J Physiol* (in press).

CHAPTER 5

Conventional echocardiography

Ole-A. Breithardt, MD

Introduction

Echocardiography has played an essential role in cardiac resynchronization therapy (CRT) ever since the first successful implants [1]. Conventional techniques, such as M-mode, two-dimensional echocardiography, spectral and color-flow Doppler, have been used widely to identify patients with systolic heart failure and helped in our understanding of the mechanisms of CRT benefit during acute testing and long-term follow-up [2–9]. Despite the impressive clinical success of CRT, with a significant improvement in functional heart failure status and a reduction in overall mortality [10–12], the therapy remains costly and challenging, mainly due to the relatively high proportion (20–30%) of non-responders [13, 14]. The measurement of QRS duration by the ECG – an electrical phenomenon which provides only a crude estimation of myocardial activation – is only poorly correlated with the presence of mechanical dyssynchrony [15, 16]. In contrast, transthoracic echocardiography allows the severity of mechanical dyssynchrony and its impact on cardiac hemodynamics to be assessed immediately online and in a quantitative manner. Echocardiography seems therefore more reliable to correctly identify suitable CRT candidates in order to reduce the number of clinical non-responders [17].

Despite the obvious advantages of this widely available bedside imaging technique, at the present time the QRS duration remains the main selection criterion for the diagnosis of the presence of mechanical dyssynchrony in clinical practice and in the currently available guidelines [18, 19]. This is mainly because the large prospective randomized trials solely relied on the QRS width as the only marker for dyssynchrony. At first glance, echocardiographic assessment of dyssynchrony seems to be more time-consuming, requires special expertise and the optimal protocol for dyssynchrony assessment is not yet defined. The new echocardiographic methods such as tissue Doppler imaging (TDI) and real-time three-dimensional echocardiography are probably the most sensitive and precise methods for the quantitative definition of dyssynchrony; however, it must be stressed that important information about the presence and severity of dyssynchrony can also be obtained from conventional echocardiographic techniques, which will be discussed in the present chapter. Most of the required parameters can be obtained from any routine study, thus little extra time has to be spent and the assessment of dyssynchrony can be easily integrated into daily routine practice.

Assessment of dyssynchrony

In the failing heart, myocardial contractility is severely reduced and highly dependent on pre- and afterload. Further impairment of left ventricular (LV) performance and energy consumption is seen with the development of an electrical conduction delay, most frequently presenting with a prolonged PQ interval and a prolonged QRS complex of left bundle branch block (LBBB)-type morphology. The LV is activated slowly through the septum from the right side and the LV endocardial activation time may exceed 100 ms [20]. Left ventricular pre-ejection pressure is lower than in the right ventricle and septal motion is abnormal. This results in an uncoordinated contraction sequence and delays LV ejection at the expense of diastolic filling [21].

The electrical conduction disturbance in patients with advanced heart failure may involve the complete conduction system from the sinus node to the Purkinje fibers. Thus, atrioventricular (AV) and ventricular conduction can be similarly affected and three different levels of dyssynchrony can be distinguished by echocardiography [8]:

• Atrioventricular dyssynchrony: Delayed ventricular activation in relation to the atria due to prolongation of the PR interval (applies only to patients in sinus rhythm).

• Interventricular dyssynchrony: Delayed onset and end of left ventricular (LV) systole due to delayed LV electrical activation in comparison to the right ventricle.

• Intraventricular dyssynchrony: Delayed activation of some LV segments in ejection period and/or prolonged contraction after aortic valve closure.

It should be stressed that in most patients these different levels of dyssynchrony are closely linked and appear typically, but not always, together. The first two levels, AV and interventricular dyssynchrony can be easily identified by Doppler echocardiography. Intraventricular dyssynchrony can be assessed by parasternal M-mode or by comparison between the timing of LV systole by Doppler and segmental motion by M-mode echocardiography.

All of these parameters are relatively robust with a low inter- and intra-observer measurement variability and can be obtained with every echo scanner, without the need for dedicated hardware or software solutions. This renders them particularly useful for routine measurements and enables accurate and meaningful follow-up measurements for comparison of CRT efficacy. Table 5.1 provides an overview of the most frequently used conventional parameters for the assessment of dyssynchrony before CRT implantation and for follow-up.

The first level: atrioventricular dyssynchrony

In patients with sinus rhythm, prolongation of the PR interval delays the onset of ventricular systole in relation to atrial filling which has a negative impact on ventricular performance due to a suboptimal preload, which is of particular importance in advanced heart failure [22, 23]. Prolongation of the interval between atrial filling and ventricular activation goes mainly at the expense of the early diastolic filling period (Fig. 5.1), a phenomenon which can easily be visualized and quantified by studying ventricular inflow with transmitral Doppler [24]. The total diastolic filling interval (dFT = E wave duration + A wave duration) is shortened, mainly due to a reduction in E wave du-

Table 5.1 Overview of the most frequently used conventional parameters for the assessment of dyssynchrony before CRT implantation and for follow-up

Method	Measure	Objective	Comment
Parasternal long-axis M-mode	SPWMD >130 ms	Intraventricular dyssynchrony (septum–posterior wall)	Often difficult to acquire, limited prospective data
2D apical four- and two-chamber view	Biplane ejection fraction and volumes	Document presence of systolic heart failure and baseline volumes for follow-up	Not a marker for dyssynchrony
CW Doppler of pulmonic and aortic overflow	RV/LV pre-ejection interval (ΔPEI) >40–50 ms	Interventricular dyssynchrony (RV vs. LV)	Robust and reproducible, affected by afterload
PW Doppler of mitral inflow	Diastolic filling time <40–45% of cycle length	Hemodynamic impact of dyssynchrony on diastole	Robust, reproducible; only indirect measure; affected by heart rate
CW Doppler of mitral regurgitation jet (if present)	Slope of regurgitant jet for estimation of LV peak +dp/dt	Non-invasive estimate of LV peak +dp/dt	Tends to underestimate invasive peak +dp/dt, only indirect measure

SPWMD, septal–posterior wall motion delay; RV, right ventricle; LV, left ventricle; CW, continuous wave; PEI, pre-ejection interval; PW, pulsed wave; peak +dp/dt, peak positive rate of pressure rise.

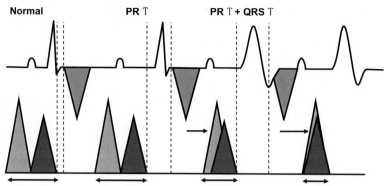

Normal   **PR ↑**   **PR ↑ + QRS ↑**

Figure 5.1 Schematic drawing illustrating the negative impact of delayed electrical activation on the timing of aortic outflow and transmitral inflow by Doppler echocardiography. Prolongation of the PR interval delays aortic flow and subsequently also the early diastolic filling wave which leads to E/A fusion and shortening of the diastolic filling time. A further deterioration of these parameters is seen during additional left ventricular dysfunction. Adapted from Cazeau *et al.* [8].

ration. In the presence of severe AV dyssynchrony, the dFT typically measures less than 40–45% of the corresponding cycle length and the E and A waves are fused (Figs 5.1 and 5.2A) [8]. With adequate AV delay optimization and ventricular resynchronization the transmitral inflow profile can be significantly improved (Figs 5.2B and 5.3). The aim is to increase the diastolic filling time to a maximum (above 50–60% of the corresponding cycle length) without early termination of atrial filling by premature mitral valve closure (Fig. 5.2B) [2, 25, 26] and to eliminate diastolic mitral regurgitation (Fig. 5.4B). The delay between atrial filling and the onset of the left ventricular pressure rise may also cause inversed AV flow during this period with the occurrence of diastolic mitral regurgitation. Ishikawa *et al.* [27] determined a critical PR interval of 0.23 ± 0.01 s, above which most patients will show some degree of diastolic mitral regurgitation, which can easily be identified by continuous wave Doppler echocardiography (Fig. 5.4A, arrow).

The second level: interventricular dyssynchrony

Normal conduction of the electrical impulse from the AV node through the Purkinje fibers causes a rapid ventricular activation which starts near the apex and propagates rapidly towards the base with the latest ventricular activation in the posterobasal LV. Total ventricular activation time in the healthy human lasts about 60–80 ms, corresponding with a QRS duration of 70–80 ms [28]. The interventricular septum is activated from left to right and LV pressure

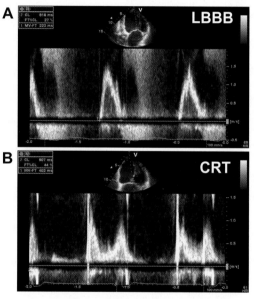

Figure 5.2 Pulsed wave transmitral inflow profile before CRT in a patient with LBBB (upper image) with fusion of the early and late filling waves and a short diastolic filling time in relation to the cycle length (27% of cycle length). CRT with AV delay optimization improves the diastolic filling time to a near normal value (44% of cycle length). The early and late diastolic filling waves are well separated during CRT. From Breithardt and Sinha [47] with permission.

rises slightly before RV pressure [29]. Under these normal conditions right and left ventricular outflow occur almost simultaneously and the interventricular mechanical delay (IVMD) between the ventricles is close to zero [30]. This parameter is defined as the

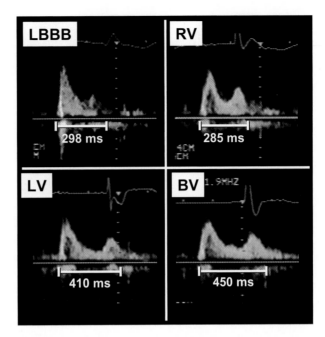

Figure 5.3 Duration of diastolic transmitral inflow measured by pulsed wave Doppler may improve significantly with CRT. In this particular example the largest increase is observed with left ventricular (LV) and biventricular (BV) VDD pacing. Conventional right ventricular (RV) VDD pacing at the same AV delay had no significant effect on filling time. From Stellbrink *et al.* [48] with permission.

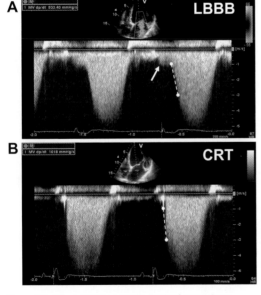

Figure 5.4 Effect of CRT on the transmitral regurgitant profile of functional mitral regurgitation by continuous wave Doppler. The onset of LV contraction is delayed due to a long PR interval and delayed ventricular activation in LBBB. Pre-systolic mitral regurgitation can be documented by continuous wave Doppler (A, arrow). Depressed LV systolic function during LBBB is indicated by the slow increase of the regurgitant velocity (A) and is significantly improved by CRT, as measured by the steeper regurgitant velocity profile (B). From Breithardt and Sinha [47] with permission.

difference between the left and right ventricular pre-ejection intervals (LV-PEI, RV-PEI), measured by standard pulsed wave Doppler echocardiography as the interval between the onset of the QRS and the onset of aortic or pulmonary outflow (Fig. 5.5). LBBB patients frequently present with values of approximately 100 ms for the RV-PEI and around 150 ms for the LV-PEI. It is important to note that always the same Doppler technique (pulsed wave or continuous wave Doppler) should be applied for both measurements and care should be taken to identify the same reference point on the ECG tracing. The IVMD correlates to QRS duration and is typically increased to more than 40 ms in patients with a QRS width of more than 150 ms [30]. In these patients it indicates the presence of significant dyssynchrony and may be used to document the effectiveness of CRT acutely and during long-term follow-up [25]. In the CARE-HF study, the median IVMD in a subgroup of 735 patients was 49.2 ms and an IVMD above the median was an independent predictor for a better outcome, defined by the primary composite endpoint (death, unplanned hospitalization, or major cardiovascular event). However, this should not imply that patients with a lesser degree of interventricular dyssynchrony by the IVMD parameter should be withheld from resynchronization therapy. In particular in patients

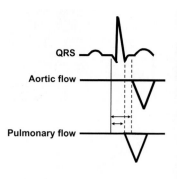 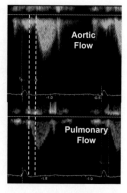

Figure 5.5 Comparison of aortic and pulmonary pre-ejection intervals for the measurement of interventricular mechanical dyssynchrony assessed by continuous wave Doppler echocardiography. The pre-ejection interval is measured from the onset of the QRS to the onset of aortic/pulmonary outflow. In a typical LBBB patient, aortic outflow occurs more than 40–50 ms later than pulmonary outflow.

with less severe QRS prolongation (<150 ms) the prognostic value of interventricular dyssynchrony is limited and in this subgroup identification of intraventricular dyssynchrony may become more important [31]. Furthermore, one study suggested that the predictive value of the interventricular delay for monitoring CRT efficacy may be limited, as the changes in the interventricular delay (assessed by pulsed wave tissue Doppler) failed to predict the hemodynamic response to CRT [32].

The third level: intraventricular dyssynchrony

Probably the most important level of dyssynchrony to be evaluated in the context of CRT is within the left ventricle. The most precise methodology for identification and quantitative assessment of this intraventricular level of dyssynchrony is probably tissue Doppler imaging, which will be discussed in another chapter. However, intraventricular dyssynchrony may also be assessed by standard echocardiographic techniques, such as M-mode and standard Doppler echocardiography.

Assessment of radial endocardial wall motion

The first step in the assessment of wall motion synchrony is the visual assessment of endocardial radial inward motion. In LBBB, the interventricular septum typically shows a characteristic abnormal relaxation pattern with biphasic motion. The experienced echocardiographer may sometimes also appreciate the delayed contraction of the posterolateral walls. Another typical feature of LBBB is the counterclockwise rocking motion of the left ventricle in the apical four-chamber view. However, in most cases the visual assessment alone is not precise enough to character-

ize dyssynchrony adequately. In an attempt to quantify dyssynchrony more precisely on the basis of radial endocardial wall motion, a semi-automated contour detection algorithm, which had been originally developed for stress echocardiography, was tested in CRT patients [33]. Septal and lateral wall motion curves were constructed by a mathematical phase analysis based on Fourier transformation and averaged over several cardiac cycles to calculate the phase angle difference between septal and lateral wall motion (Fig. 5.6). The presence of significant septal–lateral dyssynchrony, defined as a septal–lateral wall motion phase angle difference below –25° or above +25°, identified hemodynamic CRT responders, defined by an increase of more than 10% in LV peak positive dP/dt ($+dP/dt$) or in pulse pressure from baseline. An obvious limitation of this approach is the restriction to a single imaging plane. Any dyssynchrony in other walls will be overlooked and thus the precise extent of dyssynchrony cannot be measured adequately. These limitations may be overcome by three-dimensional (3D) echocardiography [34].

Septal–posterior wall motion delay by parasternal M-mode

The parasternal M-mode provides not only essential information about ventricular dimensions but may also help to quantify the severity of intraventricular dyssynchrony. Septal motion can be directly compared to the posterior wall and the temporal delay can be measured with high temporal resolution. The septal–posterior wall motion delay (SPWMD) is measured between the first maximum of systolic inward motion of the septum and the maximum inward motion of the posterior wall (Fig. 5.7, left). In a small pilot study

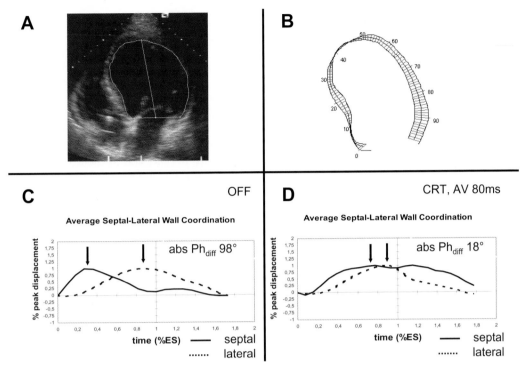

Figure 5.6 Semi-automatic endocardial border delineation was performed in the apical four-chamber view (A) and regional endocardial wall motion was calculated by a centerline method in 100 myocardial segments (B). Regional movement curves were calculated from 3–7 consecutive loops by averaging 40 adjacent septal and lateral segments. In the present example phase analysis resulted in a phase angle difference of 98° (C) and was reduced by CRT to 18° (D). In a non-simultaneous invasive measurement, LV peak dP/dt increased by more than 17% compared with no pacing. Adapted from Breithardt *et al.* [33].

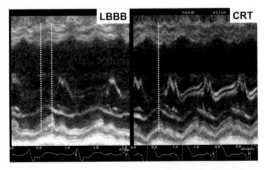

Figure 5.7 Parasternal M-mode recorded during intrinsic conduction (LBBB, left) and during CRT (right). During LBBB, a biphasic septal motion pattern with early inward motion is observed (left). Posterior wall contraction is delayed by approximately 240 ms. During biventricular CRT both walls show simultaneous inward motion (right). From Breithardt and Sinha [47] with permission.

by Pitzalis *et al.* [5] baseline SPWMD >130 ms predicted the CRT-related LV reverse remodeling effect with a specificity of 63% and a positive pre-dictive value of 80% [5]. In a subsequent analysis a baseline SPWMD >130 ms was also a predictor of long-term clinical improvement [6]. Effective CRT should reduce the SPWMD below the cut-off value of 130 ms, frequently the SPWMD will be close to zero (Fig. 5.7, right). A clear limitation is the one-dimensional characteristic of this parameter and the often impaired parasternal image quality. In the presence of very advanced heart failure and low ejection fraction the inward motion of the walls is often severely reduced, which makes clear identification of peak inward motion difficult.

Longitudinal motion by apical M-mode echocardiography

As an alternative to tissue Doppler echocardiography, longitudinal motion may also be assessed by M-mode echocardiography from the apical views [35]. Atrioventricular plane displacement (AVPD) correlates to global LV systolic function and can be improved by CRT. In a small study on 16 patients, mean septal–lateral AVPD increased significantly from 6.8 ± 1.9 mm to 7.5 ± 2.2 mm (P < 0.05). Most of the improvement was confined to the interventricular septum (5.2 ± 2.4, LBBB vs. 7.6 ± 2.1, CRT, P < 0.001), while the lateral wall improved only slightly (8.3 ± 2.1, LBBB vs. 9.0 ± 2.6, CRT, P = n.s.) [36]. A direct comparison of the longitudinal AVPD patterns identifies dyssynchrony and allows monitoring of the resynchronization effect (Fig. 5.8).

Systolic–diastolic overlap

One of the manifestations of intraventricular dyssynchrony is characterized by the coexistence of post-systolic contraction (i.e. contraction after aortic valve closure) and diastolic relaxation. Late activated segments may still contract while early activated segments already begin to relax. Thus, ventricular filling coincides with post-systolic contraction, and an overlap between systole (defined by the latest contracting segment) and diastole (defined by the onset of ventricular filling) may occur [8]. This phenomenon can be most elegantly visualized by tissue Doppler echocardiography, but may – in extreme cases – also be documented by comparing Doppler and M-mode recordings if TDI is not available. The onset of ventricular filling is measured by transmitral pulsed wave Doppler as the interval from the first detected QRS signal on the ECG to the onset of LV diastolic filling (Q-E). This time interval is then compared with the timing of apical motion of the posterolateral segments by M-mode echocardiog-

raphy, where in normal situation the time from the QRS to peak motion should not exceed the Q-E interval. The diagnostic value of this comparison has not yet been prospectively established, thus any pathologic finding should be confirmed by further investigations (e.g. by more advanced TDI studies).

A possible pitfall is the comparison of two time measurements from different echo techniques: pulsed wave Doppler and M-mode. An inherent delay between the displayed QRS signal and the pulsed wave Doppler signal may be apparent in some echo scanners, while this is usually not observed for M-mode recordings. This may lead to an underestimation of the severity of dyssynchrony. Our experience suggests that only very few patients with extreme dyssynchrony will show a significant systolic–diastolic overlap when M-mode recordings and transmitral Doppler recordings are compared.

Additional measurements: valvular and hemodynamic assessment

The non-invasive evaluation of valvular function and cardiac hemodynamics is an essential part of every echo exam before CRT and during follow-up. Any possible indication for valvular surgery has to be ruled out before initiation of CRT and the hemodynamic evaluation goes beyond the routine measurements of biplane LV ejection fraction and RV systolic pressure. Left ventricular end-diastolic and end-systolic cavity volumes should be documented and taken into consideration before a final decision

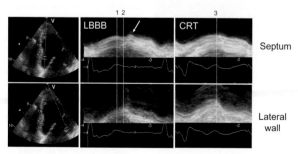

Figure 5.8 Septal–lateral longitudinal motion assessed by M-mode echocardiography from the apical four-chamber view. Before pacing during intrinsic conduction (LBBB) clear dyssynchrony between the septum (upper row) and the lateral wall (lower row) can be appreciated. An early septal peak (1) is followed by a small notch (2) which coincides with peak motion in the lateral wall and is followed by post-systolic septal shortening (arrow). During CRT, both walls show an improved atrioventricular plane displacement with simultaneous peak apical motion (3).

on CRT initiation is made. Although very advanced dilatation (i.e. end-diastolic volumes above 350–400 mL) is not a contraindication by itself, such patients may respond less favorably to CRT in the long term [3] and may therefore be more suitable for alternative treatments, such as cardiac transplantation. In a well-recompensated patient the hemodynamic data may reveal only mild signs of impairment at rest despite a very low ejection fraction, but typically the non-invasively determined measures such as LV peak positive dP/dt and cardiac output (see below) are severely impaired. Knowledge on these baseline measures enables comparison during follow-up and identification of hemodynamic responders.

Left ventricular systolic performance by dP/dt

The steepness of the continuous wave Doppler regurgitant jet allows an estimate for LV systolic function to be obtained by measuring the time difference between 1 m/s and 3 m/s on the regurgitant slope. This corresponds to the time that is required for the LV pressure to rise by 32 mmHg ($36 - 4 = 32$ mmHg) and can be recalculated to 1 s, thus providing the LV rate of pressure rise (LV peak +dP/dt) in millimeters of mercury per second [37]. An improvement in the estimated LV peak +dP/dt may serve as an indicator for the hemodynamic improvement by CRT (Fig. 5.4). Quantification of LV peak +dP/dt at baseline and during CRT may enable later comparison during follow-up and allows characterization of hemodynamic responders [25, 38].

Left ventricular performance by the myocardial performance index and isovolumic contraction time

The myocardial performance index (MPI) is a combined systolic and diastolic Doppler-derived index for the assessment of global LV performance which correlates well with invasive measurements of LV systolic and diastolic function [39]. It represents the sum of the isovolumic contraction time (IVCT) and the isovolumic relaxation time (IVRT) divided by LV ejection time. The sum of IVCT and IVRT is obtained by subtracting LV ejection time from the interval between cessation and onset of the mitral inflow profile (Fig. 5.9). In patients with normal

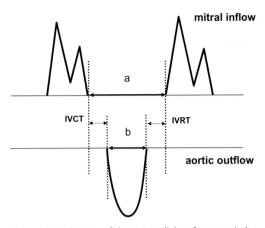

Figure 5.9 Evaluation of the myocardial performance index by Doppler echocardiography of mitral inflow and aortic outflow. The interval between cessation and onset of mitral inflow (a) minus the LV ejection time (b) represents the sum of the isovolumic time intervals (IVCT + IVRT). Myocardial performance index (MPI) = (a – b)/b [49].

LV function the MPI measures less than 0.5, values above 0.8 indicate significantly depressed LV performance. In a series of 32 heart failure patients recruited from the PATH-CHF I trial [40] the average MPI during intrinsic conduction (mostly LBBB) was 1.21 ± 0.5 and correlated to baseline peak positive LV dP/dt in a non-simultaneous measurement (Fig. 5.10). Biventricular CRT resulted in an immediate reduction of the MPI to 0.85 ± 0.3. Hemodynamic responders showed a significantly higher improvement in MPI than hemodynamic non-responders. More recently Porciani *et al.* [41] reported similar effects of simultaneous biventricular CRT with a reduction of the MPI from 1.1 ± 0.4 before CRT to 0.8 ± 0.2 during CRT. In addition, they could also demonstrate a further reduction to 0.6 ± 0.1 with tailored sequential CRT and proposed the use of MPI for individual optimization. However, calculation of the MPI is relatively time consuming and the improvement is mainly caused by a reduction in the IVCT – in the PATH-CHF I trial from 128 ± 62 ms to 89 ± 51 ms [2] – while the IVRT and the LV ejection time do not change significantly. Therefore, it seems sufficient (and probably more appropriate) to measure the IVCT directly instead of the MPI. For optimization it would be desirable to aim for an optimized IVCT within the physiologic range of 70–80 ms by conventional Doppler or pulsed wave tissue Doppler echocardiography [42].

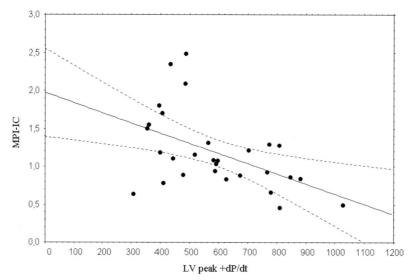

Figure 5.10 Correlation between baseline myocardial performance index during intrinsic conduction (mostly LBBB) (MPI-IC) and baseline peak positive LV d*P*/d*t* in 29 patients from the PATH-CHF I trial. From Breithardt *et al.* [2] with permission.

Functional mitral regurgitation

As discussed above, patients with a long AV interval (>0.23 s) may show diastolic mitral regurgitation (Fig. 5.4A) [27]. In relation to atrial contraction, the onset of the LV pressure rise is delayed and during this prolonged "isovolumic" contraction interval (precisely the interval between the completion of the A wave and mitral valve closure) diastolic mitral regurgitation may occur. A shorter AV delay during pacing will prevent the occurrence of diastolic mitral regurgitation (Fig. 5.4B). Besides the reduction in diastolic mitral regurgitation, CRT may also reduce the severity of the predominant systolic component by several interdependent mechanisms:

• *increased closing force [4];*
• *improved coordination of papillary muscles [43];*
• *long-term reverse remodeling [25].*

Immediately after the onset of successful resynchronization a significant reduction in functional mitral regurgitation can be observed (Fig. 5.11) [44], which is dependent on the improved coordination of the papillary muscles and the surrounding segments [43] and the simultaneous improvement in the LV rate of pressure rise (d*P*/d*t*) (Fig. 5.12) [4].

An additional reduction in the severity of mitral regurgitation may be observed in the long term, which goes along with the frequently observed reduction

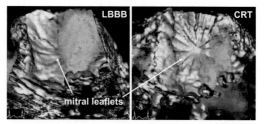

Figure 5.11 Three-dimensional transesophageal reconstruction of the transmitral regurgitant jet by color-Doppler (orange-green) in a patient with severe heart failure and cardiac dyssynchrony. Cranial view of the left atrium at mid-systole facing the closed mitral leaflets (arrows). A clear reduction of the crescent-shaped mitral regurgitant jet is seen during biventricular CRT (right) compared with intrinsic conduction with LBBB (left). The related video clips are available online at http://heart. bmjjournals.com/cgi/content/full/88/4/440/DC1?eaf. Adapted from Breithardt *et al.* [44].

in LV volume (reverse remodeling) [25]. It must be stressed that these relationships are only valid for true functional mitral regurgitation and not in the presence of structural valvular disease. In the presence of, for example, mitral valve prolapse, the increased LV rate of pressure rise may not reduce but rather increase the severity of regurgitation, thus any structural pathology must be ruled out before CRT and the severity of mitral regurgitation should be quanti-

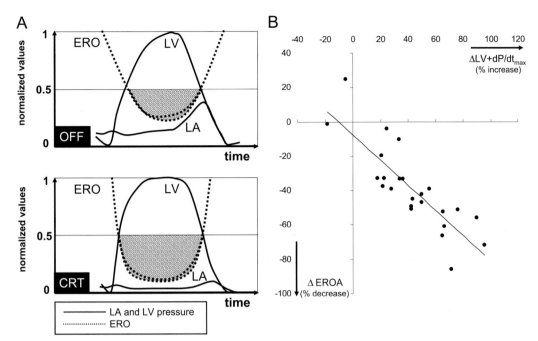

Figure 5.12 (A) Relationship between dynamic changes in transmitral pressure gradient (TMP) and effective regurgitant orifice area by the PISA method (ERO) before (OFF) and during CRT. Before CRT (A, upper panel) the impaired LV contractility results in a slow rise in left ventricular pressure (low peak LV dP/dt_{max}). TMP remains low throughout systole. Therefore, ERO remains large for a relatively long period in systole. With CRT (A, bottom panel) LV contractility improves, TMP rises faster and reaches a higher maximum earlier during systole. This leads to an earlier and more pronounced fall of ERO. The shaded area represents the time in systole during which ERO is below 50% of its initial value. (B) The decrease in ERO, displayed as the percentage change between OFF and CRT, correlates to the increase in LV systolic function, as measured by the percentage increase in LV $+dP/dt_{max}$. Reprinted from Breithardt *et al.* [4] with permission of the American College of Cardiology. Copyright 2003. The American College of Cardiology Foundation.

fied before CRT and reassessed during long-term follow-up, preferably with the PISA method [45].

Stroke volume and cardiac output

Stroke volume and cardiac output can be measured non-invasively (e.g. by pulsed wave Doppler echocardiography from the LV outflow tract) and may be applied to follow the acute hemodynamic improvement in CRT. Invasive and non-invasive studies demonstrated that successful CRT acutely increases aortic stroke volume by 10–15% [2]. This effect can be accurately measured by pulsed wave Doppler and has been evaluated in several trials. However, calculation of stroke volume is relatively time consuming, because it requires careful positioning of the pulsed wave Doppler sample volume at the level of the LV outflow tract, measurement of the LV outflow tract diameter and averaging of several beats, which makes it less attractive in daily routine. Alternatively, in patients with a stable heart rate the velocity–time integral ("stroke distance") by aortic continuous wave Doppler can be used to compare the acute changes with CRT.

Summary

A careful echocardiographic evaluation is one of the most important steps used to select good clinical responders before implantation. A variety of conventional echocardiographic parameters help to identify dyssynchrony and its hemodynamic consequences. The assessment of dyssynchrony by conventional echocardiography can be easily integrated in every routine examination of patients with symptomatic heart failure and allows improved identification of suitable patients for CRT independent of the QRS duration. The precise diagnostic value of these parameters (diagnostic sensitivity and specificity) is difficult to determine, since most parameters have only been evaluated retrospectively or in small series and the results of ongoing prospective studies are not yet available [46]. Currently, the best-validated parameter is the IVMD, as documented by the results of the recently published CARE-HF study [10]. However, the available clinical experience suggests that the diagnostic sensitivity of this parameter might be limited. Therefore patients with normal IVMD should be screened for further evidence of dyssynchrony by additional conventional or tissue Doppler examinations.

All described parameters show significant changes during resynchronization and may be used to document the hemodynamic and contractile improvement during follow-up. For this purpose it is particularly useful to compare the follow-up findings directly to the pre-implant recordings or to perform a comparison between on and off pacing. The latter comparison can be performed during reprogramming of the device to on and off pacing, as most parameters exhibit immediate changes (except benefits related to LV reverse remodeling) as a beat to beat effect.

References

1 Cazeau S, Ritter P, Lazarus A *et al.* Multisite pacing for end-stage heart failure: early experience. *Pacing Clin Electrophysiol* 1996; **19**: 1748–1757.

2 Breithardt OA, Stellbrink C, Franke A *et al.* Acute effects of cardiac resynchronization therapy on left ventricular Doppler indices in patients with congestive heart failure. *Am Heart J* 2002; **143**: 34–44.

3 Stellbrink C, Breithardt OA, Franke A *et al.* Impact of cardiac resynchronization therapy using hemodynamically optimized pacing on left ventricular remodeling in patients with congestive heart failure and ventricular conduction disturbances. *J Am Coll Cardiol* 2001; **38**: 1957–1965.

4 Breithardt OA, Sinha AM, Schwammenthal E *et al.* Acute effects of cardiac resynchronization therapy on functional mitral regurgitation in advanced systolic heart failure. *J Am Coll Cardiol* 2003; **41**: 765–770.

5 Pitzalis MV, Iacoviello M, Romito R *et al.* Cardiac resynchronization therapy tailored by echocardiographic evaluation of ventricular asynchrony. *J Am Coll Cardiol* 2002; **40**: 1615–1622.

6 Pitzalis MV, Iacoviello M, Romito R *et al.* Ventricular asynchrony predicts a better outcome in patients with chronic heart failure receiving cardiac resynchronization

therapy. *J Am Coll Cardiol* 2005; **45**: 65–69.

7 Achilli A, Sassara M, Ficili S *et al.* Long-term effectiveness of cardiac resynchronization therapy in patients with refractory heart failure and 'narrow' QRS. *J Am Coll Cardiol* 2003; **42**: 2117–2124.

8 Cazeau S, Bordachar P, Jauvert G *et al.* Echocardiographic modeling of cardiac dyssynchrony before and during multisite stimulation: a prospective study. *Pacing Clin Electrophysiol* 2003; **26**: 137–143.

9 John Sutton MG, Plappert T, Abraham WT *et al.* Effect of cardiac resynchronization therapy on left ventricular size and function in chronic heart failure. *Circulation* 2003; **107**: 1985–1990.

10 Cleland JG, Daubert JC, Erdmann E *et al.* The effect of cardiac resynchronization on morbidity and mortality in heart failure. *N Engl J Med* 2005; **352**: 1539–1549.

11 Cazeau S, Leclercq C, Lavergne T *et al.* Effects of multisite biventricular pacing in patients with heart failure and intraventricular conduction delay. *N Engl J Med* 2001; **344**: 873–880.

12 Auricchio A, Stellbrink C, Sack S *et al.* Long-term clinical effect of hemodynamically optimized cardiac resynchronization therapy in patients with heart failure and ventricular conduction delay. *J Am Coll Cardiol* 2002; **39**: 2026–2033.

13 Fox DJ, Fitzpatrick AP, Davidson NC. Optimisation of cardiac resynchronisation therapy: Addressing the problem of "non-responders". *Heart* 2005; **91**: 1000–1002.

14 Reuter S, Garrigue S, Barold SS *et al.* Comparison of characteristics in responders versus nonresponders with biventricular pacing for drug-resistant congestive heart failure. *Am J Cardiol* 2002; **89**: 346–350.

15 Bleeker GB, Schalij MJ, Molhoek SG *et al.* Relationship between QRS duration and left ventricular dyssynchrony in patients with end-stage heart failure. *J Cardiovasc Electrophysiol* 2004; **15**: 544–549.

16 Yu CM, Yang H, Lau CP *et al.* Regional left ventricle mechanical asynchrony in patients with heart disease and normal QRS duration: implication for biventricular pacing therapy. *Pacing Clin Electrophysiol* 2003; **26**: 562–570.

17 Bax JJ, Ansalone G, Breithardt OA *et al.* Echocardiographic evaluation of cardiac resynchronization therapy: ready for routine clinical use? A critical appraisal. *J Am Coll Cardiol* 2004; **44**: 1–9.

18 Gregoratos G, Abrams J, Epstein AE *et al.* ACC/AHA/NASPE 2002 Guideline Update for Implantation of Cardiac Pacemakers and Antiarrhythmia Devices – summary article: a report of the American College of Cardiology/American Heart Association Task Force on Practice Guidelines (ACC/AHA/NASPE Committee to Update the 1998 Pacemaker Guidelines). *J Am Coll Cardiol* 2002; **40**: 1703–1719.

19 Hunt SA, Abraham WT, Chin MH *et al.* ACC/AHA 2005

Guideline Update for the Diagnosis and Management of Chronic Heart Failure in the Adult: summary article: a Report from the American College of Cardiology/American Heart Association Task Force on Practice Guidelines (Writing Committee to Update the 2001 Guidelines for the Evolution and Management of Heart Failure). *J Am Coll Cardiol* 2005; **46**: 1116–1143.

20 Vassallo JA, Cassidy DM, Marchlinski FE *et al.* Endocardial activation of left bundle branch block. *Circulation* 1984; **69**: 914–923.

21 Grines CL, Bashore TM, Boudoulas H, Olson S, Shafer P, Wooley CF. Functional abnormalities in isolated left bundle branch block. The effect of interventricular asynchrony. *Circulation* 1989; **79**: 845–853.

22 Chevalier S, Basta M, Leitch JW. The importance of the left atrioventricular interval during atrioventricular sequential pacing. *Pacing Clin Electrophysiol* 1997; **20**: 2958–2966.

23 Auricchio A, Ding J, Spinelli JC *et al.* Cardiac resynchronization therapy restores optimal atrioventricular mechanical timing in heart failure patients with ventricular conduction delay. *J Am Coll Cardiol* 2002; **39**: 1163–1169.

24 Kindermann M, Fröhlig G, Doerr T, Schieffer H. Optimizing the AV delay in DDD pacemaker patients with high degree AV block: mitral valve Doppler versus impedance cardiography. *Pacing Clin Electrophysiol* 1997; **20**: 2453–2462.

25 Yu CM, Chau E, Sanderson JE *et al.* Tissue doppler echocardiographic evidence of reverse remodeling and improved synchronicity by simultaneously delaying regional contraction after biventricular pacing therapy in heart failure. *Circulation* 2002; **105**: 438–445.

26 Cazeau S, Gras D, Lazarus A, Ritter P, Mugica J. Multisite stimulation for correction of cardiac asynchrony. *Heart* 2000; **84**: 579–581.

27 Ishikawa T, Kimura K, Miyazaki N *et al.* Diastolic mitral regurgitation in patients with first-degree atrioventricular block. *Pacing Clin Electrophysiol* 1992; **15**: 1927–1931.

28 Prinzen FW, Peschar M. Relation between the pacing induced sequence of activation and left ventricular pump function in animals. *Pacing Clin Electrophysiol* 2002; **25**: 484–498.

29 Little WC, Reeves RC, Arciniegas J, Katholi RE, Rogers EW. Mechanism of abnormal interventricular septal motion during delayed left ventricular activation. *Circulation* 1982; **65**: 1486–1491.

30 Rouleau F, Merheb M, Geffroy S *et al.* Echocardiographic assessment of the interventricular delay of activation and correlation to the QRS width in dilated cardiomyopathy. *Pacing Clin Electrophysiol* 2001; **24**: 1500–1506.

31 Bader H, Garrigue S, Lafitte S *et al.* Intra-left ventricular electromechanical asynchrony. A new independent predictor of severe cardiac events in heart failure patients. *J Am Coll Cardiol* 2004; **43**: 248–256.

32 Bordachar P, Lafitte S, Reuter S *et al.* Echocardiographic parameters of ventricular dyssynchrony validation in patients with heart failure using sequential biventricular pacing. *J Am Coll Cardiol* 2004; **44**: 2157–2165.

33 Breithardt OA, Stellbrink C, Kramer AP *et al.* Echocardiographic quantification of left ventricular asynchrony predicts an acute hemodynamic benefit of cardiac resynchronization therapy. *J Am Coll Cardiol* 2002; **40**: 536–545.

34 Kapetanakis S, Kearney MT, Siva A, Gall N, Cooklin M, Monaghan MJ. Real-time three-dimensional echocardiography: a novel technique to quantify global left ventricular mechanical dyssynchrony. *Circulation* 2005; **112**: 992–1000.

35 Alam M, Rosenhamer G. Atrioventricular plane displacement and left ventricular function. *J Am Soc Echocardiogr* 1992; **5**: 427–433.

36 Breithardt OA, Stellbrink C, Sinha AM, Hoffmann R, Franke A, Hanrath P. Biventricular pacing acutely improves longitudinal myocardial function in severe heart failure. *Eur Heart J* 2001 (abstract).

37 Bargiggia GS, Bertucci C, Recusani F *et al.* A new method for estimating left ventricular dP/dt by continuous wave Doppler-echocardiography. Validation studies at cardiac catheterization. *Circulation* 1989; **80**: 1287–1292.

38 Oguz E, Dagdeviren B, Bilsel T *et al.* Echocardiographic prediction of long-term response to biventricular pacemaker in severe heart failure. *Eur J Heart Failure* 2002; **4**: 83–90.

39 Tei C, Nishimura RA, Seward JB, Tajik AJ. Noninvasive Doppler-derived myocardial performance index: correlation with simultaneous measurements of cardiac catheterization measurements. *J Am Soc Echocardiogr* 1997; **10**: 169–178.

40 Auricchio A, Stellbrink C, Sack S *et al.* The Pacing Therapies for Congestive Heart Failure (PATH-CHF) study: rationale, design, and endpoints of a prospective randomized multicenter study. *Am J Cardiol* 1999; **83**: 130D–135D.

41 Porciani MC, Dondina C, Macioce R *et al.* Echocardiographic examination of atrioventricular and interventricular delay optimization in cardiac resynchronization therapy. *Am J Cardiol* 2005; **95**: 1108–1110.

42 Gessner M, Blazek G, Kainz W, Gruska M, Gaul G. Application of pulsed-Doppler tissue imaging in patients with dual chamber pacing: the importance of conduction time and AV delay on regional left ventricular wall dynamics. *Pacing Clin Electrophysiol* 1998; **21**: 2273–2279.

43 Kanzaki H, Bazaz R, Schwartzman D, Dohi K, Sade LE, Gorcsan J, III. A mechanism for immediate reduction in mitral regurgitation after cardiac resynchronization therapy: insights from mechanical activation strain mapping. *J Am Coll Cardiol* 2004; **44**: 1619–1625.

44 Breithardt OA, Kuhl HP, Stellbrink C. Acute effects of re-synchronisation treatment on functional mitral regurgitation in dilated cardiomyopathy. *Heart* 2002; **88**: 440.

45 Bargiggia GS, Tronconi L, Sahn DJ *et al.* A new method for quantitation of mitral regurgitation based on color flow Doppler imaging of flow convergence proximal to regurgitant orifice. *Circulation* 1991; **84**: 1481–1489.

46 Yu CM, Abraham WT, Bax J *et al.* Predictors of response to cardiac resynchronization therapy (PROSPECT) – study design. *Am Heart J* 2005; **149**: 600–605.

47 Breithardt OA, Sinha AM. Verbesserte Identifizierung geeigneter Kandidaten für die kardiale Resynchronisationstherapie mittels transthorakaler Echokardiographie. *Herzschrittmacherther Elektrophysiol* 2005; **16**: 10–19.

48 Stellbrink C, Breithardt OA, Hanrath P. Biventrikuläre Stimulation bei Herzinsuffizienz. *Internist (Berl)* 2000; **41**: 261–268.

49 Tei C, Ling LH, Hodge DO *et al.* New index of combined systolic and diastolic myocardial performance: a simple and reproducible measure of cardiac function – a study in normals and dilated cardiomyopathy. *J Cardiol* 1995; **26**: 357–366.

CHAPTER 6

Newer echocardiographic techniques for the assessment of cardiac resynchronization therapy

Cheuk-Man Yu, MBChB(CUHK), MRCP(UK), MD(CUHK), FHKCP, FHKAM(Medicine), FRACP, FRCP(Edin), *Qing Zhang,* BM, MM & *Jeffrey Wing-Hong Fung,* MBChB(CUHK), MRCP(UK), FHKCP, FHKAM(Medicine), FRCP(Edin)

Introduction

The development of cardiac resynchronization therapy (CRT) also consolidated a multidisciplinary approach in the management of heart failure patients by cardiologists of various subspecialties, which typically involves heart failure physicians for medical therapy, electrophysiologists for device implantation and programming, as well as echocardiographic specialists for cardiac assessment. The unique role of echocardiographic assessment of CRT is widely accepted by virtue of its easy accessibility, non-invasive nature, lack of irradiation and because it permits serial assessment after device implantation. In past years further strength was added with the enhancement of quantitative analysis and development of new tools that allow assessment of regional cardiac function and mechanical dyssynchrony. In conjunction with incorporation of advanced technologies, the followings are the unique roles of echocardiography in the CRT era:

- Assessment of mechanical dyssynchrony (or asynchrony) in heart failure patients
- Understanding the mechanism of benefit of CRT from the mechanical perspective
- Differentiating responders from non-responders of CRT
- Predicting responders of CRT from indices of systolic dyssynchrony

- Potential selection of heart failure patients for CRT in whom QRS duration is normal but who have accompanied systolic dyssynchrony
- Optimization of device programming, in particular the optimization of atrioventricular and interventricular intervals.

To achieve the above tasks, a few echocardiographic technologies are potentially useful. The role of conventional echo tools has been described in Chapter 5, such as M-mode, two-dimensional, Doppler and color-Doppler echocardiography. However, new echocardiographic technologies have permitted a more comprehensive and quantitative assessment of global and regional cardiac function, in particular systolic dyssynchrony. These include spectral pulse tissue Doppler imaging (TDI), color-TDI, and post-processing imaging techniques of color-TDI such as strain, strain rate, tissue tracking, displacement, and tissue synchronization imaging (TSI). Another new technology is three-dimensional echocardiography. Table 6.1 summarizes the techniques, roles, advantages, and disadvantages of the new echocardiographic tools for the assessment of systolic dyssynchrony in CRT.

Echocardiographic technologies

Tissue Doppler imaging

TDI is a special form of Doppler echocardiography used to detect the direction and velocity of the con-

Table 6.1 Summary of various new echocardiographic tools for the assessment of systolic dyssynchrony

Echo technology	Methods of assessing dyssynchrony	Views	Indices of systolic dyssynchrony	Strength	Limitations
Pulse TDI [41]	Time to peak systolic velocity in ejection phase	Apical four-chamber	Septolateral wall delay (could include more views and sites theoretically)	Predict +ve response Robust as based on fundamental data	Less comprehensive by two segments (can be improved by incorporating more segments) Not true offline analysis Time consuming during online patient scanning
Color TDI [8, 13]	Time to peak systolic velocity in ejection phase (T_s) of six basal, six mid LV segments	Apical four-, two-, and three-chamber	T_s-SD (12 segments) Maximal difference in T_s (12 segments) The above two methods can apply for six basal LV segments	Predict +ve response Allows offline analysis Highly comprehensive Robust Can determine indices of dyssynchrony during offline post-processing imaging Can transform into other	Learning curve
Tissue tracking [17]	Tissue tracking illustrates systolic displacement as color codes	Apical four-, two-, and three-chamber	N/A	Correlates with gain in systolic function	Semi-quantitative May not differentiate isovolumic from ejection phase contraction in the color image Use motion as indirect marker of dyssynchrony
Displacement imaging [15, 16]	Time to maximal systolic displacement (T_d)	Apical or short-axis views	The "SD" or "maximal difference" methods can be applied for T_d		

Technique	Method	Views	Number of LV segments	Advantages	Disadvantages
DLC or post-systolic shortening [17]	+ve and dominant velocity after AV closure by TDI, and -ve strain rate by SRI	Apical four-, two-, and three-chamber	Number of LV segments with DLC	Correlates with gain in systolic function	Semi-quantitative Time consuming Learning curve
Strain [15, 26]	Time to peak -ve strain (T_{str})	Apical views	The "SD" or "maximal difference" methods can be applied for T_{str}	Change in regional strain may reflect change in dyssynchrony	Role of time to peak -ve strain unsure Relatively large variability Learning curve Technically demanding
Strain rate imaging [15, 26]	Time to peak -ve strain rate (T_{sr})	Apical views	SD of T_{sr} and maximal difference in T_{sr} (of two or multiple LV segments)	Differentiate translational motion "theoretically"	Role of time to peak -ve strain rate not confirmed Large observer variability Learning curve Strong technical demand
Tissue synchronization imaging (TSI) [19, 20]	Time to peak +ve myocardial velocity sampled automatically	Apical views	Same as TDI methods for velocity assessment	Quick visual appreciation of regional wall dyssynchrony Faster than TDI method "theoretically" Both quantitative and qualitative	Setting of beginning and end of TSI is critical Intrinsic problems of automated sampling of T_s Learning curve Technically demanding
Three-dimensional echo [22, 23]	Use time to minimal regional volume (T_{mrv}) in multiple segments to calculate indices of dyssynchrony	Apical views	SD of T_{mrv} and maximal difference in T_{mrv} (of six basal, 12 or 16 LV segments) SD of "% T_{mrv} of cardiac cycle" of 16 LV segments	Accurate volumetric measurement Potentially most comprehensive Quantitative and qualitative Assess dyssynchrony within single LV reconstruction loop	Relatively low spatial resolution Time consuming for semi-automatic offline analysis (but significantly improved in new generation hardware/software)

DLC, delay longitudinal contraction; SRI, strain rate imaging.

tracting or relaxing myocardium. This is achieved by suppressing the high-pass filter but setting the threshold filter so that the low-frequency, high-amplitude myocardial signals will be detected while the high-frequency, low-amplitude red blood cell signals will be neglected for analysis [1]. TDI is a robust and reproducible echocardiographic tool to detect regional function and timing of cardiac events in the myocardium [2]. In application of TDI, two-dimensional TDI images are generated, and "myocardial velocity curves" are constructed from the 2D color-coded TDI images by placing the sampling window into the region of interest, typically the myocardium within a particular segment of the ventricle.

The myocardial velocity curve can be either constructed online by spectral pulse TDI or reconstituted offline from the 2D color-TDI image. To assess cardiac function and dyssynchrony, TDI can be performed on apical four-chamber, two-chamber and three-chamber (or apical long-axis) views to examine the long-axis motion of the heart; or alternatively the parasternal short-axis views for circumferential fiber function. The examination of long-axis motion is recommended, as substantiated by the anatomical architecture of the ventricle. It has been known for decades that the majority of the myocardial fibers, in particular the endocardial and epicardial layers, are aligned longitudinally and only a small proportion of middle layer fibers are aligned circumferentially [3]. Furthermore, the continuous work from Torrent-Guasp *et al.* illustrated in human dissection that the ventricles are wrapped by a continuous piece of myocardium in an oblique fashion forming a helical structure [4, 5]. As a result, the main axis of contraction of the heart is in the longitudinal direction. However, in the event of heart failure with left ventricular (LV) dilatation,

the helical heart will criss-cross in a more horizontal manner. This implies the potential importance of examining circumferential motion.

In apical views, the myocardial velocity curve consists of systolic myocardial velocities indicative of an isovolumic contraction phase and an ejection phase, both of which are positively or apically directed. During diastole, it consists of an isovolumic relaxation phase (negative or biphasic profiles), and early diastolic and late diastolic relaxation, which are negatively directed.

Spectral pulse tissue Doppler imaging

Spectral pulse TDI has a good temporal resolution with highly robust signals. TDI signals are generated online from 2D color-TDI images when the Doppler sampling window is placed on the region of interest (Fig. 6.1) [6]. This allows a quick online assessment of cardiac function and regional synchronicity. As myocardial velocity curves have to be created online, assessment of just one segment is possible at a time. This precludes simultaneous comparison of multiple sites. Furthermore, repeated sampling from offline analysis is not possible and the assessment of multiple segments is cumbersome if it is performed during the time of scanning.

Offline 2D-color tissue Doppler imaging

The 2D-color TDI cine loops of multiple beats can be stored digitally for offline analysis (Fig. 6.2). This allows the comparison of multiple segments from each view simultaneously, and is a much quicker way of assessing myocardial function and synchronicity. This method can also reduce the time for online image acquisition and hence scanning time of the patient is reduced. The offline analysis can be performed in a blinded fashion to provide an objec-

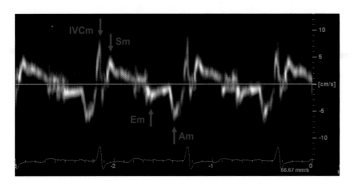

Figure 6.1 Spectral pulse tissue Doppler imaging from basal septal segment in apical four-chamber view. The sampling window is placed at the basal septal segment and myocardial velocity curve is created online that contains positive myocardial isovolumic (IVCm) and ejection phase (Sm) contraction velocities and negative early (Em) and late (Am) diastolic velocities. The time to peak Sm (T_s) is measured to assess systolic dyssynchrony.

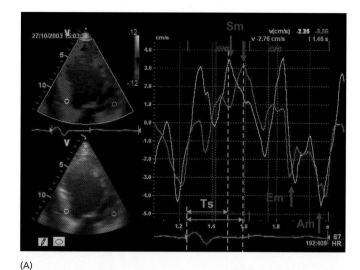

(A)

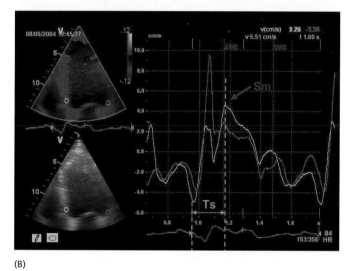

(B)

Figure 6.2 Color 2D tissue Doppler imaging (TDI) in the apical four-chamber view. Movement of the myocardium towards the probe (during contraction) is shown in red while away from the probe (during relaxation) is shown in blue. Multiple sampling windows are placed at septal and lateral segments at both basal and mid levels offline to reconstitute myocardial velocity curves similar to that of online spectral pulse TDI. The time to peak myocardial systolic velocities in the ejection phase (T_s) is measured to assess systolic dyssynchrony. There was systolic dyssynchrony with delay of T_s at the basal lateral segment for 120 ms relative to the septal segment (A). Such delay was totally abolished after CRT (B).

tive way of assessment in which repeated measurements by different persons are possible. However, adequate technical attention is mandatory in order to obtain optimal image quality, including gain, color saturation, sector size and depth, high frame rate as well as pulse repetitive frequency. For both spectral Doppler and 2D-color TDI methods, the QRS complex is often referenced when systolic mechanical dyssynchrony is assessed [7–9].

Color M-mode tissue Doppler imaging

From the 2D-color images, interrogation of regional motion can be performed by creating the M-mode image through the line of interest, the

so-called color M-mode TDI image (Fig. 6.3). Although this method has been employed to identify regional dyssynchrony [10, 11], it is largely a qualitative technique to identify regional dyssynchrony and is largely superseded by the quantitative TDI methods based on spectral pulse Doppler and offline 2D-color TDI technologies.

Indices of mechanical dyssynchrony by tissue Doppler imaging

A number of indices of mechanical dyssynchrony have been proposed in the literature and the list is continuing to increase. However, the principles of these indices are to examine for variation of tim-

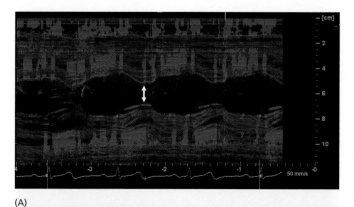

(A)

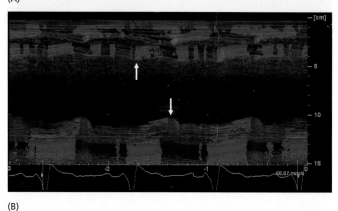

(B)

Figure 6.3 Color M-mode of tissue Doppler imaging (TDI). A patient without systolic dyssynchrony showing normal color codes on myocardium (A), with red signifies movement towards the probe and blue away from the probe. Despite the presence of LV hypertrophy, the contraction and relaxation of the anteroseptal and posterior walls occurs at the same time. The color codes are different in both walls because the movement is opposite to each other with respect to the Doppler direction. A heart failure patient with systolic dyssynchrony (B). The anteroseptal motion is paradoxical with red color in systole and blue in diastole (opposite to the normal color) (arrow). The posterior wall is likely to exhibit post-systolic shortening and therefore "contracts" (red color coding) during early diastole (arrow).

ing of contraction in different regions of the LV (*intra*ventricular dyssynchrony) or between the left and right ventricle (*inter*ventricular dyssynchrony). Technically the following principles of quantitative assessment of dyssynchrony can be considered:

- The time from the beginning of the QRS complex to the onset of systolic velocity.
- The time from the beginning of the QRS complex to peak systolic velocity in the ejection phase (T_s).
- The time from the beginning of the QRS complex to peak post-systolic shortening velocity.

Although "systolic" velocity usually refers to ejection phase (period between aortic valve opening and closure) in most of the studies, some researchers examine post-systolic shortening (positive myocardial velocity occurring after aortic valve closure and typically greater than the ejection peak, at the global timing of isovolumic relaxation phase or early diastole). Based on the above principles, one can establish indices of systolic dyssynchrony from simple (e.g. septolateral delay, septoposterior delay), inter-

mediate (six basal LV segments, septal vs. free wall segments in basal and mid levels) or more comprehensive (e.g. six basal, six mid LV segments) models of mechanical dyssynchrony [12–14].

Displacement imaging and tissue tracking

Displacement imaging is derived from the temporal integration of myocardial velocity curve (i.e. velocity–time integral) from TDI data. It illustrates the cumulated amount of myocardial excursion during different periods of the cardiac cycle and presents it on a "curve" format throughout a cardiac cycle (Fig. 6.4) [15, 16]. When the amount of myocardial displacement is presented semi-quantitatively by transforming into color codes (each represent an increment of displacement of 2 cm) and overlay onto the 2D images, it is called "tissue tracking" (Fig. 6.5). To assess systolic dyssynchrony quantitatively, the time to maximal systolic displacement can be measured from displacement

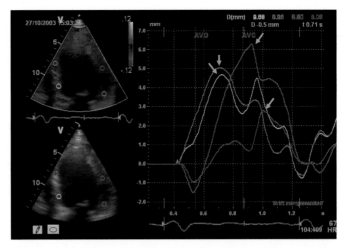

(A)

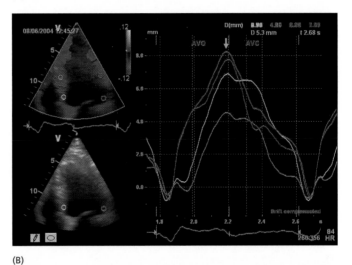

Figure 6.4 Displacement imaging at apical four-chamber (A and B), apical two-chamber (C and D) and apical long-axis (E and F) views before (A, C, and E) and after (B, D, and F) CRT. Normal systolic displacement at these views occurs with the largest amplitude at the basal LV segments which move towards the apex. Therefore, the apex is relatively stationary with respect to long-axis motion. The displacement mapping is cumulative and therefore it increases in amplitude during systole and reaches the maximal amplitude at end-systole (arrows). In this patient, systolic dyssynchrony is illustrated by the unusually early maximal displacement at some segments (e.g. septum), and delayed displacement in others which extend beyond the aortic valve closure (e.g. lateral, anterior and posterior walls). After CRT, improvement is reflected by the realignment of maximal systolic displacement in most of the segments to the same timing before aortic valve closure.

(B)

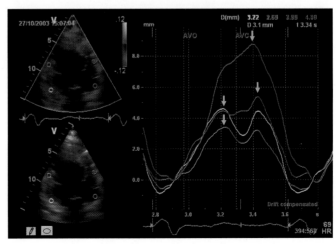

(C)

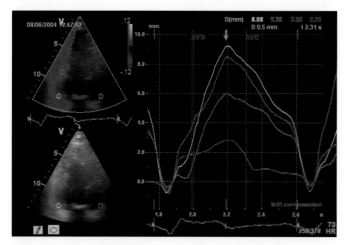

(D)

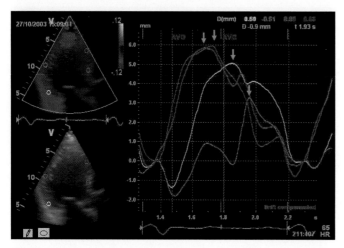

(E)

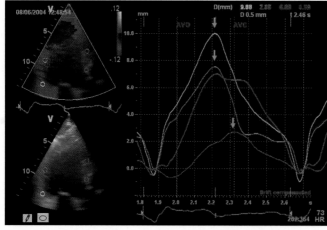

(F)

Figure 6.4 (*Continued*)

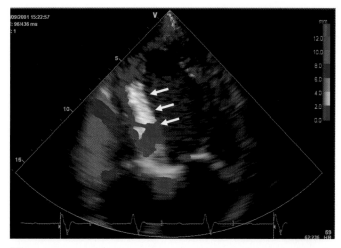

(A)

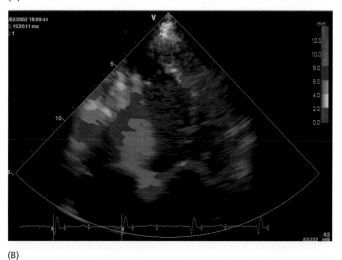

(B)

Figure 6.5 Tissue tracking on apical four-chamber (A and B), apical two-chamber (C and D) and apical long-axis (E and F) views before (A, C, and E) and after (B, D, and F) CRT. Cumulated positive systolic displacement is represented as color codes, each representing an increment of 2 cm. Poor systolic displacement is illustrated by the absence of color code (e.g. septum), or red to yellow color codes (inferior wall) (arrows). Increase in displacement has been described as a surrogate marker of improved systolic dyssynchrony, which is illustrated by the different color codes after CRT. Note that in Fig. 6.4, the improvement in displacement is shown by the values on the y-axis.

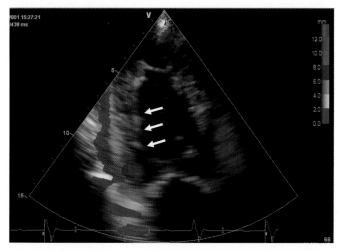

(C)

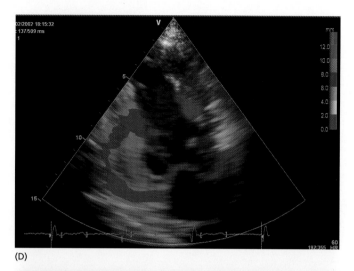

(D)

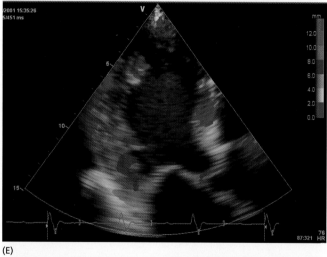

(E)

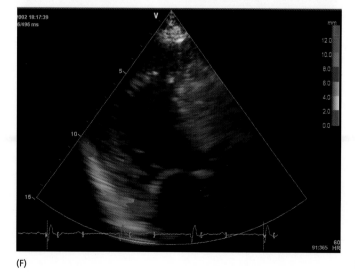

(F)

Figure 6.5 (*Continued*)

imaging at either apical or parasternal views [15, 16]. It has been suggested that the improvement of displacement in tissue tracking can serve as a surrogate marker of reduced systolic dyssynchrony [17, 18]. However, the superiority of displacement mapping to tissue velocity in assessing patients with CRT has not been confirmed.

Strain imaging

Strain mapping is another post-processing mapping of TDI data that calculates the amount of myocardial deformation in a cumulated manner throughout the cardiac cycle. Tissue strain was calculated by the formula $\varepsilon = (L - L_0)/L_0 \times 100\%$. In order to assess systolic dyssynchrony, the time to minimal

strain at different regions can be measured (Fig. 6.6) [15].

Strain rate imaging

Strain rate imaging reflects the rate of change of strain in the cardiac cycle (i.e. the first derivative or slope of the strain curve). Therefore, strain rate imaging is a measure of the rate of deformation of the myocardium (Fig. 6.7). Theoretically, both strain and strain rate imaging are superior to tissue velocities and displacement mapping as translational motion from passive motions can be eliminated, such as respiration and tethering of adjacent segments. However, current technical limitations outweigh the theoretical advantages of strain rate imaging

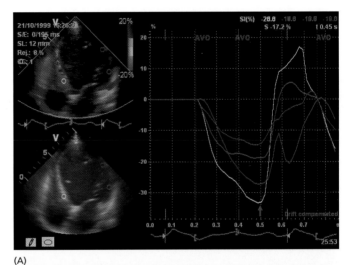

Figure 6.6 Strain imaging on apical four-chamber (A and B), apical two-chamber (C and D), and apical long-axis (E and F) views before (A, C, and E) and after (B, D, and F) CRT. Normal systolic strain in apical views is negative with the largest cumulated values occurring during end-systole. In this patient, systolic dyssynchrony is illustrated by the paradoxical direction of strain curve (e.g. positive during systole in septal, anterior and posterior walls) as well as the delay in maximal negative strain beyond the aortic valve closure (e.g. anterior, anteroseptal, and posterior walls) (arrows). However, improvement in systolic strain is only observed in some segments (e.g. anterior–septal and posterior segments at apical long-axis view), but worsened in other segments (e.g. septal and lateral segments at apical four-chamber view).

(A)

(B)

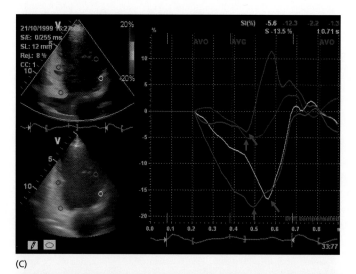

(C)

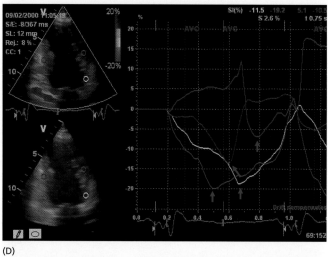

(D)

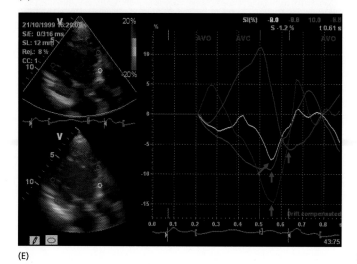

(E)

Figure 6.6 (*Continued*)

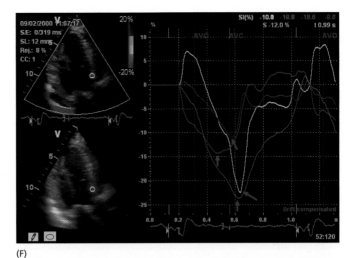

Figure 6.6 (*Continued*)   (F)

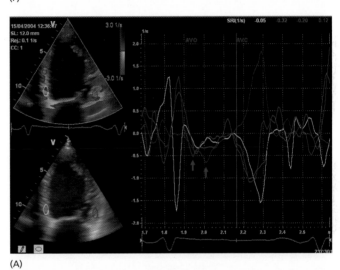

(A)

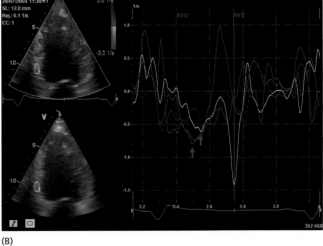

Figure 6.7 Strain rate imaging at apical four-chamber (A and B) and apical two-chamber (C and D) views before (A and C) and after (B and D) CRT. Normal systolic strain rate at apical views is negative in ejection period (arrows) and with two positive peaks during early and late diastolic phases. Although the time to peak negative systolic strain rate at baseline is obviously dyssynchronous, no improvement is discernible after CRT, which may limit the use of strain rate imaging as a tool to assess dyssynchrony. Note the presence of significant background noises in these curves.   (B)

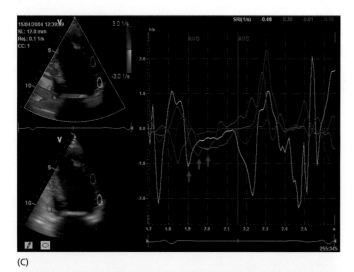

(C)

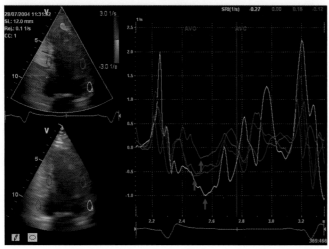

(D)

Figure 6.7 (*Continued*)

which include artifacts and random noises. The use of time to peak negative strain rate has been attempted to measure systolic dyssynchrony, though it was found to be significantly inferior to tissue velocity in a comparative study [13].

Tissue synchronization imaging

TSI portrays regional dyssynchrony on two-dimensional images by transforming the timing of regional peak positive velocity of TDI data into color codes which allows immediate visual identification of regional delay in systole by comparing the color mapping of orthogonal walls (Fig. 6.8) [19–21]. In addition, quantitative measurement of regional delay is possible. Since this imaging modality is derived from TDI data, indices of systolic dyssynchrony similar to that of TDI can be generated. At present, it is recommended that quantitative analysis should be carried out by performing measurement of the myocardial velocity curve (which is same as those from TDI) rather than directly from the color-coded TSI images to avoid technical errors during sampling.

Three-dimensional echocardiography

Three-dimensional echocardiography is another technology that provides a comprehensive model of assessing systolic dyssynchrony in multiple regions of the left ventricle in a "wide-angle" volume-

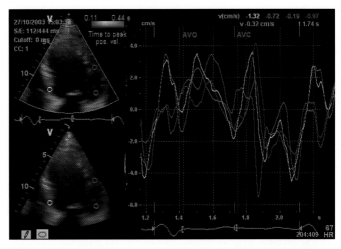

(A)

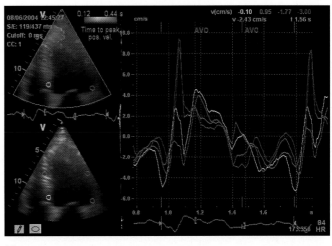

(B)

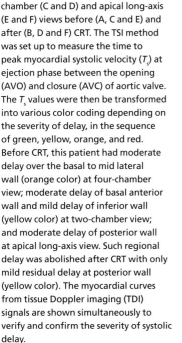

Figure 6.8 An example of tissue synchronization imaging (TSI) at apical four-chamber (A and B), apical two-chamber (C and D) and apical long-axis (E and F) views before (A, C and E) and after (B, D and F) CRT. The TSI method was set up to measure the time to peak myocardial systolic velocity (T_s) at ejection phase between the opening (AVO) and closure (AVC) of aortic valve. The T_s values were then be transformed into various color coding depending on the severity of delay, in the sequence of green, yellow, orange, and red. Before CRT, this patient had moderate delay over the basal to mid lateral wall (orange color) at four-chamber view; moderate delay of basal anterior wall and mild delay of inferior wall (yellow color) at two-chamber view; and moderate delay of posterior wall at apical long-axis view. Such regional delay was abolished after CRT with only mild residual delay at posterior wall (yellow color). The myocardial curves from tissue Doppler imaging (TDI) signals are shown simultaneously to verify and confirm the severity of systolic delay.

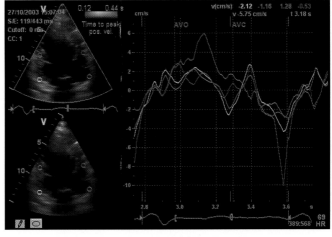

(C)

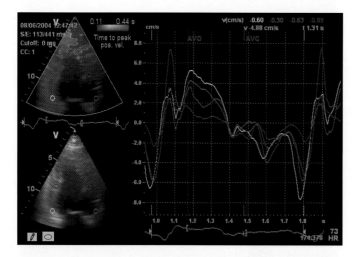

(D)

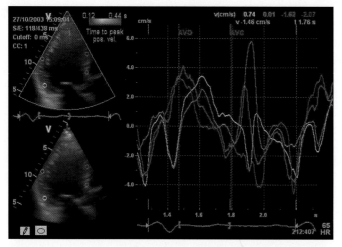

(E)

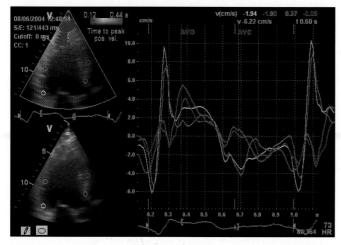

(F)

Figure 6.8 (*Continued*)

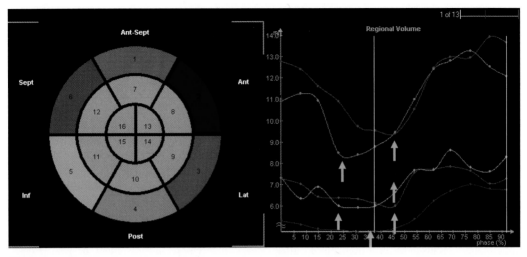

(A)

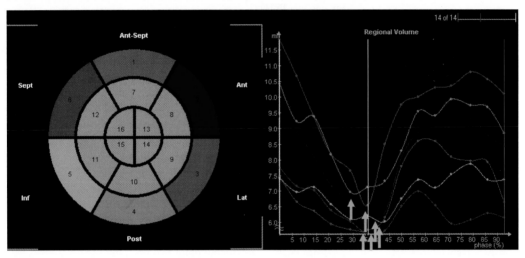

(B)

Figure 6.9 3D-Echocardiography in a patient before (A) and after (B) CRT. Regional volumetric curves of the six basal LV segments show dyssynchronous LV contraction in CRT-off mode, as reflected by scattered timings to minimal regional volume (arrows). There was improvement of LV systolic dyssynchrony in CRT-on mode, with more congregated points of minimal regional volume (arrows).

rendered cine loop that is captured from only a few beats (Fig. 6.9). Assessment of systolic dyssynchrony is based on the offline reconstruction of regional volumetric curves in a 16- (or recently 17-) segmental model as defined by the American Society of Echocardiography. From the regional volumetric curves, the time to minimal regional volume can be measured, and indices of systolic dyssynchrony was calculated from 6-basal, 12- (6-basal, 6-mid) or 16-segmental models [22, 23].

Assessment of systolic dyssynchrony in heart failure patients receiving cardiac resynchronization therapy

Most of the studies that applied advanced echocardiographic technologies to patients receiving CRT focus on the assessment of systolic dyssynchrony, as electromechanical delay resulting in regional dyssynchrony is believed to be the primary abnormality in heart failure with prolongation of QRS duration. In these patients, three levels of mechanical dyssynchrony have been described that underlie the development of electrical abnormalities, namely interventricular dyssynchrony, intraventricular dyssynchrony, and atrioventricular dyssynchrony. The first two phenomena are related to the prolongation of QRS duration that delays the electrical propagation of the ventricle(s), while atrioventricular dyssynchrony occurs in first-degree atrioventricular block that jeopardizes LV diastolic filling, reduces cardiac output and leads to the occurrence of diastolic mitral regurgitation [24].

It is speculated that when the culprit abnormal mechanical event is corrected by CRT, reversal of such abnormalities results in the improvement of cardiac function, such as gain in ejection fraction, reduction of LV size (or LV reverse remodeling) and alleviation of mitral regurgitation. Table 6.2 summarizes the representative studies based on new echocardiographic techniques that have assessed mechanical dyssynchrony correlated with improvement of cardiac function after CRT. CRT increases septal inward excursion, as illustrated by contrast variability imaging which examined endocardial excursion in a very small arc of 15° in the LV in 10 patients [25]. In this study, the lateral wall excursion was unchanged, though systolic function was increased as a result of improved systolic dyssynchrony [25]. The study by Sogaard *et al.* examined "delayed longitudinal contraction" (which is the same as post-systolic shortening) in 20 patients receiving CRT [17]. The delayed longitudinal contraction in the basal LV segments was reduced from 18.7% to 8.1% at one-year follow-up, which correlated with the improvement in ejection fraction [17].

There are other mechanical phenomena described after CRT. For example, there is reversal of mid-septal and mid-lateral wall peak strain and strain rate values after CRT, which became higher in the septum than in the lateral wall after treatment [26]. Such a change, however, does not explain why cardiac function was favorably improved as reported in other studies. Sun *et al.* described a different finding that the pre-pacing septal strain rate was higher than the lateral wall, and the improvement occurred in the lateral wall during biventricular pacing and in both walls during LV pacing [15]. Also, reduction in the differences in timing of maximal long-axis displacement between septolateral wall or antero-

inferior wall was observed after CRT [15]. Whether such changes explained the gain in systolic function has not been explored.

Mechanical dyssynchrony can be assessed more comprehensively by TDI through examination of multiple segments in multiple views. Yu *et al.* [8] looked for potential predictor(s) of LV reverse remodeling in 30 patients receiving CRT, which included demographic, clinical, and echocardiographic parameters. LV reverse remodeling was defined as a reduction of LV end-systolic volume (LVESV) >15%, which was observed in 57% of patients. Improvement of New York Heart Association (NYHA) class was observed in all the responders of LV reverse remodeling, but in only 54% of non-responders. Furthermore, improvement of peak oxygen uptake, maximal metabolic equivalent by treadmill exercise test and 6-Minute Hall-Walk distance was only observed in the responders [8]. The "Asynchrony Index" was calculated by calculating the standard deviation of time to peak myocardial systolic velocity in ejection phase (T_s-SD) of the 12 LV segments by TDI from the three apical (four-chamber, two-chamber, and long-axis) views (Appendix 1)[8]. The Asynchrony Index at baseline was found to correlate closely with the degree of LV reverse remodeling. Furthermore, a cut-off value of Asynchrony Index of 32.6 ms, which was derived from 88 normal controls, was able to differentiate responders from non-responders of reverse remodeling [8].

The study by Bordachar *et al.* examined a number of echocardiographic indices of systolic dyssynchrony by spectral pulse TDI from the 12 LV segments that examined the maximal difference in time to onset or peak systolic velocity as well as the T_s-SD [27]. This study observed that the changes of cardiac output and mitral regurgitation after optimized sequential biventricular pacing correlated with the improvement of TDI indices of systolic dyssynchrony by all the three TDI indices ($r = -0.64$ to -0.67, all $P < 0.001$). This was superior to other methods that examined delayed longitudinal contraction, septo-posterior wall delay by M-mode echocardiography or Doppler method of interventricular mechanical delay [27].

Three-dimensional echocardiography is another evolving echocardiographic tool for the assessment of systolic dyssynchrony. An acute study examined the acute changes of LV synchronicity in 13 patients during the CRT "on" and "off" periods [22]. There

Table 6.2 Echocardiographic tools to assess mechanical dyssynchrony before and after CRT

Author	Sample size	Echo technique	Echo parameters of systolic dyssynchrony	Follow-up period	Findings
Kawaguchi [25]	10	Contrast echo	Septal and lateral wall motion	9 ± 12 months	↑ Septal inward motion, ↓ spatial and temporal dyssynchrony in LV by 40%, and correlated with ↑ EF
Ansalone [11]	31	TDI	TDI at septal, lateral, inferior, posterior, and anterior walls	Acute	Pacing at site with longest regional contraction plus isovolumic relaxation had more ↑ EF
Yu [8]	30	TDI	T_s-SD of six basal, six mid LV segments (ejection phase)	3 months	T_s-SD was the single independent predictor of LV reverse remodeling by a cut-off value of 32.6ms
Bordachor [27]	41	M-mode, Doppler and TDI	T_s-SD, Maximal difference in time to onset or peak of 12 LV segments, DLC, SPWMD, IVMD	3 months	↑ Cardiac output and ↓mitral regurgitation correlated with the improvement of all 3 TDI parameters, and was superior to DLC and SPWMD or IVMD
Sogaard [17]	20	TDI and SRI	TDI and SRI for delayed longitudinal contraction	12 months	Number of basal segments with delayed longitudinal contraction predicted ↑ EF
Popović [67]	22	Strain	Septal and lateral wall strain	1–12 months	↑ Global LV peak strain, ↓coefficient of change in LV strain, no change in septal or lateral wall displacement
Breithardt [26]	18	Strain and SRI	Strain and SRI at septal & lateral wall	Acute	Baseline – lateral wall strain and strain rate more than septal; CRT – reversal of such relationship
Sun [15]	34	Strain, SRI and displacement	Strain, SRI, and displacement at septal and lateral wall	Acute	↑ EF and ↑ peak strain rate at lateral wall by CRT, ↑ septal and inferior wall displacement by LV pacing
Zhang [22]	13	3D Echocardiography compared with TDI	Standard deviation (or maximal difference) of absolute time to minimal regional volume of six basal, 12 or 16 LV segments	Acute	↑ LV volume ↓ EF during CRT "off" period; indices of 16 LV segments by 3D echo closely correlated with T_s-SD by TDI
Kapetanakis [23]	26	3D Echocardiography	SDI, by standard deviation of % time to minimal regional volume of 16 LV segments	10 ± 1 month	Clinical responders (17/23) had larger baseline SDI than non-responders, but similar EF; LV reverse remodeling was observed only in responders

DLC, delayed longitudinal contraction; EF, ejection fraction; IVMD, interventricular mechanical delay by Doppler echocardiography; SDI, systolic dyssynchrony index; SRI, strain-rate imaging; SPWMD, septo-posterior wall motion delay by M-mode echocardiography; TDI, tissue Doppler imaging; T_s-SD, standard deviation of time to peak myocardial systolic velocity.

was immediate worsening of indices of systolic dyssynchrony derived from six basal, 12 and 16 LV segments by calculating either the standard deviation or maximal difference in time to minimal regional volume [22]. A good correlation between the 16-segment models of 3D-echocardiography and Asynchrony Index (or T_s-SD) of TDI was observed ($r = 0.739$ and 0.809, both $P < 0.05$) [22]. Another study by Kapetanakis *et al.* examined 26 patients before and after CRT by 3D-echocardiography for a mean duration of 10 ± 1 months [23]. The Systolic Dyssynchrony Index was derived from the standard deviation of % time to minimal regional volume of 16 LV segments. It was observed that patients with long-term clinical response had significantly larger values of baseline Systolic Dyssynchrony Index than clinical non-responders, and had evidence of LV reverse remodeling [23].

Understanding the mechanism of benefit of cardiac resynchronization therapy from mechanical perspectives

The mechanisms of benefits of CRT can be examined from a mechanical perspective. In a study by Yu *et al.*, 25 patients who underwent CRT were studied sequentially for three months by echocardiography with TDI [7]. Measurement of T_s was performed at six basal and six mid LV segments and the two right ventricular (RV) segments. LV dyssynchrony was il- lustrated by the widespread regional variation of T_s among various segments. TDI achieved systolic syn- chronicity by homogeneously delaying those early contracting segments to a timing similar to the de- layed segments (Fig. 6.10) [7]. As a result, not only septolateral delay was abolished, other patterns of delay were also corrected (Fig. 6.11). The septal-to-RV free wall delay was also abolished after CRT. Further- more, echocardiographic improvement were pacing dependent, which included LV reverse remodeling, increase in ejection fraction or $+dP/dt$, reduction of mitral regurgitation and increase in LV diastolic filling time. When CRT was temporarily withheld, there was no immediate worsening of systolic func- tion or enlargement of LV. However, all the observed echocardiographic benefits were gradually lost in the next four weeks without CRT (Fig. 6.12) [7]. This is also the first study to illustrate the contrasting effect of pacing "on" and "off", and confirmed the independ- ent benefit of pacing on cardiac function. Further- more, the chronic benefit of pacing on cardiac func- tion is progressive and is additive to the acute benefits on cardiac function which are observed within 48 h after device implantation [28, 29].

Improvement of mitral regurgitation is another cardinal echocardiographic feature in CRT. With reduction of regurgitant volume into the left atri- um, atrial filling pressure is reduced and LV volume overload is decreased. This enhances the process of LV reverse remodeling. Mechanisms for the reduc- tion of mitral regurgitation are likely related to the

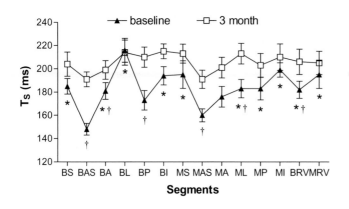

Figure 6.10 Changes in the time to peak myocardial systolic velocity in the ejection phase (T_s) before (triangles) and after (squares) CRT. At baseline, there was marked regional variation in T_s among the LV segments. The T_s was earliest in the basal anteroseptal segment and latest in the basal lateral segment. After CRT, the T_s values were homogeneously delayed to a timing close to that of the basal lateral segment so that regional variation in T_s was abolished. *$P < 0.05$ vs. basal anteroseptal segment at baseline. †$P < 0.05$ when comparing the same segment before and after pacing therapy. B, basal; M, mid; A, anterior; AS, anteroseptal; I, inferior; L, lateral; P, posterior; S, septal; RV, right ventricle.

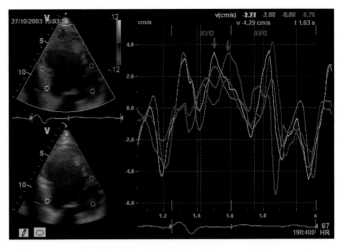

(A)

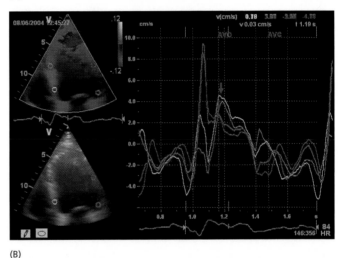

(B)

Figure 6.11 Color TDI with myocardial velocity curves reconstructed at apical four-chamber (A and B), apical two-chamber (C and D) and long-axis (E and F) views before (A, C, and E) and after (B, D, and F) CRT. The use of three apical views can establish the six basal, six mid segmental model to examine for systolic asynchrony. Aortic valve opening (AVO) and closure (AVC) markers are tagged relative to the ECG signal to provide a temporal guidance on "ejection" period. Delay in the time to peak systolic velocity is evident in the lateral, anterior and posterior walls at baseline (arrows). After CRT, there is realignment of the contractile profile, in particular in the ejection phase where the peak contractions occur at about the same time (arrows). The Asynchrony Index (or T_s-SD) of the six basal, six mid segmental model decreased from 41 ms before CRT to 28 ms after the therapy.

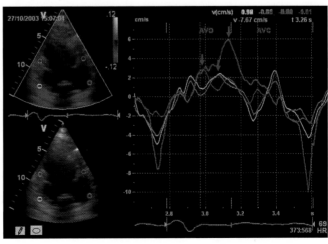

(C)

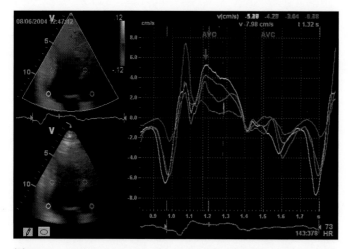

(D)

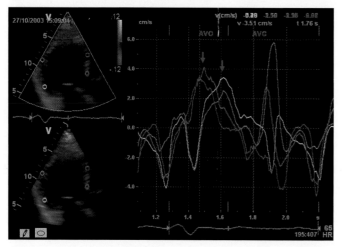

(E)

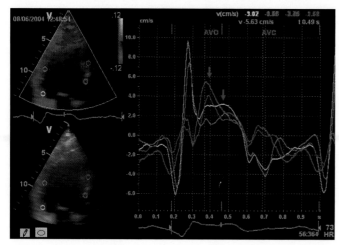

(F)

Figure 6.11 (*Continued*)

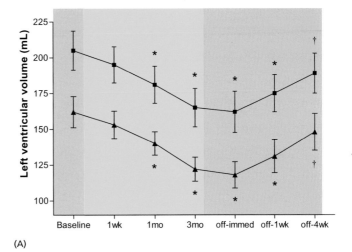

(A)

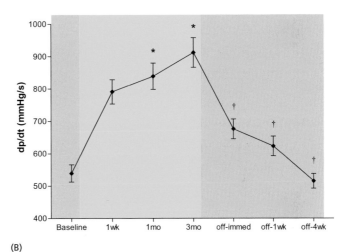

(B)

Figure 6.12 Changes in LV end-diastolic and end-systolic volumes (A), +dP/dt (B), isovolumic contraction time (C), ejection fraction (D), mitral regurgitation (E), and LV filling time (F) before and after CRT for three months, as well as when pacing was suspended for four weeks. The period in pink indicates when there was no pacing while those in yellow are periods with CRT. * indicates significant difference vs. baseline, † indicates significant difference vs. biventricular pacing for three months.

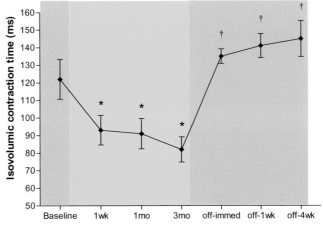

(C)

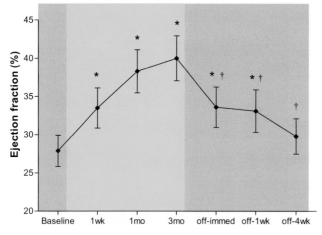

(D)

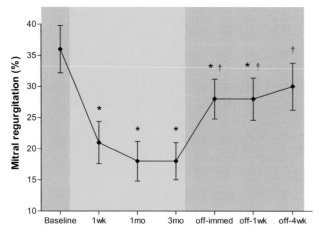

(E)

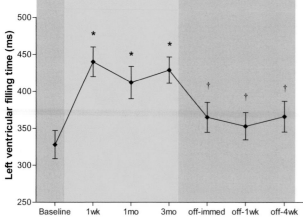

(F)

Figure 6.12 (*Continued*)

improvement of systolic dyssynchrony, which also affects the movement of papillary muscle that distorts the normal timing of movement of mitral apparatus. This was demonstrated by the study from Kanzaki *et al.* in which interpapillary muscle delay was present by measuring the time to peak strain in the short-axis view. Such delay was greatly reduced after CRT, which correlated with reduction in mitral regurgitant fraction ($r = 0.77, P < 0.001$) [30].

Non-responders to cardiac resynchronization therapy

Although the clinical and echocardiographic benefits of CRT have been well demonstrated, about one-third of patients did not respond to the therapy; the so-called non-responders [13, 31–37]. A number of methods have been used to characterize these non-responders, including investigation of hemodynamic, clinical, and echocardiographic variables. An acute hemodynamic response was defined as ≥5% increase in pulse pressure by invasive manometry, and non-responders were observed to comprise 12/39 (31%) patients in a study [31]. However, methods envisaged to assess acute response have limitations: the acute hemodynamic response has not been shown to predict the long-term benefits of CRT; and some patients who have no or minimal acute changes in any assessment modality (such as hemodynamic parameters, cardiac function, LV volume and clinical status) may show gradual and delayed improvement after a few months [19]. Another definition of non-responders is based on clinical status; defined by a lack of improvement of NYHA functional class, exercise capacity, heart failure-related quality of life, or the occurrence of events such as heart failure hospitalization or mortality, or based on the clinical composite score [38]. Non-responder rates range from 18% to 52% [33–36].

Obviously, the limitation of this definition at present is the lack of consensus on what clinical criteria should be selected to define non-responders. Furthermore, some clinical endpoints are subjected to the placebo effect, as exemplified by multicenter trials [35, 36]. Another way of assessing responders relies on the assessment of change in LV size and cardiac function. A commonly used parameter is LV reverse remodeling as assessed by the change in LVESV. In CRT trials, using a vigorous definition of reduction of LVESV >15%, volumetric non-re-

sponders were observed in about 40% of patients in four previous studies [8, 37, 39, 40]. The advantage of assessing LV reverse remodeling is related to its objectivity, since it reflects the improvement of cardiac structure and function. LVESV can also be assessed offline in a blinded fashion, and is less subject to the placebo effect. Studies have also found that patients who are volumetric responders showed greater improvement in clinical status [8, 41].

There are two major factors that determine the failure to respond favorably to CRT, namely the placement of an LV lead at a suboptimal location and the limitation of ECG-based patient selection criteria. Placement of the LV lead at a location that resynchronizes the electrical and mechanical activation sequence of the LV to provide better coordination during systole is crucial for successful CRT. It is recommended that the LV lead should be positioned at the LV free wall, which corresponds to the anatomical region of the lateral or posterio-lateral cardiac vein [35, 42, 43]. In the PATH-CHF II study, 30 patients with either LV or biventricular pacing were assessed in the acute phase. LV free wall pacing resulted in a larger gain in pulse pressure (9% vs. 5%, $P < 0.001$) and +dP/dt (12% vs. 5%, $P < 0.001$) when compared with LV anterior wall pacing [44]. Due to anatomical and technical limitations, up to one-third of patients may not have the LV lead implanted in the free wall [43, 45].

Currently, patient selection criteria for CRT are based on QRS duration as an indicator of electromechanical delay. Left bundle branch block (LBBB) and left intraventricular conduction delay (IVCD) are patterns that signify a conduction abnormality within the left ventricle. As CRT has been shown to improve intraventricular dyssynchrony within the left ventricle [46] it is likely that the therapy will benefit patients with LBBB and IVCD. However, there are no definite data on the benefit of CRT for patients with right bundle branch block (RBBB). Most clinical studies did not address this issue. From the MIRACLE study, it appears that patients with RBBB will benefit less than those with LBBB or IVCD. The study from Garrigue *et al.* demonstrated that in patients with RBBB those with accompanying intraventricular dyssynchrony in the LV as shown by TDI were more likely to benefit from CRT than those without [47].

In heart failure patients with prolonged QRS duration, electrical delay in the LV may not be present, which was illustrated by studies based on 3D non-contact mapping electrograms [48]. In the same line, absence of mechanical dyssynchrony was also observed in about 27–36% of heart patients with QRS >120 ms when TDI was performed to examine intraventricular dyssynchrony from the six basal, six mid segmental model by the Asynchrony Index and maximal difference in T_s among the 12 LV segments [9]. This observation was further confirmed by another study that examined intraventricular dyssynchrony in multiple segments by TDI in 158 heart failure patients with normal, mildly prolonged (120–150 ms) and severely prolonged (>150 ms) QRS duration [49]. Although a slightly different method of assessing dyssynchrony was employed, absence of systolic intraventricular dyssynchrony was observed in 43% of patients in the mildly prolonged QRS duration group and 29% in the group with QRS duration >150 ms [49].

Based on these data, it appears that the surface ECG is not a sensitive marker to predict the presence or absence of LV electrical activation delay. In general, prolonged QRS duration on surface ECG may be caused by interventricular and/or intraventricular delay [50, 51]. However, a few researchers have suggested that the correctional effect of CRT on interventricular delay probably plays only a secondary role [13, 27, 50]. This probably accounts for the lack of benefit from CRT in some patients with wide QRS complex. As new echocardiographic techniques are powerful tools to assess ventricular dyssynchrony, it is likely that a proper use of these technologies will help to predict responders to CRT.

Predicting responders to cardiac resynchronization therapy from indices of systolic dyssynchrony

In order to predict and differentiate responders from non-responders of CRT, echocardiographic assessment of systolic asynchrony has a unique role. A number of echocardiographic techniques and their derived indices of asynchrony have been proposed. However, to apply an echocardiographic index of systolic asynchrony in clinical practice, a cut-off value needs to be identified objectively to determine if systolic dyssynchrony is clinically relevant. Furthermore, a good index needs to be able to predict a favorable response with a high sensitivity in order to be incorporated as a screening test; and a high

specificity as a "rule in" test to ascertain the presence of systolic asynchrony. Table 6.3 summarizes the key studies that examined systolic dyssynchrony by TDI and its post-processing technologies, which also derived a cut-off value for predicting a favorable response to CRT [6, 8, 13, 19, 20, 40, 41].

Bax *et al.* [41] evaluated 25 patients with color-coded TDI by a two-basal segmental model in an acute study. In these patients, LV ejection fraction increased from $22 \pm 5\%$ to $31 \pm 10\%$ and the septolateral delay decreased from 71 ± 38 ms to 36 ± 34 ms after CRT. Acute responders were defined as those with an increase in LV ejection fraction of ≥5%. Only responders of systolic function showed an improvement in clinical status, which included NYHA class, quality of life and 6-Minute Hall-Walk distance. A septolateral delay at baseline ≥60 ms has a sensitivity of 76% and specificity of 87.5% of predicting an increase in LV ejection fraction [41]. Subsequently, the same group examined 85 patients for a follow-up period of one year to determine the non-responder rate and the value of assessing septolateral delay [52]. When chronic responders were defined as an improvement in NYHA functional class of ≥1 score and a gain of ≥25% in 6-Minute Hall-Walk distance, the prevalence was 73%. This landmark study observed that a septolateral delay ≥65 ms predicts the clinical response with a sensitivity and specificity of 80%. Importantly, patients who were above this cut-off value had a lower mortality than those who were below [52].

Notobartolo *et al.* examined the myocardial velocity curve from offline 2D-color TDI analysis by choosing the highest peak velocity in either ejection phase or post-systolic shortening among the six basal LV segments from the three apical views [40]. The index of systolic dyssynchrony was calculated from the maximal difference in time to peak velocity among these six segments, called the "peak velocity difference". In 49 patients who received the therapy, a peak velocity difference of >110 ms at baseline predicted LV reverse remodeling (defined as a reduction of LVESV >15%) at three-month follow-up with a sensitivity of 97%, though the specificity was only 55% [40]. On the other hand, examination of ejection phase velocity seems to provide a better trade-off between sensitivity and specificity. When Asynchrony Index (or T_s-SD) of the six basal, six mid segmental model

Table 6.3 Published criteria of systolic asynchrony by TDI that predict a favorable echocardiographic response to CRT

Author	Sample size	Criteria	Follow-up period	Definition of responders	Cut-off value	Sensitivity	Specificity
Bax [41]	25	Septal-to-lateral delay in T_s (ejection phase)	Acute (within 24 h)	Absolute ↑EF ≥5%	>60 ms	76%	87.5%
Bax [52]	85	Septal-to-lateral delay in T_s (ejection phase)	(1) 12 months (2) 6 months (echo)	(1) Clinical: ↓ NYHA ≥1 and ↑ 6MHW ≥25% (2) ↓LVVs >15%	≥65 ms	(1) 80% (2) 92%	(1) 80% (2) 92%
Yu [13]	54	T_s-SD of six basal, six mid LV segments (ejection phase)	3 months	↓LVVs >15%	>31.4 ms	96%	78%
Yu [53]	(1) QRS >120–150 ms: 27 (2) QRS >150 ms: 31	T_s-SD of six basal, six mid LV segments (ejection phase)	3 months	↓LVVs >15%	>32.6 ms (derived from normal population)	1. 83% 2. 100%	1. 86% 2. 78%
Penicka [6]	49	T_s (onset) of BS, BL, BP and BRV by summation of inter- and intraventricular delay	6 months	Relative ↑EF ≥25%	>102 ms	96%	71%
Notabartolo [40]	49	Maximal difference in T_s in six basal segments (both ejection phase and post-systolic shortening)	3 months	↓LVVs >15%	>110 ms	97%	55%
Gorcsan [19]	29	Septoposterior delay (both ejection phase and post-systolic shortening)	Acute (within 48 h)	↑Stroke volume ≥15%	>65 ms	87%	100%
Yu [20]	56	(1) Lateral wall delay (2) T_s-SD of six basal, six mid LV segments (ejection phase)	3 months	↓LVVs >15%	(1) Qualitative (2) >34.4 ms	(1) 47% (2) 87%	(1) 89% (2) 81%

BS, basal septal; BL, basal lateral; BP, basal posterior; BRV, basal right ventricular; LVVs, left ventricular end-systolic volume; TDI, tissue Doppler imaging; TSI, tissue synchronization imaging, T_s, time to peak myocardial systolic velocity; T_s (onset), time to onset of myocardial systolic velocity; T_s-SD, standard deviation of time to peak myocardial systolic velocity; EF, ejection fraction; NYHA, New York Heart Association; 6MHW, 6-Minute Hall-Walk.

was employed with a cut-off value of 32.6 ms, it was able to segregate responders from non-responders of LV reverse remodeling [8]. Since the degree of QRS prolongation might have impacted on the response rate to CRT, a further study was conducted to examine whether such a difference exists between patients with QRS >120–150 ms and those with QRS >150 ms [53]. This study showed that the response rate of LV reverse remod-eling was lower in the less wide QRS group (46%) than those with QRS >150 ms (68%).

TDI provides an important insight into the reason for the lack of favorable response. In fact, only responders suffered from significant systolic dyssynchrony, with large values of Asynchrony Index which were improved after CRT. On the other hand, the non-responders had mild systolic dyssynchrony (Fig. 6.13). Intriguingly, CRT in these patients actually worsens

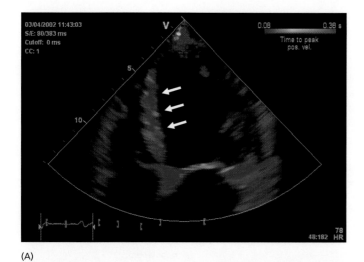

(A)

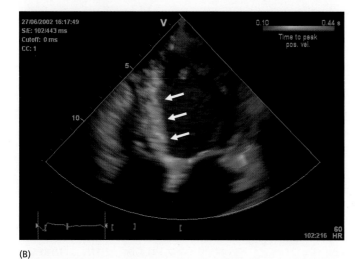

(B)

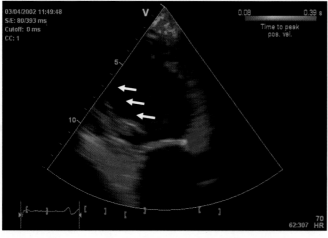

(C)

Figure 6.13 Tissue synchronization imaging (TSI) of a non-responder to CRT. Apical views at baseline (A, C, and E) show no evidence of systolic dyssynchrony despite prolonged QRS duration. The same views after CRT (B, D, and F) illustrated worsening of systolic synchronicity, with delay in septal and inferior walls (arrows).

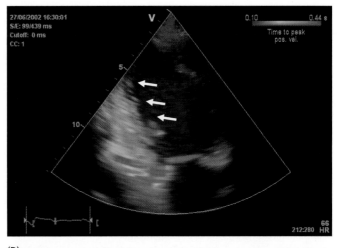

(D)

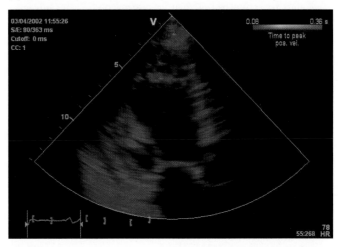

(E)

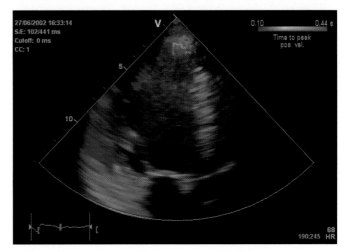

Figure 6.13 (*Continued*)   (F)

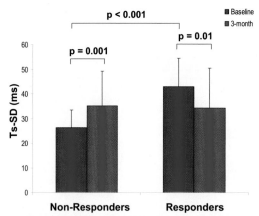

Figure 6.14 Comparison of Asynchrony Index (T_s-SD) before and three months after CRT in responders and non-responders of LV reverse remodeling. Responders had significantly higher baseline T_s-SD than non-responders which was decreased after biventricular pacing. In contrast, the non-responders had low T_s-SD which was worsened after the therapy. Intriguingly, the final values of Asynchrony Index were similar between the two groups.

mechanical dyssynchrony, as shown by the increase in Asynchrony Index (Fig. 6.14) [53]. Therefore, this study showed the potential importance of echocardiography in accurately predicting the response to CRT, and advised caution in the implantation of devices for those who do not have significant systole mechanical dyssynchrony as there might be further worsening of cardiac function. Furthermore, the predictive value of LV reverse remodeling response is lower in patients with QRS >120–150 ms than those with QRS >150 ms (sensitivity of 83% vs. 100%) [53].

Another way of assessing systolic dyssynchrony is to measure the time to onset of mechanical contraction in ejection phase. The work by Penicka *et al.* employed pulse Doppler TDI at three basal LV segments at septal, lateral, and posterior wall as well as basal RV segment by apical four-chamber and apical long-axis views [6]. This method defined intraventricular dyssynchrony as the maximal electromechanical delay among the three basal LV segments, and interventricular dyssynchrony as the maximal delay between the RV segment and the three LV sites. The result observed that adding intra- and interventricular dyssynchrony has a high predictive value for CRT response, which was defined as a relative increase in ejection fraction by 25%. A cut-off value of 102 ms derived from the study population reported an accuracy of 88% [6].

Only few studies compared multiple echocardiographic indices of systolic asynchrony at the same time. When this was attempted in two studies [13, 20], it was concluded that Asynchrony Index (or T_s-SD) has the highest predictive value for LV reverse remodeling when compared with indices that were derived from a smaller number of segments (e.g. only two to eight LV segments). In one study where 18 echocardiographic parameters derived from TDI or strain rate imaging were compared for their predictive value for LV reverse remodeling three months after CRT, Asynchrony Index had the greatest value of correlation coefficient ($r = -0.74$, $P < 0.001$) and area of receiver operating characteristics (ROC) curve (area = 0.94, $P < 0.001$) (Figs 6.15 and 6.16) [13]. Furthermore, for the same

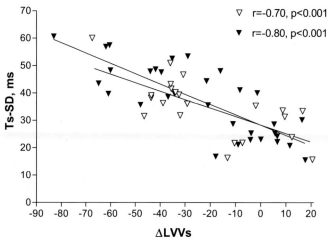

(A)

Figure 6.15 A scatterplot of the change in LV end-systolic volume (ΔLVVs) and severity of systolic asynchrony as measured by: standard deviation of the time to peak myocardial systolic velocity of the 12 LV segments (T_s-SD) (A), number of segments with post-systolic shortening among the 12 left ventricular segments (PSS-12) (B), maximal difference in time to peak myocardial systolic velocity among the six basal LV segments (T_s-6 basal) (C), and difference in time to peak systolic velocity between basal septal and basal posterior segment (T_s-sep-post) (D). The regression lines for patients with ischemic (▽) and non-ischemic (▼) etiologies are shown separately in each graph.

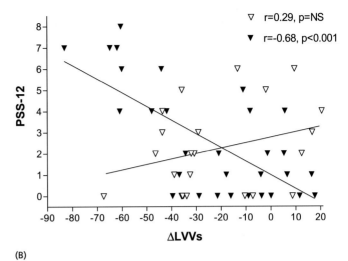

(B)

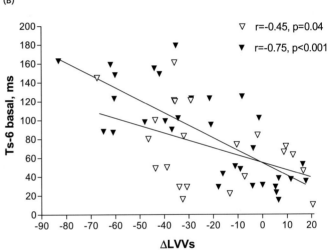

(C)

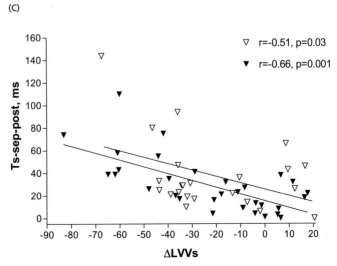

Figure 6.15 (*Continued*)

(D)

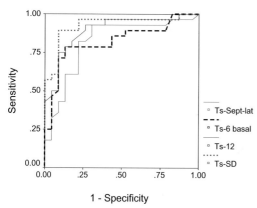

Figure 6.16 The receiver operating characteristics curves for identification of LV reverse remodeling in all the patients receiving CRT for the following parameters: standard deviation of the time to peak myocardial systolic velocity of the 12 LV segments (T_s-SD), maximal difference in time to peak myocardial systolic velocity among the 12 (T_s-12) or six basal (T_s-6 basal) LV segments as well as difference between the time to peak myocardial systolic velocity between basal septal and lateral segment (T_s-sept-lat).

index, the predictive value is consistently highly in non-ischemic than ischemic patients, presumably related to the more homogeneous pattern of mechanical dyssynchrony in non-ischemic cardiomyopathy [13]. Also, improvement of interventricular dyssynchrony appears to be a secondary event which does not predict LV reverse remodeling [13]. From the receiver operating characteristics curve, a cut-off value of 31.4 ms was derived, which is very close to the value derived from normal population of 32.6 ms [8]. This cut-off value gives a sensitivity of 96% and specificity of 78% [13].

Another evolving technique of measuring systolic dyssynchrony is TSI. As explained, it transforms positive T_s into color mapping that allows a quick qualitative estimation of regional delay, in addition to quantitative assessment of myocardial velocity curves. The study by Gorscan *et al.* examined regional wall delay quantitatively by TSI in 29 patients receiving CRT [19]. This acute study defined a positive response as an increase in stroke volume for ≥15% within 48 h after CRT. The TSI timing window of assessing dyssynchrony was adjusted to begin with the pre-ejection period and end in early diastolic period which included the possible occurrence of post-systolic shortening. A delay between anterior septum and posterior wall of >65 ms pre-

dicted the gain in stroke volume with a sensitivity of 87% and specificity of 100% [19]. Another larger study by Yu *et al.* employed TSI to examine only the ejection phase by tagging the beginning and the end of TSI to aortic valve opening and closure, respectively [20]. In 56 patients, qualitative analysis illustrated that the most severe delay region occurring at the lateral wall is a specific finding which predicted a favorable LV reverse remodeling response, although the sensitivity is low. However, qualitative analysis from the six basal, six mid segmental model yielded a sensitivity and specificity of 87% and 81%, respectively [20]. In fact, the predictive values by TSI appeared to be lower than that of TDI when the same indices were compared, as were the ROC curve areas [20]. Therefore, TSI may be a useful adjunctive tool to provide a quick qualitative screening of systolic dyssynchrony. In cases where severe lateral wall delay is observed, the patient will have a high probability of responding to CRT. When such delay is not present or other regions of delay are suspected, a detailed quantitative assessment by myocardial velocity curve is advisable.

Clinical importance of assessing left ventricular reverse remodeling as the echocardiographic endpoint of the cardiac resynchronization therapy response

A number of studies that examined the improvement of cardiac function selected LV reverse remodeling as an echocardiographic endpoint [7, 13, 14, 39, 40, 54]. A commonly used parameter is the change in LVESV by the biplane Simpson's equation. This is particularly common in studies in which the predictive values of systolic dyssynchrony indices were compared with echocardiographic responses to CRT [13, 14, 39, 40]. In fact, LV reverse remodeling represents the composite effect of favorable geometric changes of the ventricle after therapy, regression of LV dilatation as well as improvement of systolic function. In drug trials, although the amplitude of LV reverse remodeling is much smaller than that observed in CRT trials, the reduction of LV end-systolic volume predicted a favorable long-term clinical outcome [55–57]. In fact, a recent clinical study of CRT also confirmed the clinical importance of LV reverse remodeling [58]. In 141 heart failure patients who received CRT, responders of LV reverse remodeling at 3–6 months were associated with a favorable long-term clinical outcome. This includes a lower all-cause mortality (6.9% vs. 30.6%, log-rank $\chi^2 = 13.26$, $P = 0.0003$), cardiovascular mortality (2.3% vs. 24.1%, log-rank $\chi^2 = 17.1$, $P < 0.0001$), heart failure event (11.5% vs. 33.3%, log-rank $\chi^2 = 8.71$, $P = 0.0032$), and the composite endpoint of all-cause mortality or cardiovascular hospitalization (Fig. 6.17) [58]. Furthermore, in the Cox regression multivariate analysis model, the reduction of LV end-systolic volume was the only independent predictor of all-cause mortality and cardiovascular mortality [58]. Although previous studies arbitrarily defined responders of LV reverse remodeling as >15% reduction in LV end-systolic

volume, the latest data from the receiver operating characteristics curve method suggest that a 10% reduction in LV end-systolic volume is clinically important to predict all-cause mortality [58].

Systolic dyssynchrony in heart failure patients with normal QRS duration – implication for cardiac resynchronization therapy

Current guidelines for CRT or CRT-D recommend the prerequisite occurrence of prolonged QRS duration [59]. This patient group constitutes only about one-quarter or less of the heart failure population according to large heart failure registries [60, 61]. The concept of electromechanical coupling delay that occurs exclusively in prolonged QRS duration was

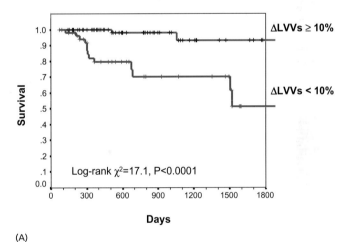

(A)

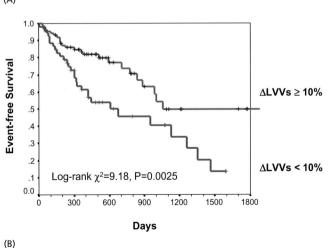

Figure 6.17 Kaplan–Meier curves for cardiovascular mortality (A) and composite end-point of all-cause mortality or cardiovascular hospitalization (B) dichotomized by the status of LV reverse remodeling. Responders are defined as a reduction of LV end-systolic volume for ≥10% while non-responders had a <10% reduction of LV end-systolic volume.

(B)

challenged by studies that examined the relationship between QRS duration and occurrence of mechanical asynchrony in heart failure patients. The first published study by Yu *et al.* examined the prevalence of systolic dyssynchrony in 67 heart failure patients with QRS duration >120 ms (in the form of LBBB or IVCD), 45 heart failure patients with QRS duration ≤120 ms and 88 normal controls [9]. By the use of TDI with a cut-off value of Asynchrony Index (or T_s-SD) >32.6 ms (derived from a normal population), systolic dyssynchrony was present in 43% of heart failure patients with narrow QRS and in 64% with wide QRS complexes [9]. When the criterion of "maximal difference in T_s" from the six basal, six mid segmental model of >100 ms was used, the preva-

lence of systolic dyssynchrony was 51% and 73% respectively (Figs 6.18 and 6.19) [9]. Three more recent reports also observed the presence of mechanical dyssynchrony in heart failure patients with narrow QRS complex by TDI technology [16,49,62]. The report by Ghio *et al.* examined 61 heart failure patients with normal QRS duration, 21 patients with LBBB and QRS between 120 and 150 ms and 76 patients with QRS duration ≥150 ms by 2D-color TDI [49]. Intraventricular dyssynchrony was assessed by apical four- and two-chamber views at basal and mid segments for maximal difference of time to onset of systolic wave, with a cut-off value of >50 ms. The prevalence of systolic intraventricular dyssynchrony in these three groups was 30%, 57%, and 71%, re-

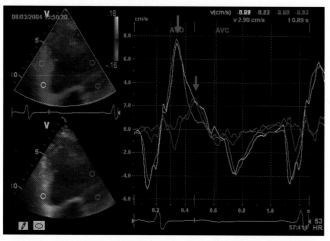

(A)

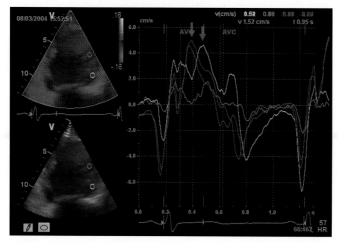

(B)

Figure 6.18 A heart failure patient with systolic mechanical dyssynchrony but has normal QRS duration. Tissue Doppler imaging (TDI) at apical four-chamber (A), apical two-chamber (B), and apical long-axis (C) views showing myocardial velocity curves of six basal, six mid LV segments. This patient has systolic delay in lateral, inferior and posterior wall as illustrated by the delay in time to peak myocardial systolic velocities in ejection phase (arrows).

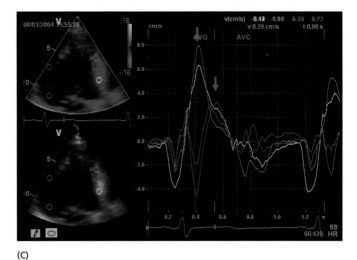

Figure 6.18 (*Continued*) (C)

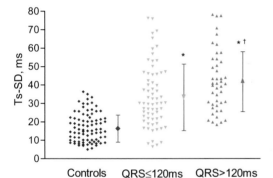

(A)

(B)

Figure 6.19 Scatterplots showing the distribution of the standard deviation of the time to peak myocardial systolic velocity (T_s-SD) (A) and maximal difference in time to peak myocardial systolic velocity (B) of all the 12 LV segments in normal controls, patients with heart failure and QRS duration ≤120 ms and patients with heart failure and QRS duration >120 ms. *$P < 0.001$ vs. controls. †$P ≤ 0.02$ vs. QRS ≤120 ms group.

spectively [49]. By use of septolateral delay >60 ms at basal LV segments, 27% of heart failure patients with QRS duration ≤120 ms were reported to have systolic dyssynchrony, and these figures were 60% and 70% respectively in those with intermediate and wide QRS complex (>150 ms) [62]. In the subset of heart failure patients caused by idiopathic dilated cardiomyopathy, tissue displacement imaging documented systolic dyssynchrony in 36% (5 out of 14) of patients who exhibited anteroseptal-to-posterior wall delay [16].

The occurrence of systolic dyssynchrony was also confirmed recently by another complementary technology, 3D-echocardiography. The study

by Kapetanakis *et al.* examined 83 patients with LV systolic dysfunction (ejection fraction <50%) by biplane Simpson's method, of whom 43 had a duration <120 ms [23]. Systolic dyssynchrony index was derived from 3D-echocardiography by calculating the standard deviation of % time to minimal regional volume of 16 LV segments, and a cut-off value of 8.3% was defined based on 3 standard deviations from normal subjects. Among those with moderate to severe LV dysfunction (ejection fraction <40%), 37% of patients had evidence of systolic dyssynchrony [23].

The identification of systolic dyssynchrony by TDI in narrow QRS population may potentially benefit more heart failure patients from CRT. There are two single-center studies that examined the benefit of CRT in such patients [63, 64]. The study by Achilli *et al.* examined 14 heart failure patients with normal QRS duration (≤120 ms). M-Mode echocardiography was performed to evaluate systolic dyssynchrony by demonstrating delayed LV wall contraction when compared with global LV diastolic filling by Doppler signals [63]. Interestingly, patients with normal QRS duration have evidence of improvement in NYHA class, 6-Minute Hall-Walk distance, reduction in LV diameter and mitral regurgitation, as well as increase in ejection fraction and LV filling time. Intriguingly, it appears that the magnitude of improvement was similar between these patients and the ones with QRS >120 ms [63]. Another study by Turner *et al.* compared the change in cardiac function in nine heart failure patients with normal QRS duration before and after CRT [65]. Dyssynchrony was measured by T_s of the six basal LV segments from three apical views. Biventricular pacing resulted in a 2.3% ($P < 0.05$) increase in LV ejection fraction. Furthermore, color TDI showed homogeneous delay in T_s in the six basal segments, leading to the abolition of regional delay in a manner similar to that observed in patients with wide QRS duration [7, 65]. In fact, acute hemodynamic improvement of cardiac output and pulmonary capillary wedge pressure was also observed in these patients receiving CRT [66].

Our recent study examined 24 heart failure patients with normal QRS duration of <120 ms but who had evidence of mechanical dyssynchrony by TDI based on Asynchrony Index (or T_s-SD) [64]. There was significant improvement of NYHA class, maximal exercise capacity, and 6-Minute Hall-Walk distance. Echocardiographic evidence of LV reverse remodeling with reduction of LV volume, gain in ejection fraction and increase in sphericity index was confirmed. There was also reduction of mitral regurgitation and gain in LV filling time [64]. By TSI mapping, improvement of systolic dyssynchrony was evident in these patients with reduction of Asynchrony Index [21].

Summary

A number of new imaging modalities have been demonstrated to be useful in the assessment systolic dyssynchrony. Among various techniques, TDI is the most frequently employed technology, providing a robust tool to quantify regional function. A number of indices have been successfully developed to assess mechanical dyssynchrony. In the early establishment phase of CRT, examination of systolic dyssynchrony helped to decode the mechanism of benefit of this new therapy by gaining insight on how resynchronization of the ventricle(s) can be achieved. Subsequently, the assessment of systolic dyssynchrony became clinically relevant as at least one-third of patients are non-responders to CRT. In heart failure patients with prolonged QRS duration of >120 ms, assessment of mechanical dyssynchrony before device implantation helps to predict responders of therapy. It is important to realize that non-responders were suffering from minimal mechanical dyssynchrony despite widening of QRS complexes; and worsening of systolic dyssynchrony is demonstrated in these patients after CRT. Furthermore, in the new echocardiographic era where mechanical dyssynchrony is demonstrated by TDI and 3D-echocardiography in 30–40% of heart failure patients with normal QRS duration, CRT may have a potential role in this selected group.

Appendix 1 Assessment of systolic Asynchrony Index (T_s-SD) by tissue Doppler imaging

From the apical four-chamber, two-chamber, and three-chamber (or apical long-axis) views, a six basal, six mid segmental model is obtained in the LV, including the septal, lateral, anterior, inferior, anteroseptal, and posterior segments at both basal and mid levels [8, 13]. The systolic myocardial velocities consist of isovolumic contraction phase and ejection phase, both of which are positively directed. During diastole, it consists of isovolumic relaxation phase (negative or biphasic profiles) as well as early and late diastolic relaxation, which are negatively directed. To calculate the Asynchrony Index, the peak myocardial systolic velocity is determined. In order to measure the time to peak systolic velocity in the ejection phase (T_s) of individual segments, the following steps are the rule-of-thumb:

- First, the use of aortic valve opening and closure markers superimposed on TDI tracings to guide for the identification of *ejection* phase is strongly recommended (from Doppler echocardiography at the LV outflow tract or aortic valve level in the apical five-chamber view).

- Measure the time from the onset of the QRS complex to the *highest* systolic peak during the *ejection* phase (between aortic value opening and closure in general).
- If there are multiple peaks in ejection phase, take the peak with highest positive velocity (not the first if it is not the highest).
- If there are two or more peaks in the ejection phase with the same amplitude in velocity, choose the earliest peak among those with the same highest velocity.
- If the segment only has a negative peak in the ejection phase, or the velocity is too noisy with very low and inconsistent velocities, neglect those particular segments and proceed with the rest of the measurable segments.
- Do not measure T_s on the isovolumic contraction phase, the isovolumic relaxation phase, or during post-systolic shortening.
- The T_s-SD is then calculated as the "standard deviation" of T_s among six basal, six mid LV segments using any standardized statistical software (e.g. SPSS or Microsoft Excel). In general, the larger the value of T_s-SD, the more severe the systolic dyssynchrony.

References

1 Gorcsan J, Gulati VK, Mandarino WA, Katz WE. Color-coded measures of myocardial velocity throughout the cardiac cycle by tissue Doppler imaging to quantify regional left ventricular function. *Am Heart J* 1996; **131**: 1203–1213.

2 Yu CM, Lin H, Ho PC, Yang H. Assessment of left and right ventricular systolic and diastolic synchronicity in normal subjects by tissue Doppler echocardiography and the effects of age and heart rate. *Echocardiography* 2003; **20**: 19–27.

3 Henein MY, Gibson DG. Normal long axis function. *Heart* 1999; **81**: 111–113.

4 Greenbaum RA, Ho SY, Gibson DG, Becker AE, Anderson RH. Left ventricular fibre architecture in man. *Br Heart J* 1981; **45**: 248–263.

5 Torrent-Guasp F, Kocica MJ, Corno A *et al.* Systolic ventricular filling. *Eur J Cardiothorac Surg* 2004; **25**: 376–386.

6 Penicka M, Bartunek J, de Bruyne B *et al.* Improvement of left ventricular function after cardiac resynchronization therapy is predicted by tissue Doppler imaging echocardiography. *Circulation* 2004; **109**: 978–983.

7 Yu CM, Chau E, Sanderson JE *et al.* Tissue Doppler echocardiographic evidence of reverse remodeling and improved synchronicity by simultaneously delaying regional contraction after biventricular pacing therapy in heart failure. *Circulation* 2002; **105**: 438–445.

8 Yu CM, Fung JWH, Lin H, Zhang Q, Sanderson JE, Lau CP. Predictors of left ventricular reverse remodeling after cardiac resynchronization therapy for heart failure secondary to idiopathic dilated or ischemic cardiomyopathy. *Am J Cardiol* 2003; **91**: 684–688.

9 Yu CM, Lin H, Zhang Q, Sanderson JE. High prevalence of left ventricular systolic and diastolic asynchrony in patients with congestive heart failure and normal QRS duration. *Heart* 2003; **89**: 54–60.

10 Ansalone G, Giannantoni P, Ricci R *et al.* Doppler myocardial imaging in patients with heart failure receiving biventricular pacing treatment. *Am Heart J* 2001; **142**: 881–896.

11 Ansalone G, Giannantoni P, Ricci R, Trambaiolo P, Fedele F, Santini M. Doppler myocardial imaging to evaluate the effectiveness of pacing sites in patients receiving biventricular pacing. *J Am Coll Cardiol* 2002; **39**: 489–499.

12 Bax JJ, Ansalone G, Breithardt OA *et al.* Echocardiographic evaluation of cardiac resynchronization therapy: ready for routine clinical use? A critical appraisal. *J Am Coll Cardiol* 2004; **44**: 1–9.

13 Yu CM, Fung JW, Zhang Q *et al.* Tissue Doppler imaging is superior to strain rate imaging and postsystolic shortening on the prediction of reverse remodeling in both ischemic and nonischemic heart failure after cardiac resynchronization therapy. *Circulation* 2004; **110**: 66–73.

14 Yu CM, Abraham WT, Bax J *et al.* Predictors of response to cardiac resynchronization therapy (PROSPECT) – study design. *Am Heart J* 2005; **149**: 600–605.

15 Sun JP, Chinchoy E, Donal E *et al.* Evaluation of ventricular synchrony using novel Doppler echocardiographic indices in patients with heart failure receiving cardiac resynchronization therapy. *J Am Soc Echocardiogr* 2004; **17**: 845–850.

16 Sade LE, Kanzaki H, Severyn D, Dohi K, Gorcsan J, III. Quantification of radial mechanical dyssynchrony in patients with left bundle branch block and idiopathic dilated cardiomyopathy without conduction delay by tissue displacement imaging. *Am J Cardiol* 2004; **94**: 514–518.

17 Sogaard P, Egeblad H, Kim WY *et al.* Tissue Doppler imaging predicts improved systolic performance and re-

versed left ventricular remodeling during long-term cardiac resynchronization therapy. *J Am Coll Cardiol* 2002; **40**: 723–730.

18 Sogaard P, Egeblad H, Pedersen AK *et al.* Sequential versus simultaneous biventricular resynchronization for severe heart failure: evaluation by tissue Doppler imaging. *Circulation* 2002; **106**: 2078–2084.

19 Gorcsan J, III, Kanzaki H, Bazaz R, Dohi K, Schwartzman D. Usefulness of echocardiographic tissue synchronization imaging to predict acute response to cardiac resynchronization therapy. *Am J Cardiol* 2004; **93**: 1178–1181.

20 Yu CM, Zhang Q, Fung JW *et al.* A novel tool to assess systolic asynchrony and identify responders of cardiac resynchronization therapy by tissue synchronization imaging. *J Am Coll Cardiol* 2005; **45**: 677–684.

21 Yu CM, Zhang Q, Fung JW. Visualization of regional left ventricular mechanical delay by tissue synchronization imaging in heart failure patients with wide and narrow QRS complexes undergoing cardiac resynchronization therapy. *Circulation* 2005; **112**: e93–e95.

22 Zhang Q, Yu CM, Fung JW *et al.* Assessment of the effect of cardiac resynchronization therapy on intraventricular mechanical synchronicity by regional volumetric changes. *Am J Cardiol* 2005; **95**: 126–129.

23 Kapetanakis S, Kearney MT, Siva A, Gall N, Cooklin M, Monaghan MJ. Real-time three-dimensional echocardiography: a novel technique to quantify global left ventricular mechanical dyssynchrony. *Circulation* 2005; **112**: 992–1000.

24 Yu CM, Fung JWH, Zhang Q *et al.* The role of repeating atrioventricular interval optimization during long-term follow up after cardiac resynchronization therapy for heart failure: comparison of echocardiography and bioimpedance methods. *J Am Soc Echocardiogr* 2004; **17**: 534.

25 Kawaguchi M, Murabayashi T, Fetics BJ et al. Quantitation of basal dyssynchrony and acute resynchronization from left or biventricular pacing by novel echo-contrast variability imaging. *J Am Coll Cardiol* 2002; **39**: 2052–2058.

26 Breithardt OA, Stellbrink C, Herbots L *et al.* Cardiac resynchronization therapy can reverse abnormal myocardial strain distribution in patients with heart failure and left bundle branch block. *J Am Coll Cardiol* 2003; **42**: 486–494.

27 Bordachar P, Lafitte S, Reuter S *et al.* Echocardiographic parameters of ventricular dyssynchrony validation in patients with heart failure using sequential biventricular pacing. *J Am Coll Cardiol* 2004; **44**: 2157–2165.

28 Bax JJ, Molhoek SG, van Erven L *et al.* Usefulness of myocardial tissue Doppler echocardiography to evaluate left ventricular dyssynchrony before and after biventricular pacing in patients with idiopathic dilated cardiomyopathy. *Am J Cardiol* 2003; **91**: 94–97.

29 Yu CM, Lin H, Fung WH, Zhang Q, Kong SL, Sanderson JE. Comparison of acute changes in left ventricular volume, systolic and diastolic functions and intraventricular synchronicity after biventricular and right ventricular pacing for heart failure. *Am Heart J* 2002; **145**: 1–18.

30 Kanzaki H, Bazaz R, Schwartzman D, Dohi K, Sade LE, Gorcsan J, III. A mechanism for immediate reduction in mitral regurgitation after cardiac resynchronization therapy: insights from mechanical activation strain mapping. *J Am Coll Cardiol* 2004; **44**: 1619–1625.

31 Auricchio A, Ding J, Spinelli JC *et al.* Cardiac resynchronization therapy restores optimal atrioventricular mechanical timing in heart failure patients with ventricular conduction delay. *J Am Coll Cardiol* 2002; **39**: 1163–1169.

32 Nelson GS, Curry CW, Wyman BT *et al.* Predictors of systolic augmentation from left ventricular preexcitation in patients with dilated cardiomyopathy and intraventricular conduction delay. *Circulation* 2000; **101**: 2703–2709.

33 Alonso C, Leclercq C, Victor F *et al.* Electrocardiographic predictive factors of long-term clinical improvement with multisite biventricular pacing in advanced heart failure. *Am J Cardiol* 1999; **84**: 1417–1421.

34 Reuter S, Garrigue S, Barold SS *et al.* Comparison of characteristics in responders versus nonresponders with biventricular pacing for drug-resistant congestive heart failure. *Am J Cardiol* 2002; **89**: 346–350.

35 Abraham WT, Fisher WG, Smith AL *et al.* Cardiac resynchronization in chronic heart failure. *N Engl J Med* 2002; **346**: 1845–1853.

36 Young JB, Abraham WT, Smith AL *et al.* Combined cardiac resynchronization and implantable cardioversion defibrillation in advanced chronic heart failure: the MIRACLE ICD Trial. *JAMA* 2003; **289**: 2685–2694.

37 Stellbrink C, Breithardt OA, Franke A *et al.* Impact of cardiac resynchronization therapy using hemodynamically optimized pacing on left ventricular remodeling in patients with congestive heart failure and ventricular conduction disturbances. *J Am Coll Cardiol* 2001; **38**: 1957–1965.

38 Packer M. Proposal for a new clinical end point to evaluate the efficacy of drugs and devices in the treatment of chronic heart failure. *J Card Failure* 2001; **7**: 176–182.

39 Pitzalis MV, Iacoviello M, Romito R *et al.* Cardiac resynchronization therapy tailored by echocardiographic evaluation of ventricular asynchrony. *J Am Coll Cardiol* 2002; **40**: 1615–1622.

40 Notabartolo D, Merlino JD, Smith AL *et al.* Usefulness of the peak velocity difference by tissue Doppler imaging

technique as an effective predictor of response to cardiac resynchronization therapy. *Am J Cardiol* 2004; **94**: 817–820.

41 Bax JJ, Marwick TH, Molhoek SG *et al.* Left ventricular dyssynchrony predicts benefit of cardiac resynchronization therapy in patients with end-stage heart failure before pacemaker implantation. *Am J Cardiol* 2003; **92**: 1238–1240.

42 Gras D, Leclercq C, Tang AS, Bucknall C, Luttikhuis HO, Kirstein-Pedersen A. Cardiac resynchronization therapy in advanced heart failure – the multicenter InSync clinical study. *Eur J Heart Failure* 2002; **4**: 311–320.

43 Cazeau S, Leclercq C, Lavergne T *et al.* Effects of multisite biventricular pacing in patients with heart failure and intraventricular conduction delay. *N Engl J Med* 2001; **344**: 873–880.

44 Butter C, Auricchio A, Stellbrink C *et al.* Effect of resynchronization therapy stimulation site on the systolic function of heart failure patients. *Circulation* 2001; **104**: 3026–3029.

45 Alonso C, Leclercq C, d'Allonnes FR *et al.* Six year experience of transvenous left ventricular lead implantation for permanent biventricular pacing in patients with advanced heart failure: technical aspects. *Heart* 2001; **86**: 405–410.

46 Gum PA, O'Keefe JH, Jr., Borkon AM *et al.* Bypass surgery versus coronary angioplasty for revascularization of treated diabetic patients. *Circulation* 1997; **96**: II-10.

47 Garrigue S, Reuter S, Labeque JN *et al.* Usefulness of biventricular pacing in patients with congestive heart failure and right bundle branch block. *Am J Cardiol* 2001; **88**: 1436–1441.

48 Fung JW, Yu CM, Yip G, Zhang Y, Chan H, Kum CC, Sanderson JE. Variable left ventricular activation pattern in patients with heart failure and left bundle branch block. *Heart* 2004; **90**: 17–19.

49 Ghio S, Constantin C, Klersy C, Serio A, Fontana A, Campana C, Tavazzi L. Interventricular and intraventricular dyssynchrony are common in heart failure patients, regardless of QRS duration. *Eur Heart J* 2004; **25**: 571–578.

50 Auricchio A, Abraham WT. Cardiac resynchronization therapy: current state of the art: cost versus benefit. *Circulation* 2004; **109**: 300–307.

51 Auricchio A, Yu CM. Beyond the measurement of QRS complex toward mechanical dyssynchrony: cardiac resynchronisation therapy in heart failure patients with a normal QRS duration. *Heart* 2004; **90**: 479–481.

52 Bax JJ, Bleeker GB, Marwick TH *et al.* Left ventricular dyssynchrony predicts response and prognosis after cardiac resynchronization therapy. *J Am Coll Cardiol* 2004; **44**: 1834–1840.

53 Yu CM, Fung JW, Chan CK *et al.* Comparison of efficacy of reverse remodeling and clinical improvement for

relatively narrow and wide QRS complexes after cardiac resynchronization therapy for heart failure. *J Cardiovasc Electrophysiol* 2004; **15**: 1058–1065.

54 Breithardt OA, Stellbrink C, Kramer AP *et al.* Echocardiographic quantification of left ventricular asynchrony predicts an acute hemodynamic benefit of cardiac resynchronization therapy. *J Am Coll Cardiol* 2002; **40**: 536–545.

55 Konstam MA, Rousseau MF, Kronenberg MW *et al.* Effects of the angiotensin converting enzyme inhibitor enalapril on the long-term progression of left ventricular dysfunction in patients with heart failure. SOLVD Investigators. *Circulation* 1992; **86**: 431–438.

56 White HD, Norris RM, Brown MA, Brandt PW, Whitlock RM, Wild CJ. Left ventricular end-systolic volume as the major determinant of survival after recovery from myocardial infarction. *Circulation* 1987; **76**: 44–51.

57 St John Sutton MG, Pfeffer MA, Plappert T *et al.* Quantitative two-dimensional echocardiographic measurements are major predictors of adverse cardiovascular events after acute myocardial infarction. The protective effects of captopril. *Circulation* 1994; **89**: 68–75.

58 Yu CM, Bleeker GB, Fung JWH *et al.* Left ventricular reverse remodeling but not clinical improvement predicts long-term survival after cardiac resynchronization therapy. *Circulation* 2005; **112**: 1580–1586.

59 Gregoratos G, Abrams J, Epstein AE *et al.* ACC/AHA/NASPE 2002 guideline update for implantation of cardiac pacemakers and antiarrhythmia devices: summary article: a report of the American College of Cardiology/American Heart Association Task Force on Practice Guidelines (ACC/AHA/NASPE Committee to Update the 1998 Pacemaker Guidelines). *Circulation* 2002; **106**: 2145–2161.

60 Baldasseroni S, Opasich C, Gorini M *et al.* Left bundle-branch block is associated with increased 1-year sudden and total mortality rate in 5517 outpatients with congestive heart failure: a report from the Italian network on congestive heart failure. *Am Heart J* 2002; **143**: 398–405.

61 Farwell D, Patel NR, Hall A, Ralph S, Sulke AN. How many people with heart failure are appropriate for biventricular resynchronization? *Eur Heart J* 2000; **21**: 1246–1250.

62 Bleeker GB, Schalij MJ, Molhoek SG *et al.* Relationship between QRS duration and left ventricular dyssynchrony in patients with end-stage heart failure. *J Cardiovasc Electrophysiol* 2004; **15**: 544–549.

63 Achilli A, Sassara M, Ficili S *et al.* Long-term effectiveness of cardiac resynchronization therapy in patients with refractory heart failure and "narrow" QRS. *J Am Coll Cardiol* 2003; **42**: 2117–2124.

64 Yu CM, Fung JWH, Zhang Q *et al.* Cardiac resynchronization therapy for heart failure patients with normal QRS duration and coexisting mechanical asynchrony. *J*

Am Coll Cardiol 2005; **45**: 160A.

65 Turner MS, Bleasdale RA, Vinereanu D *et al.* Electrical and mechanical components of dyssynchrony in heart failure patients with normal QRS duration and left bundle-branch block: impact of left and biventricular pacing. *Circulation* 2004; **109**: 2544–2549.

66 Turner MS, Bleasdale RA, Mumford CE, Frenneaux MP, Morris-Thurgood JA. Left ventricular pacing improves haemodynamic variables in patients with heart failure with a normal QRS duration. *Heart* 2004; **90**: 502–505.

67 Popovic ZB, Grimm RA, Perlic G *et al.* Noninvasive assessment of cardiac resynchronization therapy for congestive heart failure using myocardial strain and left ventricular peak power as parameters of myocardial synchrony and function. *J Cardiovasc Electrophysiol* 2002; **13**: 1203–1208.

CHAPTER 7

Value of non-echocardiographic imaging techniques in cardiac resynchronization therapy

Jeroen J. Bax, MD, PhD, *Gabe B. Bleeker,* MD &
Martin J. Schalij, MD, PhD

Introduction

Over recent years, cardiac resynchronization therapy (CRT) has contributed significantly to the treatment of patients with end-stage, drug-refractory heart failure. The clinical benefits of CRT will be discussed in Chapter 13. In essence, eight large, randomized, clinical trials including a total of 4017 patients have demonstrated an improvement in New York Heart Association (NYHA) class, quality of life score and 6-minute walking distance [1–8]. Among these trials, three have clearly demonstrated an improvement in prognosis [3, 5, 6]. Performing cardiovascular imaging also has its unique role in the CRT era. As discussed in the previous chapter, echocardiography is useful to demonstrate the improvement in left ventricular (LV) systolic function (LV ejection fraction), a reduction in LV volumes (indicating LV reverse remodeling) and a reduction in mitral regurgitation. Based on the available evidence the current ACC/AHA/NASPE guidelines indicate that CRT is beneficial in patients with heart failure, severe systolic LV dysfunction, and wide QRS complex (level of evidence class IB). Although the results of these large trials are promising, analysis of individual patient response to CRT reveals that a substantial percentage of patients (up to 30%) do not respond to this therapy. Accordingly, intensive effort has been invested in optimization of selection of potential responders to CRT prior to device implantation.

Assessment of cardiac dyssynchrony

Response to CRT has been related to the presence of cardiac dyssynchrony [9], in which cardiovascular imaging has a major role. In the target heart failure population, three forms of dyssynchrony exist, namely atrioventricular dyssynchrony, interventricular dyssynchrony, and intra (left) ventricular dyssynchrony.

- Atrioventricular dyssynchrony (a delay between atrial and ventricular contraction) results in mitral valve incompetence with occurrence of late diastolic regurgitation and a reduced ventricular filling time (limiting diastolic stroke volume). Moreover, atrial systole can occur simultaneously with early passive filling, with further reduction of ventricular filling.
- Interventricular dyssynchrony, as present during left bundle branch block (LBBB), results in right ventricular (RV) events preceding LV events, locally different contraction patterns, abnormal distribution of LV mechanical work, deficiencies in regional perfusion and decreased mechanical performance [10]. The delayed LV contraction and relaxation induces interventricular dyssynchrony and affects mainly the interventricular septal motion which reduces LV ejection. Conversely, the earlier onset of RV contraction results in RV ejection occurring during the LV end-diastolic phase.

Moreover, the higher RV pressure reverses the trans-septal pressure gradient and displaces the septum into the LV.

- Intra (left) ventricular dyssynchrony induces regions with early and delayed contraction that will contribute to a reduction of systolic performance, an increase in end-systolic volume and wall stress, a delayed relaxation and a reduction in LV efficiency [11].

All three forms of cardiac dyssynchrony contribute to reduced LV performance and heart failure, and CRT may (partially) correct these dyssynchronies. However, which of these dyssynchronies best predicts response to CRT is unclear.

As already discussed in previous chapters, echocardiography is currently considered the optimal technique to assess cardiac dyssynchrony, and the majority of studies have demonstrated that the presence of LV dyssynchrony (and to a lesser extent interventricular dyssynchrony) is most predictive for response to CRT [9]. This chapter concerns the value of non-echocardiographic imaging techniques in selection and evaluation of patients undergoing CRT.

Which non-echocardiographic imaging techniques are available?

Various non-echocardiographic techniques are of value in patients undergoing CRT, including nuclear imaging techniques, magnetic resonance imaging (MRI), and computed tomography (CT) techniques. These techniques (except CT) allow assessment of cardiac dyssynchrony, but also provide additional information that is useful in the selection of patients for CRT, including identification of scar tissue and viable myocardium in the target region for the LV pacing lead. Moreover, nuclear imaging techniques can measure other effects of CRT (e.g. changes in perfusion, (oxidative) metabolism, and innervation).

Finally, CT techniques permit non-invasive imaging of the venous anatomy, which may be useful in the decision whether LV lead implantation can be performed transvenously or whether a surgical approach is needed. In the following paragraphs, the merits of these different non-invasive imaging techniques in the selection and evaluation of patients undergoing CRT are discussed.

Nuclear imaging to assess cardiac dyssynchrony

The available nuclear imaging techniques that have been used in selection and evaluation of CRT include radionuclide angiography, single photon emission computed tomography (SPECT), and positron emission tomography (PET).

Radionuclide angiography is a technique that has been used extensively for the assessment of LVEF, but can also be used for evaluation cardiac dyssynchrony [12, 13]. Fourier analysis provides a functional image (a parametric map of sequential contraction) which permits precise quantification of inter- and intra (left) ventricular dyssynchrony, with high reproducibility [12, 13]. Fauchier and co-workers [14] reported normal values using this technique, based on data derived from a control group. Based on the mean values ± 2 SD of the control subjects, the upper limits of normal for interventricular synchrony were set at 40 ms, and at 45 ms for intra (LV) dyssynchrony. Application of these normal values to a cohort of 103 patients with heart failure demonstrated that intra (LV) dyssynchrony was frequently observed in patients with wide QRS complex and LBBB configuration, but was also present in 41% of heart failure patients with a normal QRS duration. The same authors [15] explored the use of radionuclide angiography with phase image analysis for prognostication of a large cohort of patients with idiopathic dilated cardiomyopathy and heart failure. Multivariate analysis demonstrated that the presence of intra (left) ventricular dyssynchrony and elevated pulmonary capillary wedge pressure were the only predictors of event-free survival. Of note, interventricular dyssynchrony was not predictive for events in this study.

Few studies have used radionuclide angiography to assess cardiac dyssynchrony before CRT and related the findings to outcome after CRT. Kerwin *et al.* [16] evaluated 13 patients with wide QRS complex (mean duration 156 ± 48 ms), dilated cardiomyopathy (LVEF <35%, mean 17 ± 7%), NYHA class II–III, and sinus rhythm. Half of these patients underwent CRT implantation as part of a multicenter clinical trial (VIGOR, CHF trial, Guidant, St Paul, Minnesota, USA); the remaining patients were referred for electrophysiology testing, during which biventricular pacing was performed. Gated equilibrium blood pool scintigraphic studies were obtained with a portable gamma camera during sinus rhythm and biventricular pacing. During biventricular pacing, the LVEF increased from $17 \pm 7\%$ to $23 \pm 8\%$ ($P < 0.05$, relative improvement 36%), and RV ejection fraction increased from $16 \pm 6\%$ to $20 \pm 5\%$ ($P = 0.01$, relative improvement 33%). From the gated blood pool studies, the inter- and intra (LV) ventricular dyssynchrony was determined during sinus rhythm and biventricular pacing. The majority of patients had some extent of inter- and intra (LV) dyssynchrony. During biventricular pacing the interventricular dyssynchrony decreased from $28 \pm 23°$ (the mean difference in phase angles) to $14 \pm 13°$ ($P = 0.01$) whereas the intra (LV) dyssynchrony showed some increase from $33 \pm 26°$ to $39 \pm 22°$ ($P = 0.02$). Of note, the reduction in interventricular dyssynchrony was directly related to the increase in LVEF during biventricular pacing.

One other study used radionuclide angiography to evaluate the inter-relationships between cardiac dyssynchrony and the effect of CRT [17]. Toussaint and colleagues [17] evaluated 34 consecutive patients with NYHA class III–IV heart failure, LV ejection fraction (LVEF) <40% (mean $20 \pm 8\%$), wide QRS complex (>150 ms, mean 179 ± 18 ms), LBBB configuration, and sinus rhythm. All patients underwent radionuclide angiography the day before CRT implantation, which was repeated one week and every six months after implantation. LVEF improved from $20 \pm 8\%$ to $23 \pm 11\%$ at one-week follow-up and to $27 \pm 12\%$ at late follow-up (mean 20 ± 7 months, $P < 0.01$). The authors also showed an immediate reduction in inter- and intra (LV) dyssynchrony at one-week follow-up, with a further reduction over time. Both baseline inter- and intra (LV) dyssynchrony were related to improvement in LVEF, but also baseline LVEF was predictive of improvement in LVEF. The combination of a baseline LVEF >15% with significant interventricular dyssynchrony was the best predictor of long-term improvement in LVEF.

These results from these two studies on radionuclide angiography to assess cardiac dyssynchrony are only partially in line with the results of echocardiographic tissue Doppler imaging; in the tissue Doppler studies a clear reduction in intra (LV) dyssynchrony is consistently shown, and this parameter

appears to best predict response to CRT [9]. Most likely, radionuclide angiography and tissue Doppler imaging do not assess completely identical parameters which may explain the discrepancy between the findings, and direct comparisons between both modalities are needed to better understand these results.

Other information derived from nuclear imaging

Positron emission tomography (PET) is the only imaging technique that allows quantitative assessment of myocardial blood flow (MBF) and metabolism. This technique has been used in various studies to evaluate the effect of CRT on MBF and metabolism. In Table 7.1, a summary of the PET studies evaluating the effect on MBF and flow reverse is provided [18–24]. In total, seven studies with 108 patients have evaluated MBF and flow reserve before and after CRT. The studies consistently demonstrate a reduced MBF in the patients with severe heart failure (compared with normal individuals), with an abnormal (heterogeneous) distribution. After CRT, none of the studies has been able to demonstrate an increase in global MBF. However, several studies showed, on a regional basis, a more balanced perfusion after CRT; for example Lindner *et al.* [24] demonstrated that before CRT regional MBF was highest in the lateral wall and lowest in the septum, whereas after CRT, MBF decreased in the lateral wall and increased in the septum resulting in a more uniform distribution.

Next, a few studies with PET and ^{11}C-acetate evaluated oxidative metabolism before and after CRT [20, 24–26]. In 42 patients with dilated cardiomyopathy, it was demonstrated that global oxidative metabolism was reduced and non-homogeneously distributed in patients with dilated cardiomyopathy and LBBB, with a higher oxygen consumption in the lateral wall compared with the septum [27]. Ukkonen *et al.* [26] performed an elegant study with eight patients in NYHA class III–IV, with depressed LV function (mean LVEF $26 \pm 9\%$), wide QRS complex (>120 ms), LBBB configuration, and sinus rhythm. These patients underwent CRT implantation and oxidative metabolism was evaluated by PET and ^{11}C-acetate with the pacemaker on and off. LV function (stroke volume index, LVEF) improved

Table 7.1 Effect of CRT on myocardial blood flow (MBF) and flow reserve (MBFR) as measured by positron emission tomography (PET)

Author	No. patients	LVEF	Technique, tracer	Effect of CRT
Neri [18]	8	27 ± 12%	PET, ^{13}N-ammonia	MBF unchanged
Nielsen [19]	14	21 ± 5%	PET, ^{13}N-ammonia	MBF unchanged
Sundell [20]	10	32 ± 8%	PET, ^{15}O-water	MBF unchanged
				MBFR unchanged
Braunschweig [21]	6	22 ± 9%	PET, ^{11}C-acetate	MBF unchanged
				MBFR unchanged
Nowak [22]	14	23 ± 13%	PET, ^{15}O-water	MBF unchanged
Knaapen [23]	14	25 ± 7%	PET, ^{15}O-water	MBF unchanged
				MBFR increased
Lindner [24]	42	22 ± 5%	PET, ^{11}C-acetate	MBF unchanged

significantly with CRT. Moreover, the improvement in LV function was not associated with an increase in global oxidative metabolism, indicating an improved myocardial efficiency. Moreover, similar to MBF in earlier studies, regional oxidative metabolism decreased in the lateral wall compared with the septum. Sundell *et al.* [20] reported similar findings in 10 patients undergoing CRT, with an improved cardiac efficiency during CRT. Moreover, during low-dose dobutamine stress, a similar trend was observed, with an improved efficiency with pacing (although the difference did not reach statistical significance) suggesting that during stress, CRT may also be beneficial (Fig. 7.1).

Myocardial glucose utilization was evaluated in two PET studies using ^{18}F-fluorodeoxyglucose, demonstrating that glucose uptake was reduced

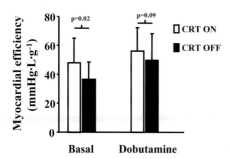

Figure 7.1 With cardiac resynchronization therapy (CRT), basal myocardial efficiency (assessed by positron emission tomography using ^{11}C-acetate) was increased (left) and a similar trend was observed during dobutamine stress (although the increase was not significant, right). Reprinted from Sundell *et al.* [20] with permission from the American College of Cardiology Foundation.

in the interventricular septum compared with the lateral wall, which homogenized during CRT [18, 28].

Another factor that is important for the success of CRT is whether scar tissue or viable myocardium is present in the region of latest activation (where the LV lead should be positioned). Recently, a case report was presented demonstrating that a beneficial response to CRT was reversed after few months when an acute infarction occurred in the region where the LV lead was positioned [29]. This case illustrates the possible need for the presence of viable myocardium in the target region for LV lead positioning. It would therefore be of interest to evaluate non-invasively, before CRT implantation, whether the target region for LV lead positioning contains viable tissue or whether scar tissue is present. This can easily be done with nuclear imaging, using PET or SPECT. An example of a patient with a large scar in the inferolateral wall on resting technetium-99m tetrofosmin SPECT is demonstrated in Fig. 7.2. However, such concept of pre-pacing assessment needs substantiation from further studies.

Finally, cardiac innervation can be assessed with nuclear imaging using PET and SPECT tracers. For example, beta-adrenergic receptor density can be measured with PET and S-[^{11}C]CGP 12177 [30], and it has been demonstrated that beta-adrenergic receptor density is reduced after acute infarction, and the severity of reduction predicts subsequent LV dilation. Cardiac innervation can also be assessed by ^{123}I-metaiodoben-zylguanidine (MIBG) imaging with SPECT, and impaired cardiac adrenergic innervation as assessed by MIBG imaging is strongly related to mortality in patients with heart

Figure 7.2 Short-axis slices obtained with resting technetium-99m tetrofosmin SPECT indicating a defect in tracer uptake in the inferolateral region, indicating scar tissue in this region. If this patient had been referred for CRT, and the preferred LV lead position had been the inferolateral region, this patient would not have been selected for CRT.

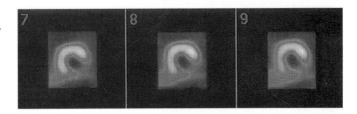

failure [31]. Preliminary data in 13 patients with heart failure undergoing MIBG imaging before and six months after CRT demonstrated favorable changes in the neurohumoral system [32].

Magnetic resonance imaging in cardiac resynchronization therapy

Minimal data are available on the use of MRI for assessment of cardiac dyssynchrony. Two studies have evaluated the feasibility of tagged MRI to assess intra (LV) dyssynchrony, in an animal model and in normal individuals [33, 34]. In an acute study by Nelson *et al.*, patients with LBBB were stimulated by LV pacing [35]. Intraventricular dyssynchrony was examined by the assessment of circumferential strains in about 80 sites throughout the LV by tagged MRI in eight patients with di-

lated cardiomyopathy and seven control subjects. Strain variance at the time of maximal shortening was used as a marker of systolic dyssynchrony, which correlated with the acute improvement of hemodynamics as reflected by the percentage change in $+\mathrm{d}P/\mathrm{d}t_{\mathrm{max}}$ [35]. Leclercq *et al.* [36] have used tagged MRI in a sophisticated animal model on heart failure. The authors demonstrated that biventricular pacing resulted in an acute improvement of hemodynamic parameters combined with an improvement in LV systolic function. Moreover, tagged MRI demonstrated an acute improvement in intraventricular (LV) dyssynchrony after biventricular pacing. Interestingly, this study also reported that improvement of mechanical dyssynchrony could be dissociated with electrical dyssynchrony which remains abnormal after LV pacing (Figs 7.3 and 7.4). In a subsequent animal study

Figure 7.3 (A) Electrical epicardial activation map of whole heart for three pacing modes. Activation time is color coded (blue early, red late). With RA pacing (LBBB), electrical activation spread from right to left, whereas LV pacing reversed the pattern but did not reduce conduction delay. BiV pacing, however, showed improved electrical synchrony. (B) Short-axis slice demonstrating that activation time at the endocardial septum was similar to that at epicardial electrodes over the same region. (C) Group data for electrical activation delay (relative to earliest activation) at various sites for three pacing modes. Only BiV pacing reduced the gradient of activation delay. (Courtesy of Christophe. Leclercq and David Kass.)

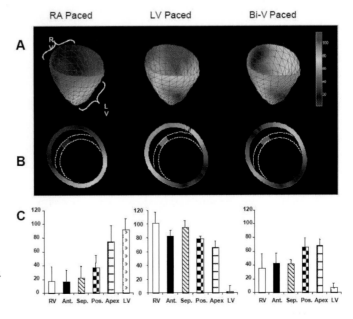

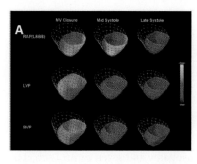

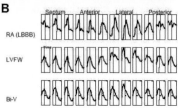

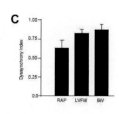

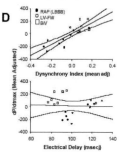

Figure 7.4 (A) Mechanical LV activation maps for 3 pacing modes. LV contraction was dyssynchronous with RA (LBBB) stimulation, with early septal shortening (blue) and LV–free wall stretch (yellow) followed by lateral shortening. For BiV and LV pacing, mechanical activation was more synchronous, with less early and late systolic dyskinesis, and mechanical maps were remarkably similar by mid–late systole. Numbers shown reflect time duration from electrical stimulation at septal and lateral sites to time when mechanical data were displayed. (B) Chamber synchrony (CURE) improved similarly with LV and BiV modes. (C) CURE positively correlated with dP/dt_{max} but not with electrical delay. dP/dt_{max} is adjusted for its mean value in each respective animal. (Courtesy of Christophe. Leclercq and David Kass.)

from the same group, it was suggested that cardiac dyssynchrony analysis may be preferred using circumferential rather than longitudinal strain maps [37]. These MRI approaches need further evaluation in patients. The main limitations of MRI techniques are the time-consuming data acquisition and analysis, and the fact that repeat analysis after CRT implantation is not possible in patients with pacemakers.

Similar to nuclear imaging, MRI is well-suited for assessment of viability and scar tissue. In particular, contrast-enhanced MRI allows precise delineation of scar tissue [38]. Shortly after intravenous administration of gadolinium-based contrast agents, regions with scar tissue show increased image intensity (white, hyperenhanced, Fig. 7.5). The mechanism underlying the hyperenhancement appears related to the interstitial space between collagen fibers, which is larger in scar tissue than in the densely packed myocytes in normal myocardium, and the contrast agent will be trapped in these areas in infarcted tissue. Kim and co-workers [39] elegantly validated contrast-enhanced MRI to detect scar tissue in animal experiments, showing a perfect agreement between the extent of scar tissue on contrast-enhanced MRI and the histological extent of necrosis using triphenyltetrazolium chloride (TTC) staining of the explanted hearts. The major advantage of con-

trast-enhanced cardiac MRI over other imaging techniques is the superb spatial resolution, making differentiation between transmural and subendocardial scar tissue possible (Fig. 7.5). This MRI approach is likely to further optimize selection of patients for CRT by excluding patients with a large scar in the target region for LV lead positioning.

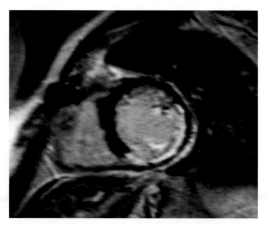

Figure 7.5 Short-axis MRI image using contrast-enhanced imaging. With this approach, scar tissue is visible as hyperenhanced regions (white); in this patient, scar tissue is present in the infero-lateral region, and (due to the excellent spatial resolution) one can appreciate that the scar formation is not completely transmural, since a small part of the epicardium is still viable (black).

Computed tomography techniques in cardiac resynchronization therapy

The CT techniques (electron beam CT (EBCT) and multislice CT (MSCT)) do not allow assessment of cardiac dyssynchrony, nor assessment of perfusion, metabolism, innervation, viability, or scar tissue. However, the CT techniques do permit non-invasive visualization of venous anatomy. Currently, venous anatomy is depicted during retrograde venography. Meisel and co-workers [40] have recently published their experience in 129 consecutive patients and confirmed that the venous anatomy is highly variable [41] and not all patients are suited for transvenous LV lead implantation. Ideally, venous anatomy should be assessed non-invasively, at the outpatient clinic, to determine whether a transvenous approach is feasible, or whether a (minimal invasive) surgical approach should be used for LV lead implantation. The feasibility of MSCT to visualize venous anatomy was recently demonstrated [42, 43]. MSCT allowed not only precise determination of coronary sinus and its tributaries, but also assessment of distances between veins and ostial size of the coronary sinus. An example of an MSCT depicting venous anatomy is shown in Fig. 7.6.

Similarly, EBCT can also provide non-invasive visualization of the venous system [44]. At present, CT techniques are not routinely used to assess venous anatomy prior to CRT implantation, and limitations exist, including the radiation dose of CT techniques. If non-invasive visualization of the venous system is ever to be clinically implemented, it should be stressed that the integration of venous anatomy with information on the site of latest electrical activation (e.g. derived from non-contact electroanatomical mapping technique) is needed to determine the preferred approach for LV lead implantation (transvenous versus surgical).

Conclusion

Various non-echocardiographic, non-invasive imaging techniques may play a role in selection of patients for CRT, in particular radionuclide angiography (with phase image analysis) and tagged MRI. The available evidence on the value of these tools to assess cardiac dyssynchrony and prediction of response to CRT is minimal, and echocardiography (in particular tissue Doppler imaging techniques) remains the technique of choice to select patients for CRT.

These non-echocardiographic techniques, however, can also provide other information on effects

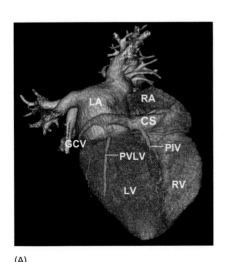

(A)

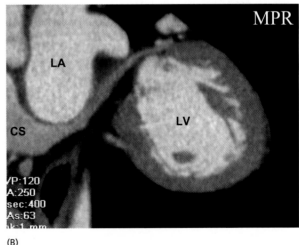

(B)

Figure 7.6 Non-invasive multi-slice computed tomography of the venous anatomy. Left panel: 3D volume rendered reconstruction. Right panel: multi-planar curved reconstruction (MPR) of the coronary sinus. Indicated on the 3D reconstruction (left panel) are the coronary sinus (CS), the posterior interventricular vein (PIV), the posterior vein of the left ventricle (PVLV), and the great cardiac vein (GCV). LA, left atrium; LV, left ventricle; RA, right atrium; RV, right ventricle. Based on Jongbloed *et al.* [42].

of CRT such as perfusion and metabolism. In addition, nuclear imaging techniques and MRI can be used to assess viability and scar tissue in the target region for LV lead positioning, which is also important for the response to CRT.

Finally, non-invasive visualization of venous anatomy is possible with CT techniques, which could be of use in deciding the optimal approach for LV lead implantation.

The non-echocardiographic techniques may have additional value in the selection and evaluation of patients undergoing CRT, but further studies are needed.

References

1 Auricchio A, Stellbrink C, Sack S et al. Pacing Therapies in Congestive Heart Failure (PATH-CHF) Study Group. Long-term clinical effect of hemodynamically optimized cardiac resynchronization therapy in patients with heart failure and ventricular conduction delay. J Am Coll Cardiol 2002; **39**: 2026–2033.

2 Cazeau S, Leclercq C, Lavergne T et al. Multisite Simulation in Cardiomyopathies MUSTIC) Study Investigators. Effects of multisite biventricular pacing in patients with heart failure and intraventricular conduction delay. N Engl J Med 2001; **344**: 873–880.

3 Abraham WT, Fisher WG, Smith AL et al. MIRACLE Study Group. Multicenter InSync Randomized Clinical Evaluation. Cardiac resynchronization in chronic heart failure. N Engl J Med 2002; **346**: 1845–1853.

4 Young JB, Abraham WT, Smith AL et al. Multicenter In-Sync ICD Randomized Clinical Evaluation (MIRACLE ICD) Trial Investigators. Combined cardiac resynchronization and implantable cardioversion defibrillation in advanced chronic heart failure: the MIRACLE ICD trial. JAMA 2003; **289**: 2685–2694.

5 Bristow MR, Saxon LA, Boehmer J et al. Comparison of Medical Therapy, Pacing and Defibrillation in Heart Failure (COMPANION) Investigators. Cardiac-resynchronization therapy with or without an implantable defibrillator in advanced chronic heart failure. N Engl J Med 2004; **350**: 2140–2150.

6 Cleland J, Daubert JC, Erdmann E et al. The effect of cardiac resynchronization on morbidity and mortality in heart failure. N Engl J Med 2005; **352**: 1539–1549.

7 Auricchio A, Stellbrink C, Butter C et al. Pacing Therapies in Congestive Heart Failure II Study Group, Guidant Heart Failure Research Group. Clinical efficacy of cardiac resynchronization therapy using left ventricular pacing in heart failure patients stratified by severity of ventricular conduction delay. J Am Coll Cardiol 2003; **42**: 2109–

2116.

8 Lozano I, Bocchiardo M, Achtelik M et al. VENTAK CHF/CONTAK CD Investigators Study Group. Impact of biventricular pacing on mortality in a randomized crossover study of patients with heart failure and ventricular arrhythmias. Pacing Clin Electrophysiol 2000; **23**: 1711–1712.

9 Bax JJ, Ansalone G, Breithardt OA et al. Echocardiographic evaluation of cardiac resynchronization therapy: ready for routine clinical use? A critical appraisal. J Am Coll Cardiol 2004; **44**: 1–9.

10 Grines CL, Bashore TM, Boudoulas H, Olson S, Shafer P, Wooley CF. Functional abnormalities in isolated left bundle branch block. The effect of interventricular asynchrony. Circulation 1989; **79**: 845–853.

11 Kass DA. Ventricular dyssynchrony and mechanisms of resynchronization therapy. Eur Heart J 2002; **4**: D23–D30.

12 Botvinick EH. Scintigraphic blood pool and phase image analysis: The optimal tool for the evaluation of resynchronization therapy. J Nucl Cardiol 2003; **10**: 424–428.

13 O'Connell JW, Schreck C, Moles M et al. A unique method by which to quantitate synchrony with equilibrium radionuclide angiography. J Nucl Cardiol 2005; **12**: 441–450.

14 Fauchier L, Marie O, Casset-Senon D, Babuty D, Cosnay P, Fauchier JP. Reliability of QRS duration and morphology on surface electrocardiogram to identify ventricular dyssynchrony in patients with idiopathic dilated cardiomyopathy. Am J Cardiol 2003; **92**: 341–344.

15 Fauchier L, Marie O, Casset-Senon D, Babuty D, Cosnay P, Fauchier JP. Interventricular and intraventricular dyssynchrony in idiopathic dilated cardiomyopathy. A prognostic study with Fourier phase analysis of radionuclide angioscintigraphy. J Am Coll Cardiol 2002; **40**: 2022–2030.

16 Kerwin WF, Botvinick EH, O'Connell JW et al. Ventricular contraction abnormalities in dilated cardiomyopathy: Effect of biventricular pacing to correct interventricular dyssynchrony. J Am Coll Cardiol 2000; **35**: 1221–1227.

17 Toussaint JF, Lavergne T, Kerrou K et al. Basal asynchrony and resynchronization with biventricular pacing predict long-term improvement of LV function in heart failure patients. Pacing Clin Electrophysiol 2003; **26**: 1815–1823.

18 Neri G, Zanco P, Zanon F, Buchberger R. Effect of biventricular pacing on metabolism and perfusion in patients affected by dilated cardiomyopathy and left bundle branch block: evaluation by positron emission tomography. Europace 2003; **5**: 111–115.

19 Nielsen JC, Bottcher M, Jensen HK, Nielsen TT, Pedersen AK, Mortensen PT. Regional myocardial perfusion during chronic biventricular pacing and after acute change of the pacing mode in patients with congestive heart fail-

ure and bundle branch block treated with an atrioventricular sequential biventricular pacemaker. *Eur J Heart Failure* 2003; **5**: 179–186.

20 Sundell J, Engblom E, Koistinen J *et al.* The effects of cardiac resynchronization therapy on left ventricular function, myocardial energetics and metabolic reserve in patients with dilated cardiomyopathy and heart failure. *J Am Coll Cardiol* 2004; **43**: 1027–1033.

21 Braunschweig F, Sorensen J, von Bibra H *et al.* Effects of biventricular pacing on myocardial blood flow and oxygen consumption using carbon-11 acetate positron emission tomography in patients with heart failure. *Am J Cardiol* 2003; **92**: 95–99.

22 Nowak B, Stellbrink C, Sinha AM *et al.* Effects of cardiac resynchronization therapy on myocardial blood flow measured by oxygen-15 water positron emission tomography in idiopathic-dilated cardiomyopathy and left bundle branch block. *Am J Cardiol* 2004; **93**: 496–499.

23 Knaapen P, van Campen LM, de Cock CC *et al.* Effects of cardiac resynchronization therapy on myocardial perfusion reserve. *Circulation* 2004; **110**: 646–651.

24 Lindner O, Vogt J, Kammeier A *et al.* Effect of cardiac resynchronization therapy on global and regional oxygen consumption and myocardial blood flow in patients with non-ischaemic and ischaemic cardiomyopathy. *Eur Heart J* 2005; **26**: 70–76.

25 Knuuti J, Sundell J, Naum A *et al.* Right ventricular oxidative metabolism assessed by PET in patients with idiopathic dilated cardiomyopathy undergoing cardiac resynchronization therapy. *Eur J Nucl Med Mol Imaging* 2004; **31**: 1592–1598.

26 Ukkonen H, Beanlands RS, Burwash IG *et al.* Effect of cardiac resynchronization on myocardial efficiency and regional oxidative metabolism. *Circulation* 2003; **107**: 28–31.

27 Lindner O, Vogt J, Baller D *et al.* Global and regional myocardial oxygen consumption and blood flow in severe cardiomyopathy with left bundle branch block. *Eur J Heart Failure* 2005; **7**: 225–230.

28 Nowak B, Sinha AM, Schaefer WM *et al.* Cardiac resynchronization therapy homogenizes myocardial glucose metabolism and perfusion in dilated cardiomyopathy and left bundle branch block. *J Am Coll Cardiol* 2003; **41**: 1523–1528.

29 Kanhai SM, Viergever EP, Bax JJ. Cardiogenic shock shortly after initial success of cardiac resynchronization therapy. *Eur J Heart Failure* 2004; **6**: 477–481.

30 Spyrou N, Rosen SD, Fath-Ordoubadi F *et al.* Myocardial beta-adrenoceptor density one month after acute myocardial infarction predicts left ventricular volumes at six months. *J Am Coll Cardiol* 2002; **40**: 1216–1224.

31 Merlet P, Benvenuti C, Moyse D *et al.* Prognostic value of MIBG imaging in idiopathic dilated cardiomyopathy. *J Nucl Med* 1999; **40**: 917–923.

32 Erol-Yilmaz A, Verberne HJ, Schrama TA *et al.* Cardiac resynchronization induces favourable neurohumoral changes. *Pacing Clin Electrophysiol* 2005; **28**: 304–310.

33 Wyman BT, Hunter WC, Prinzen FW, Faris OP, McVeigh ER. Effects of single- and biventricular pacing on temporal and spatial dynamics of ventricular contraction. *Am J Physiol Heart Circ Physiol* 2002; **282**: H372–H379.

34 Zwanenburg JJM, Gotte MJW, Kuijer JPA, Heethaar RM, Van Rossum AC, Marcus JT. Timing of cardiac contraction in humans mapped by high-temporal-resolution MRI tagging: early onset and late peak of shortening in lateral wall. *Am J Physiol Heart Circ Physiol* 2004; **286**: H1872–H1880.

35 Nelson GS, Curry CW, Wyman BT *et al.* Predictors of systolic augmentation from left ventricular preexcitation in patients with dilated cardiomyopathy and intraventricular conduction delay. *Circulation* 2000; **101**: 2703–2709.

36 Leclercq C, Faris O, Tunin R *et al.* Systolic improvement and mechanical resynchronization does not require electrical synchrony in the dilated failing heart with left bundle-branch block. *Circulation* 2002; **106**: 1760–1763.

37 Helm RH, Leclercq C, Faris O *et al.* Cardiac dyssynchrony analysis using circumferential versus longitudinal strain: implications for assessing cardiac resynchronization. *Circulation* 2005; **111**: 2760–2767.

38 Kaandorp TAM, Lamb HJ, Van der Wall EE, De Roos A, Bax JJ. Cardiovascular MR to access myocardial viability in chronic ischaemic LV dysfunction. *Heart* 2005; **91**: 1359–1365.

39 Kim RJ, Fieno DS, Parrish TB *et al.* Relationship of MRI delayed contrast enhancement to irreversible injury, infarct age, and contractile function. *Circulation* 1999; **100**: 1992–2002.

40 Meisel E, Pfeiffer D, Engelmann L *et al.* Investigation of coronary venous anatomy by retrograde venography in patients with malignant ventricular tachycardia. *Circulation* 2001; **104**: 442–447.

41 Singh JP, Houser S, Heist K, Ruskin JN. The coronary venous anatomy. A segmental approach to aid cardiac resynchronization therapy. *J Am Coll Cardiol* 2005; **46**: 68–74.

42 Jongbloed MR, Lamb HJ, Bax JJ, Schuijf JD, De Roos A, Van der Wall EE, Schalij MJ. Noninvasive visualization of the cardiac venous system using multislice computed tomography. *J Am Coll Cardiol* 2005; **45**: 749–753.

43 Abbara S, Cury RC, Nieman K *et al.* Noninvasive evaluation of cardiac veins with 16-MDCT angiography. *Am J Roentgenol* 2005; **185**: 1001–1006.

44 Mao S, Shinbane JS, Girsky MJ *et al.* Coronary venous imaging with electron beam computed tomographic angiography: Three-dimensional mapping and relationship with coronary arteries. *Am Heart J* 2005; **150**: 315–322.

SECTION 3

Pulse generators

CHAPTER 8

Device-specific features in cardiac resynchronization therapy

Martin J. Schalij, MD, PhD, *Lieselot van Erven,* MD, PhD,
Gabe B. Bleeker, MD *& Jeroen J. Bax,* MD, PhD

Introduction

Since the introduction of cardiac resynchronization therapy (CRT) for selected patients with advanced heart failure, now more than 10 years ago, technical progress has been impressive [1, 2]. In CRT, electrical pacing of the heart is applied to correct mechanical dyssynchrony of ventricular contraction. In recent years numerous randomized and nonrandomized trials have demonstrated improvement in clinical parameters following CRT including New York Heart Association (NYHA) class, quality of life, and 6-minute walking distance [1–10]. The summary of clinical trials is discussed in Chapter 13. In essence, reduction of all-cause mortality has been demonstrated by large clinical trials of both CRT and CRT-defibrillator devices [7, 8]. Based on these outcome trials, current selection criteria for CRT include NYHA functional class III–IV, left ventricular ejection fraction (LVEF) <35%, and a QRS width of >120 ms [4–8].

Electrical stimulation is aimed at correcting the three identified forms of dyssynchrony as discussed previously, namely (1) atrioventricular dyssynchrony, resulting in mitral valve incompetence and a reduced ventricular filling time; (2) interventricular dyssynchrony, as present in left bundle branch block (LBBB), during which the right ventricular (RV) contraction precedes that of the left ventricle; and (3) intraventricular dyssynchrony, which refers to the occurrence of dyssynchrony within the left ventricle [11–17]. In some patients, however, dys-synchrony is caused by a combination of two or more forms of dyssynchrony. Typically CRT utilizes three different pacing leads (and positions) to correct dyssynchrony: one lead will be inserted in the right atrium, one in the RV apex and the other one will be placed through the coronary sinus into one of the posterolateral tributaries of the coronary sinus (or by a minimally invasive surgical technique inserted directly on the left ventricular (LV) epicardial region of interest) [2, 18, 19]. These three leads will be connected to a biventricular pacing device and in this way dyssynchrony on different levels can be corrected.

The first CRT pacing devices implanted were standard dual chamber pacemakers connecting the two ventricular leads to the RV pacing port of the pacemaker through a Y-connector [1]. Consequently, although programming of different pacing and timing parameters was possible, parameters including sensing threshold, capture output, and timing values in the right and left ventricles could not be programmed independently. This approach, although effective in most patients, could result in serious sensing problems because of fusion of RV and LV signals. Only in the case of permanent atrial fibrillation could the LV lead be connected to the atrial port and the RV lead to the ventricular port of the DDD pacemaker, thereby enabling to a certain extent independent programming of sensing and pacing levels.

The introduction of pacemakers with specific ports for each individual lead and the possibility of independent programming of nearly all RV and LV parameters solved most of these problems. Furthermore, as CRT optimization may include sequential timing of RV and LV stimuli, with most current CRT devices it is possible to program the interventricular interval (the time difference between the RV and LV pacing) [2, 18, 19].

Furthermore, the current generation of CRT pacemakers (CRT-P) combines sophisticated pacing features with multiple monitoring tools and even telemetric monitoring options, reflecting the functional status of the patients. As both atrial and ventricular arrhythmias are frequently observed in heart failure patients, current CRT-P also incorporates arrhythmia monitoring tools [6, 7, 10]. As ventricular arrhythmias are a serious threat to heart failure patients and several studies have shown that, in patients with a low ejection fraction, mortality can be lowered by implanting a cardioverter defibrillator (ICD), combining CRT-P with a defibrillator backup (i.e. CRT-D) may have a cumulative positive effect on all-cause mortality. However, until now no randomized studies have been performed demonstrating an additional effect of CRT-D over CRT-P.

All pacing and monitoring features incorporated in the current CRT devices offer the unique opportunity to closely follow patients with advanced heart failure and data collected by the device may serve as early warning signals triggering interventions before actual deterioration of the clinical situation occurs [19]. It can be expected that future devices will evolve into multimodality treatment and monitoring platforms and that more monitoring-only systems will become available for patients without an indication for CRT. In this review some of the most important issues concerning CRT devices will be addressed.

Pacemaker functions

As the effects of CRT are, by definition, the result of electrical resynchronization of ventricular contraction, every effort should be directed at ensuring 100% RV and LV stimulation. Furthermore, besides standard pacemaker features like programmable rate, sensing and output levels, careful programming of atrioventricular delay and interventricular delay is of importance [19, 20].

Specific features like lead configurations and related issues such as integrated or true bipolar LV pacing (which may cause erroneous anodal pacing of the RV) are beyond the scope of this chapter.

Programming issues

Rate

In general, rate settings will be in line with more traditional pacemaker settings. The use of rate response devices may be advantageous in patients with severe cardiac disease as they may be chronotropic incompetent (due to, for example, beta blockers). However, under normal circumstances, the system will be programmed in a VDD (stimulation in the ventricles only) or DDD (stimulation in right atrium and both ventricles) mode and the atrial lead will only be used for sensing. In the case of a VDD mode, in our institution, the lower rate will be programmed between 30 and 50 beats/min and when programmed in the DDD mode the lower rate will be programmed at 50–60 beats/min. When the unit is programmed to the VDD mode, even with a relatively slow sinus rhythm (slower than the programmed lower rate) due to modification by medical treatment, pacing will be delivered to the ventricles only. In most patients a DDD mode will be preferable. In patients with chronotropic incompetence, the unit will be programmed to a DDDR mode. Normally, the upper rate limit will be set at 140–150 beats/min. In patients with a CRT-D device the upper rate will be limited by the cut-off value programmed for the detection of VT/VF as overlapping zones cannot be programmed in the current generation devices.

Sensing

In the first devices it was not possible to program LV and RV parameters independently. Consequently a less than optimal setting for each lead had to be accepted which sometimes resulted in serious complications. For example, atrial signals sensed by the LV lead (atrioventricular cross-talk) could result in double counting and inhibition of ventricular stimulation. In earlier generation CRT-D devices atrioventricular cross-talk also occurred frequently which even could result in inappropriate shock therapy [20–22]. In addition, double counting of ventricular signals could occur, which may also result in inappropriate therapy delivery. Atrioventricular cross-talk can normally be prevented by programming a shorter atrioventricular delay, whereas double counting of ventricular signals and subsequent inappropriate therapy delivery can be prevented by increasing the detection time (duration criteria) or by adding additional stability criteria [21,22]. In the current generations of CRT-P and CRT-D devices, sensing and pacing thresholds can be evaluated for each individual lead, thereby allowing the programming of RV/LV-specific sense and output settings. With these additional features atrioventricular and interventricular cross-talk can be managed.

Another issue is that of the filters used in the different devices in relation to the implanted leads. When a small bipole is used for sensing, as with true bipolar ICD leads, filter specifications can be less strict. However, when integrated bipolar leads with larger sensing areas are combined with that filter, oversensing may occur. Thus, combining leads and ICDs from different vendors that manufacture leads with different physical properties may create serious sensing problems.

Pacing

Evaluation of pacing output thresholds is often a challenging task. Knowledge of the different pacing settings and the effect of these settings on ventricular function is therefore mandatory. Careful ex-

amination of the surface ECG and, if available, the intracardiac signals may reveal loss of capture [23]. Ammann *et al.* recently described a robust electrogram-based algorithm to detect loss of LV capture during CRT (Fig. 8.1). This algorithm can be used in clinical practice with a high sensitivity and specificity if intracardiac signals are not available to detect loss of capture [23].

Atrioventricular delay

It is well recognized that the atrioventricular delay is of crucial importance in optimizing the benefit of CRT [2,9,18,24]. As demonstrated by several studies, relatively short atrioventricular delays should be programmed to improve LV systolic function. The principle of atrioventricular optimization is to ensure as close to 100% ventricular pacing as possible by programming a relatively short atrioventricular delay. By programming the atrioventricular delay to the time when atrial filling is just completed, it will provide a maximal period for LV diastolic filling, eliminating the "presystolic" time as well as preventing the occurrence of diastolic mitral regurgitation. Optimal atrioventricular interval can be calculated by the help of echocardiography based on the method described by Ritter or Ishikawa, or by measuring intracardiac delay of electrogram signals as described in the PATH-CHF studies. The technical details and methodologies

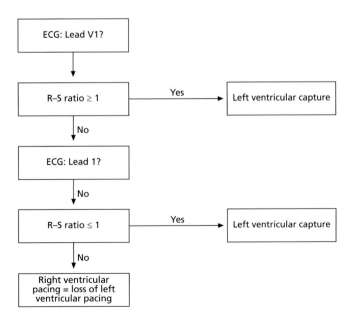

Figure 8.1 Careful examination of the surface ECG and, if available, the intracardiac signals may reveal loss of capture. This electrogram-based algorithm may be used to detect loss of left ventricular capture during CRT. Adapted from Ammann *et al.* [23].

of optimizing atrioventricular interval will be described elsewhere. Recently Sharf *et al.* demonstrated that in contrast to normal pacemaker patients the short atrioventricular delay at baseline should be prolonged during exercise to achieve an optimal systolic performance [25]. If this interesting concept can be confirmed in larger studies, dynamic lengthening of the atrioventricular delay is a desirable feature in the next generation of CRT devices, which may replace the dynamic shortening of the atrioventricular delay option available in the current units. A potential negative effect of dynamic lengthening of the atrioventricular delay is the inherent limitation of the programmable upper rate of the pacemaker (as this feature is directly dependent on the atrioventricular delay). However, until this feature becomes available it may be advisable to program the dynamic shortening of the atrioventricular delay in CRT devices off [25].

Interventricular optimization

To improve the benefit of CRT, sequential RV and LV pacing may be necessary. Several studies demonstrated that on top of an optimal programmed atrioventricular delay, interventricular timing may have a positive effect in some patients. However, the independent benefit of interventricular optimization has not been confirmed by case–control study or randomized controlled study that has another group of patients without optimization of interventricular delay. Furthermore, "fine-tuning" of a CRT device is time-consuming and, unlike optimal atrioventricular interval, interventricular delay settings cannot be predicted electrically or by "quick" echocardiographic calculation and echocardiography is necessary to evaluate the results of the programmed settings. A commonly described method is based on the calculation of cardiac output from the LV outflow tract by means of spectral pulse Doppler echocardiography (Fig. 8.2). This and other potential methods of assessing optimal interventricular delay will be discussed later in this book. Although echocardiography may not be available in all patients in the daily clinical practice, adjusting the interventricular delay should at least be performed in the group of non-responders in order to maximize the benefits of CRT.

Arrhythmia detection
Atrial arrhythmias

Atrial fibrillation develops in 20–40% of all CHF patients and may worsen the functional status of the patient, causing heart failure decompensation. Additionally, in CRT patients episodes of atrial fibrillation may result in loss of (bi-)ventricular pacing, resulting in a sudden worsening of the clinical situation, as during atrial fibrillation 100% ventricular stimulation cannot be ensured due to high or irregular intrinsic ventricular rates. Standard pacing algorithms, such as mode switching or ventricular rate regulation, proven to be effective in lowering symptoms of patients with atrial fibrillation, will not be effective in CRT patients [26–28]. Furthermore, mode switch problems such as inappropriate backswitching may occur due to special timing of atrial and ventricular signals (Fig. 8.3). Ventricular rate regulation algorithms aimed at regulating the ventricular rate during atrial fibrillation, although effective in regulating the ventricular rate, are also not effective in ensuring 100% biventricular pacing [27].

As several studies have now demonstrated that CRT is effective in patients with atrial fibrillation, strict rate regulation ensuring ventricular stimulation is important. In our own series of patients with atrial fibrillation (>80 CRT patients), ventricular pacing occurred for approximately 80% of the time [29]. This may at least partly explain the somewhat lower response rate to CRT (compared to patients with sinus rhythm). To increase this relatively low number all efforts should be directed towards converting atrial fibrillation to sinus rhythm. If sinus rhythm cannot be maintained, rate regulation is important. First choice treatment remains rate regulation by drugs (such as beta blockers and digoxin); however, if this is not successful, a catheter ablation of the atrioventricular node should be considered.

Ventricular arrhythmias

Numerous studies have demonstrated that patients with LV dysfunction and low ejection fractions are at risk of sudden cardiac death due to ventricular arrhythmias [30–40]. Several large, randomized trials have demonstrated that implantation of an ICD in patients with a low LV ejection fraction reduces all-cause mortality. Recently, the SCD-

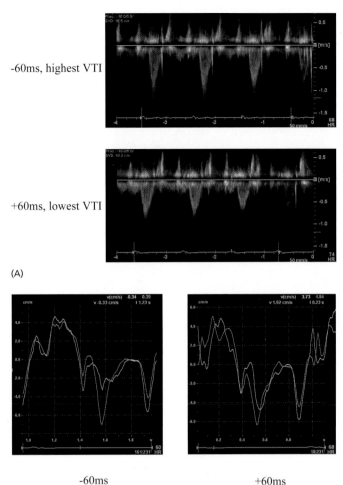

Figure 8.2 Interventricular interval optimization in a 48-year-old male using transthoracic echocardiography. Seven different V–V intervals are programmed on the CRT device from –60 ms (i.e. LV pacing 60 ms before RV pacing), –40 ms, –20 ms, 0 ms, 20 ms, 40 ms to 60 ms (i.e. RV pacing 60 ms before LV pacing). In each setting the aortic velocity time integral (VTI) is measured using pulsed wave Doppler echocardiography and the V–V interval which yields the highest aortic VTI is considered the optimal setting (A). In addition, tissue Doppler imaging can be used to evaluate the effects of different V–V intervals on LV dyssynchrony (B). In this patient a V–V interval of –60 ms resulted in the highest aortic VTI and a perfect LV systolic synchronicity. The lowest aortic VTI and the highest level of LV dyssynchrony were found at a V–V interval of 60 ms.

HeFT trial demonstrated, for the first time, that ICD therapy in patients with symptomatic heart failure and a low LV ejection fraction, regardless of the underlying cause, has a positive effect on all-cause mortality. It is therefore challenging to speculate that combining CRT with ICD therapy may have a significant additional mortality effect and should be considered in all patients with a depressed LV function. However, until now, no large randomized trials comparing the efficacy of CRT only with CRT-D have been conducted [41]. Although the COMPANION trial reported only a significant mortality effect in the CRT-D group compared with optimal medical therapy, the difference between CRT-D and CRT-P patients was not significant [7].

Technically the combination of CRT with ICD therapy creates potential problems. This is especially the case with the earlier generation devices with sensing problems that resulted in double counting of ventricular events and inappropriate shock therapy. Furthermore, atrioventricular cross-talk in the LV lead may also result in double counting and inappropriate shock therapy [21, 22]. With continuous technical improvement, independent programming of LV and RV sensing parameters and incorporation of new diagnostic algorithms, these problems become much less common.

As patients with a CRT-P device are not protected against malignant ventricular arrhythmias and it is well known that sudden cardiac death is one of the two commonest causes of mortality in

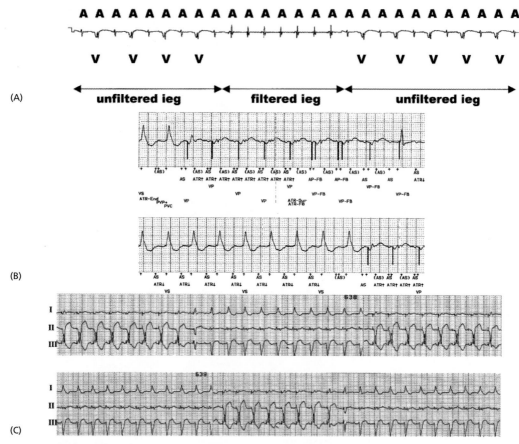

Figure 8.3 (A) Intracardiac atrial electrograms, unfiltered and filtered, as recorded by the PSA. Atrial electrograms (A) reveal atrial tachyarrhythmia. Far-field R waves (V) can be discerned in the unfiltered parts of the registration. Note the simultaneous occurrence of every second atrial deflection with the far-field ventricular signal. (B) Pacemaker tracing (continuous): surface ECG lead I and marker annotations. The cyclic character of the tracing is noteworthy. After two intrinsic beats (to be explained below), nine ventricular beats are paced in DDD mode with tracking of the atrium in a 2:1 fashion. Sensing of the atrial tachyarrhythmia is reflected in the marker annotations as "(AS)" and "AS," referring to an atrial sensed event either or not in the post-ventricular atrial refractory period (PVARP), respectively. The markers show "ATR↑," reflecting the process of counting up until the programmed number of atrial deflections fulfill the onset criteria for atrial tachycardia (programmed to 8). When the duration is also reached ("ATR-Dur") pacing in the fallback mode is started ("ATR-FB"). The pacemaker now switches to DDI pacing in the fallback mode, slowly decelerating to its programmed rate (similar to rate smoothing), with dynamic AV delay on. The first two beats in the fallback mode show atrial pacing ("AP-FB") as well as ventricular pacing ("VP-FB") since the sensed atrial events fall in the PVARP ["(AS)"]. The fourth "VP-FB" is a fusion beat of ventricular pacing and intrinsic conduction and therefore has a different configuration. From that beat on, the intrinsic rate is higher than the pacemaker rate, inhibiting DDI pacing. The atrial rhythm is misinterpreted as sinus rhythm, since due to their nearly simultaneous occurrence, every second flutter wave falls in the blanking period of the ventricular deflection. The other atrial deflections are sensed and followed by the ventricle ("VS"). The marker channel shows "ATR↓" representing the counting down of atrial deflections, after which sinus rhythm is supposedly present ("ATR-End"). Inappropriate back switching to the DDD mode occurs during which the atrial tachyarrhythmia is sensed again ("ATR↑"). (C) Surface ECG: leads I, II, and III. This continuous tracing illustrates the unusual cyclic character of repeatedly mode switching and back switching. After appropriate mode switching, the atrial tachyarrhythmia was conducted to the ventricle in a 2:1 fashion. Due to simultaneous occurrence of each second atrial flutter wave and the intrinsic ventricular deflection, the atrial channel was blanked at the second flutter wave. The atrial rate was interpreted by the pacemaker as being below the cut-off rate for mode switching. This led to inappropriate back switching to DDD mode after at least eight conducted beats (duration) establishing tracking of the atrial arrhythmia in a 2:1 fashion again and leading to cyclic mode switching. Adapted from van Erven L, Molhoek SG, van der Wall EE, Schalij MJ. Cyclic appropriate mode switching and inappropriate back switching of a biventricular pacemaker during atrial tachyarrhythmia. *Pacing Clin Electrophysiol* 2004; **27**: 249.

heart failure, it may be an option to add an audible warning signal in case of non-sustained ventricular tachycardia, allowing for an upgrade to a CRT-D unit.

Device follow-up

Heart failure patients require continued intense monitoring after CRT as device therapy is complementary to, but does not replace, pharmacological treatment. Furthermore, after implantation of a CRT device drug regimens should be adapted according to factors such as an improved hemodynamic profile. In order to monitor these patients, a structured heart failure program should be operational, in which all disciplines involved collaborate closely [20]. Although regular monitoring of these heart failure patients remains the cornerstone of successful treatment, device-based monitoring of the functional status of the patients may help to adjust medication ahead of deteriorating hemodynamic situation, thereby preventing hospitalization for decompensated heart failure.

With respect to device settings it is important to recognize the dynamic nature of the clinical syndrome of heart failure. Sudden changes in device settings may cause a deterioration of the clinical situation. However, a recurrence of heart failure symptoms may also be caused by loss of LV lead capture due to lead dislodgement or suboptimal device programming. In addition, the "non-responders" to CRT should be evaluated carefully to optimize device settings. It is therefore possible that adjusting the atrioventricular or interventricular delay as guided by echocardiography may convert a non-responder into a responder.

Output settings/automatic optimization of voltage output

The burden on the battery of a CRT device is much higher than that of standard pacemakers for a number of reasons. First, as successful CRT relies on 100% biventricular pacing on two out of three output channels, this continuous drain may shorten the device longevity significantly. Second, the LV pacing threshold is usually higher or less reliable than the RV apical lead, and therefore manual output programming will tend to set the output to a higher level than strictly necessary. Third, as thresholds may vary over time, to ensure capture, output levels will be programmed with a higher safety margin than regular pacemakers for brady-indications. Fourth, heart failure patients have less favorable electrical characteristics and anisotropy which require more frequent checking of pacing and sensing levels; this may also have resulted in higher pacing output settings [42]. All these factors will contribute to the relatively short longevity of these devices. Limiting the output and improving the longevity of these devices can be achieved by incorporating automatic optimization of voltage output algorithms. This pacemaker algorithm functions by automatic device measurements of the evoked response.

In CRT, automatic optimization of voltage output of either the RV or LV lead can be influenced by the evoked response of the other pacing site. In other words, the RV lead can sense a LV response theoretically and vice versa. Some preliminary studies, using standard DDD devices in patients with chronic atrial fibrillation (connecting the LV lead to the atrial port), demonstrated that automatic optimization of voltage output may be a feasible option for future devices [43, 44]. These automatic features may in theory increase both the longevity and safety by capture verification during biventricular pacing.

As longevity is also a cost issue besides its importance for the patient therapy, automatic optimization of voltage output may ideally lower the costs of CRT and increase its cost-effectiveness. Although automated pacing output optimization may in the future be a safe alternative to manual programming of fixed output settings, potential dangerous drawbacks of automated output settings prohibit a widespread introduction into the current CRT devices [45].

Monitoring

With the increasing numbers of patients receiving more complex devices for the treatment of a variety of different cardiac conditions, follow-up and monitoring of the clinical status becomes a challenging task. Current devices incorporate numerous tools to check both device integrity and response to therapy [46, 47]. However, it is well known that only a fraction of the available tools is currently utilized for various reasons. First, due to the increasing number of patients receiving device therapy the technical staff may have insufficient time to cope with the increasing demands for detailed device interrogation and reprogramming. Second, devices are becoming more complex, requiring advanced technical and medical skills to utilize all different options. To deal with these problems, intelligent systems should be developed to provide the technical and medical staff with the most relevant information concerning the device and the status of the patients.

Monitoring the hemodynamic profile of the patient should be focused on detecting signs of worsening heart failure at an early stage, thereby providing time to intervene and to change the medical regimen or the device settings in order to prevent hospital admissions. Currently several tools are offered by the different systems available.

Heart rate and activity logs

Changes in mean heart rate may reflect changes in the fluid status and hemodynamic situation of the patients. Both the daytime heart rate, and in particular the night heart rate, will be increased in patients with deterioration of heart failure condition. By monitoring these parameters on a regular basis detection of worsening heart failure may be possible before the patient experiences physical complaints and before a hospital admission becomes necessary.

Intrathoracic impedance monitoring and heart rate variability

Device-based technologies of intrathoracic impedance and heart rate variability for monitoring of heart failure will be described in detail in subsequent chapters.

Activity log

The activity log can provide information about the functional status of the patient. These activity logs are obtained from the accelerometer in the pacemaker and updated on a regular basis. Several devices now make it possible to retrieve these data, allowing assessment of functional status. As expected, in patients with worsening of heart failure status, daytime activity will be reduced. These data may also be helpful in optimizing device settings and may confirm the lack of a favorable response even after implantation of CRT, as reflected by the lack of increase in activity log.

Telemetric monitoring

With the increasing number of patients receiving devices and with the increasing choices of monitoring tools offered by these devices, telemetric monitoring becomes a desirable option (Fig. 8.4). Not only will this hopefully limit the number of outpatient visits, it may also offer the possibility of intervention at an earlier stage, such as alteration of medical treatment. Currently device manufacturers offer differ-

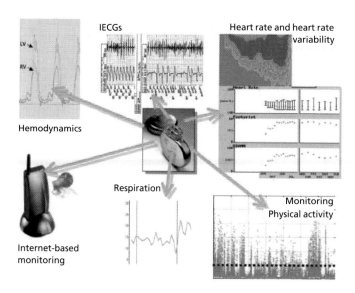

Figure 8.4 Device-based monitoring of vital signs offer the possibility of closely monitoring heart failure patients even by telemetry. Adapted from: Auricchio and Abraham [19].

ent telemetric systems. Some systems even offer the option of transmitting intracardiac electrograms, which is, of course, a unique feature allowing monitoring of device activity at a distance.

Telemetric monitoring has a number of advantages [48]. If device measurements are available on a daily basis it becomes possible to study trends in the hemodynamic profile which allows early adjustment of medical therapy before the patient experiences worsening of heart failure symptoms. Furthermore, atrial arrhythmias resulting in less biventricular pacing may be detected at an earlier stage, thus enabling reprogramming of the device or changing the regimen of antiarrhythmic and/or rate control drugs. Loss of biventricular pacing during fast paroxysmal atrial fibrillation can be a reason for rapid clinical deterioration. Therefore, early diagnosis and management with the adjunctive tool of telemetric monitoring is crucial in order to avoid heart failure decompensation. Furthermore, ventricular arrhythmia episodes can be diagnosed early and action taken accordingly.

With telemetric monitoring, device integrity can be monitored on a daily basis, ensuring a proper function of the device. This may have a reassuring effect on both the patient and the physician. In addition, if it is possible to check the device activity on a regular basis by telemetry, the routine technical checks may be scheduled at a longer time interval.

Privacy protection

Although all kinds of data are already available to the device industry, the new telemetric monitoring systems, making use of central database facilities, may evoke new questions concerning the protection of the privacy of the individual patient. This is especially true in the light of current information technology development, which offers rather unrestricted access to electronic data systems. It may be questionable whether data from patients all over the world should be stored in central database facilities in a few countries. In fact, other options may be appropriate, and it may be necessary to encourage device vendors to create database facilities in all different countries that comply with individual national privacy protection laws. Until now this issue has been relatively neglected. As we are just at the beginning of the widespread introduction of these

sophisticated monitoring devices with telemetry capabilities, it is imperative to discuss this issue seriously.

Future devices

Ideally future devices should be small (around 30 cm^3), have a longevity of approximately seven years and multimodality monitoring capabilities [49]. It is expected that in the group of patients with advanced heart failure, monitoring of vital signs may offer the possibility to prevent worsening heart failure symptoms at an earlier stage, thereby preventing unnecessary hospital admissions. Concerning the longevity of the current devices, from a recent analysis by Hauser *et al.*, it becomes clear that newer devices tend to have a shorter service life than previous models [50]. Besides this potentially negative impact on individual patients (every replacement bears a risk of complications), a shorter service life also increases costs and therefore exerts more stress on the already overloaded health care system in most places. Furthermore, in the light of the recent cascade of serious device recalls, every effort should be directed at increasing device integrity [51].

Therefore, new devices ideally should combine longevity and integrity with multiple programming and monitoring options that allow patient-tailored settings and effective disease monitoring.

Conclusions

Since the introduction of cardiac resynchronization therapy technical progress has been impressive. With all the options offered by current devices, patient-tailored therapy has become possible. It can be expected that CRT devices will evolve into multimodality diagnostic and therapeutic platforms offering the possibility of detection and treatment of a variety of different cardiac conditions. Special monitoring devices without pacing options may become available for patients without an indication for CRT.

References

1 Bakker PF, Meijburg HW, de Vries JW *et al.* Biventricular pacing in end-stage heart failure improves functional ca-

pacity and left ventricular function. *J Interv Card Electrophysiol* 2000; **4**: 395–404.

2 McAlister FA, Ezekowitz JA, Wiebe N *et al.* Systematic review: cardiac resynchronization in patients with symptomatic heart failure. *Ann Intern Med* 2004; **141**: 381–390.

3 Auricchio A, Stellbrink C, Sack S *et al.* Pacing Therapies in Congestive Heart Failure (PATH-CHF) Study Group. Long-term clinical effect of hemodynamically optimized cardiac resynchronization therapy in patients with heart failure and ventricular conduction delay. *J Am Coll Cardiol* 2002; **39**: 2026–2033.

4 Cazeau S, Leclercq C, Lavergne T *et al.* Multisite Simulation in Cardiomyopathies MUSTIC) Study Investigators. Effects of multisite biventricular pacing in patients with heart failure and intraventricular conduction delay. *N Engl J Med* 2001; **344**: 873–880.

5 Abraham WT, Fisher WG, Smith AL *et al.* MIRACLE Study Group. Multicenter InSync Randomized Clinical Evaluation. Cardiac resynchronization in chronic heart failure. *N Engl J Med* 2002; **346**: 1845–1853.

6 Young JB, Abraham WT, Smith AL *et al.* Multicenter InSync ICD Randomized Clinical Evaluation (MIRACLE ICD) Trial Investigators. Combined cardiac resynchronization and implantable cardioversion defibrillation in advanced chronic heart failure: the MIRACLE ICD trial. *JAMA* 2003; **289**: 2685–2694.

7 Bristow MR, Saxon LA, Boehmer J *et al.* Comparison of Medical Therapy, Pacing and Defibrillation in Heart Failure (COMPANION) Investigators. Cardiac-resynchronization therapy with or without an implantable defibrillator in advanced chronic heart failure. *N Engl J Med* 2004; **350**: 2140–2150.

8 Cleland J, Daubert JC, Erdmann E *et al.* The effect of cardiac resynchronization on morbidity and mortality in heart failure. *N Engl J Med* 2005; **352**: 1539–1549.

9 Auricchio A, Stellbrink C, Butter C *et al.* Pacing Therapies in Congestive Heart Failure II Study Group, Guidant Heart Failure Research Group. Clinical efficacy of cardiac resynchronization therapy using left ventricular pacing in heart failure patients stratified by severity of ventricular conduction delay. *J Am Coll Cardiol* 2003; **42**: 2109–2116.

10 Kies P, Bax JJ, Molhoek SG *et al.* Comparison of effectiveness of cardiac resynchronization therapy in patients with versus without diabetes mellitus. *Am J Cardiol* 2005; **96**: 108–111.

11 Bax JJ, Ansalone G, Breithardt OA *et al.* Echocardiographic evaluation of cardiac resynchronization therapy: ready for routine clinical use? A critical appraisal. *J Am Coll Cardiol* 2004; **44**: 1–9.

12 Grines CL, Bashore TM, Boudoulas H, Olson S, Shafer P, Wooley CF. Functional abnormalities in isolated left bundle branch block. The effect of interventricular asynchrony. *Circulation* 1989; **79**: 845–853.

13 Kass DA. Ventricular dyssynchrony and mechanisms of resynchronization therapy. *Eur Heart J* 2002; **4**: D23–D30.

14 Bader H, Garrigue S, Lafitte S *et al.* Intra-left ventricular electromechanical asynchrony. *J Am Coll Cardiol* 2004; **43**: 248–256.

15 Kerwin WF, Botvinick EH, O'Connell JW *et al.* Ventricular contraction abnormalities in dilated cardiomyopathy: Effect of biventricular pacing to correct interventricular dyssynchrony. *J Am Coll Cardiol* 2000; **35**: 1221–1227.

16 Toussaint JF, Lavergne T, Kerrou K *et al.* Basal asynchrony and resynchronization with biventricular pacing predict long-term improvement of LV function in heart failure patients. *Pacing Clin Electrophysiol* 2003; **26**: 1815–1823.

17 Leclercq C, Faris O, Tunin R *et al.* Systolic improvement and mechanical resynchronization does not require electrical synchrony in the dilated failing heart with left bundle-branch block. *Circulation* 2002; **106**: 1760–1763.

18 Kalinchak DM, Schoenfeld MH. Cardiac resynchronization: a brief synopsis part II: implant and follow-up methodology. *J Cardiovasc Electrophysiol* 2003; **9**: 163–166.

19 Auricchio A, Abraham WT. Cardiac resynchronization therapy: current state of the art. Cost versus benefit. *Circulation* 2004; **109**: 300–307.

20 Vardas PE. Pacing follow-up techniques and trouble shooting during biventricular pacing. *J Cardiac Electrophysiol* 2003; **9**: 183–187.

21 Tarieb J, Benchaa T, Foltzer E *et al.* Atrioventricular cross-talk in biventricular pacing: a potential cause of ventricular standstill. *Pacing Clin Electrophysiol* 2002; **25**: 929–935.

22 Liu BC, Villareal RP, Harihan R *et al.* Inappropriate shock delivery and biventricular pacing cardiac defibrillators. *Tex Heart Inst J* 2003; **30**: 45–49.

23 Ammann P, Sticherling C, Kalusche D *et al.* An electrogram-based algorithm to detect loss of left ventricular capture during cardiac resynchronization therapy. *Ann Intern Med* 2005; **142**: 968–973.

24 Auricchio A, Stellbrink C, Block M *et al.* Effect of pacing chamber and atrioventricular delay on acute systolic function of paced patients with congestive heart failure. *Circulation* 1999; **99**: 2993–3001.

25 Sharf C, Li P, Muntwyler J *et al.* Rate-dependent AV delay optimization in cardiac resynchronization therapy. *Pacing Clin Electrophysiol* 2005; **28**: 279–284.

26 Erven L, Molhoek SG, van der Wall EE, Schalij MJ. Cyclic appropriate mode switching and inappropriate back switching of a biventricular pacemaker during atrial tachyarrhythmia. *Pacing Clin Electrophysiol* 2004; **27**: 249.

27 Melenovsky V, Hay I, Fetics BJ *et al.* Functional impact of rate irregularity in patients with heart failure and atrial fibrillation receiving resynchronization therapy. *Eur*

Heart J 2005; **26**: 705–711.

28 Tse HF, Newman D, Ellenbogen KA, Buhr T, Markowitz T, Lau CP. Effects of ventricular rate regularization pacing on quality of life and symptoms in patients with atrial fibrillation (Atrial fibrillation symptoms mediated by pacing to mean rates [AF SYMPTOMS Study]). *Am J Cardiol* 2004; **94**: 938–941.

29 Kies P, Leclercq C, Bleeker GB *et al.* Cardiac resynchronization therapy in chronic atrial fibrillation: impact on left atrial size and reversal to sinus rhythm. *Heart* 2005; e-pub ahead of print.

30 The MERIT-HF investigators. Effect of metoprolol CR/XL in chronic heart failure: Metoprolol CR/XL Randomised Intervention Trial in Congestive Heart Failure (MERIT-HF). *Lancet* 1999; **353**: 2001–2007.

31 Randomised trial of low-dose amiodarone in severe congestive heart failure. Grupo de Estudio de la Sobrevida en la Insuficiencia Cardiaca en Argentina (GESICA) *Lancet* 1994; **344**: 493–498.

32 Singh S, Fletcher R, Gisher S, Singh B *et al.* Amiodarone in patients with congestive heart failure and asymptomatic ventricular arrhythmia. *N Engl J Med* 1995; **333**: 77–82.

33 Julian D, Camm A, Frangin G, Janse M *et al.* Randomised trial of effect of amiodarone on mortality in patients with left ventricular dysfunction after recent myocardial infarction: EMIAT. *Lancet* 1997; **349**: 667–674.

34 The Antiarrhythmic Versus Implantable Defibrillator (AVID) Investigators. A comparison of antiarrhythmic-drug therapy with implantable defibrillators in patients resuscitated from near-fatal ventricular arrhythmias. *N Engl J Med* 1997; **337**: 1576–1583.

35 Connolly S, Gent M, Roberts RS *et al.* Canadian Implantable Defibrillator Study (CIDS): A randomized trial of the implantable cardioverter defibrillator against amiodarone. *Circulation* 2000; **101**: 1297–1302.

36 Moss A, Hall J, Cannom D *et al.* for the MADIT Investigators. Improved survival with an implanted defibrillator in patients with coronary disease at high risk of ventricular arrhythmias. *N Engl J Med* 1996; **335**: 1933–1940.

37 Buxton A, Lee K, Fisher J, Josephson M, Prystowsky E, Hafley G, for the Multicenter UnSustained Tachycardia Trial (MUSTT) Investigators. A randomized study of the prevention of sudden death in patients with coronary artery disease. *N Engl J Med* 1999; **341**: 1882–1890.

38 Moss A, Zareba W, Hall WJ, Klein H *et al.* Prophylactic implantation of a Defibrillator in patients with myocardial infarction and reduced ejection fraction. *N Engl J*
Med 2002; **346**: 877–883.

39 Kadish A, Dyer A, Daubert J *et al.* Prophylactic defibrillator implantation in patients with nonischemic dilated cardiomyopathy. *N Engl J Med* 2004: **350**: 2151–2158.

40 Bardy G, Lee K, Mark D *et al.* Amiodarone or an implantable cardioverter-defibrillator for congestive heart failure. *N Engl J Med* 2005; **352**: 225–237.

41 Ghosh J, Kaye G, Cleland JG. Cardiac resynchronization therapy with or without an implantable defibrillator: only indicated when everything else has failed? *Card Electrophysiol Rev* 2003; **7**: 421–429.

42 Schuchert A, Aydin MA, Israel C, *et al.* Atrial pacing and sensing characteristics in heart failure patients undergoing cardiac resynchronization therapy. *Europace* 2005; **7**: 165–169.

43 Biffi M, Boriani G, Bertini M, Silvestri P, Martignani C, Branzi A. Pacing with capture verification in candidates for resynchronization therapy: a feasibility study. *Europace* 2005; **7**: 255–265.

44 Suri R, Harthorne JW, Galvin J. Automated optimizing pacing output: an excellent idea, but with potentially lethal pitfalls. *Pacing Clin Electrophysiol* 2001; **24**: 520–523.

45 Diotallevi P, Ravazzi PA, Gostolli E. *et al.* An algorithm for verifying biventricular capture based on evoked-response morphology. *Pacing Clin Electrophysiol* 2005; **28**: S15–S18.

46 Braunschweig F, Linde C, Eriksson MJ *et al.* Continuous haemodynamic monitoring during withdrawal of diuretics in patients with congestive heart failure. *Eur Heart J* 2002; **23**: 59–69.

47 Kadhiresan K, Carlson G. The role of implantable sensors for management of heart failure. *Stud Health Technol Inform* 2004; **108**: 219–227.

48 Coletta AP, Nikitin N, Clark AL, Cleland JG. Clinical trials update from the American Heart Association meeting: PROSPER, DIAL, home care monitoring trials, immune modulation therapy, COMPANION and anaemia in heart failure. *Eur J Heart Failure* 2003; **5**: 95–99.

49 Rosario S, Schwarz ER, Ahmad M *et al.* Benefits, unresolved questions and technical issues of cardiac resynchronization therapy for heart failure. Am J Cardiol 2005; **96**: 710–717.

50 Hauser RG. The growing mismatch between patient longevity and the service life of implantable cardioverter-defibrillators. *J Am Coll Cardiol* 2005; **45**: 2022–2025.

51 Hauser RG, Maron BJ. Lessons from the failure and recall of an implantable cardioverter-defibrillator. *Circulation* 2005; **112**: 2040–2042.

CHAPTER 9

Programming and diagnostic features of cardiac resynchronization therapy devices

Osnat Gurevitz, MD, *David Luria,* MD *& Michael Glikson,* MD

Programming cardiac resynchronization therapy devices

Programming standard parameters common to pacemakers and implantable cardioverter defibrillators (ICDs) are covered in other major textbooks. However, there are pacing features that are specifically designed for cardiac resynchronization therapy (CRT) devices which will be discussed in this chapter. In addition, programming issues that are unique to CRT patients rather than pacemaker and ICD patients, as well as ICD issues that are specific to the CRT-D patient will be discussed. The issues of atrioventricular and V-V programming and optimization and of expert systems to support this programming are discussed elsewhere in this book.

Use of basic programming parameters in cardiac resynchronization therapy devices
Lower rate programming and should the atria be paced?
The issue of recommended lower rate in CRT patients has not been resolved. Whereas older literature, based mainly on acute studies of ventricular-paced patients, demonstrated optimal cardiac output at rates between 70 and 90 bpm [1] it is not entirely clear whether long-term programming of lower rates in this range is beneficial in patients with congestive heart failure. Potential advantages of relatively rapid pacing include increased cardiac

output as well as suppression of atrial fibrillation when pacing the atria [2]. Disadvantages of more rapid pacing may include decreased battery longevity due to both the faster paced rate, as well as the need to pace the atrium, increased metabolic demand on the failing myocardium and derangement of atrioventricular synchronization and diastolic filling when the atria are mostly paced rather than sensed.

In an elegant acute hemodynamic study, Bernheim *et al.* demonstrated the superiority of atrial sensed (VDD) pacing over atrial paced (DDD) mode in CRT patients by providing better left ventricular (LV) synchronization, longer diastolic filling times and improved myocardial performance [3]. This effect was mainly due to artificially delayed activation of the left atrium, when the right atrium was paced, as well as to fusion activation of the LV between intrinsic- and biventricular-paced rhythms that was caused by "pace compensation" (programmed uniform longer atrioventricular delay while pacing the atrium). These mechanisms are demonstrated in Fig. 9.1. The authors conclude that CRT with intrinsic atrial activation has acute hemodynamic advantages over atrial paced CRT, at least in the acute settings at rest.

Notably, most controlled trials that demonstrated benefits of CRT on morbidity and mortality used VDD or DDD pacing at relatively low [4–6] or intermediate [7] rates. No studies thus far have compared slow to more rapid pacing over long-term fol-

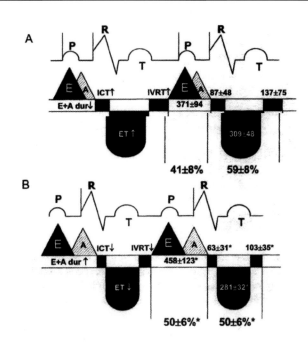

Figure 9.1 Time periods of the entire cardiac cycle (ECG and Doppler flow) in DDD pacing mode (A) compared with VDD pacing mode (B). Note the prolongation of the mitral inflow time (E + A duration) secondary to the shorter isovolumic contraction time (ICT), isovolumic relaxation time (IVRT), and aortic ejection time (ET) in the VDD as compared to the DDD pacing mode. Data of timing intervals are presented as the mean value (ms) ± SD. *$P < 0.01$ VDD vs. DDD. ECG labeling: P, P wave; R, R wave; T, T wave. Doppler inflow labeling: A, A wave (late transmitral inflow during left atrial contraction); E, E wave (early transmitral flow). Reproduced from Bernheim *et al.* [3], with permission.

low-up. Therefore, the jury is still out regarding the best lower rate for most CRT patients and further studies are needed to resolve this issue. So far we have empirically programmed CRT patients that are chronotropically competent to DDD at a lower rate of 50 ppm, and programmed DDDR at a lower rate of 70 ppm in patients with spontaneous or drug-induced sinus node dysfunction. During follow-up, device diagnostics such as heart rate histograms, % atrial pacing and information on atrial fibrillation episodes may assist in selecting the best programmed lower rate that will maintain intrinsic atrial activity at acceptable rates and may help to avoid atrial fibrillation. With a high percentage of atrial paced beats the use of rate improvements, such as rate hysteresis and search hysteresis, to further enhance intrinsic atrial activity in patients whose own rate is close to the programmed lower rate, may be considered. If atrial pacing percentage remains high, despite the use of these enhancements, the patient probably has sinus node dysfunction, where atrial pacing cannot be avoided, and programming of higher basic rate and/or rate response should be considered. When using atrial fibrillation suppression algorithms (such as Guidant's atrial pacing preference (APP)) and Proact (available in atrial/ventricular devices), the effect of decreased intrinsic atrial activity and increased average pacing rate should be noted. The

same applies to aggressive rate response that may result in a higher percentage of atrial pacing.

Upper rate programming and adaptive atrioventricular delays

Upper rate selection helps to maintain physiological heart rate response to exercise in patients with sinus node dysfunction (paced upper rate) and to prevent excessive ventricular rates in atrial tachyarrhythmias that are being tracked by the pacemaker to the ventricle (sensed upper rate or maximal tracking rate).

An in-depth discussion on selection and tailoring of age-appropriate upper rate is beyond the scope of this chapter. However, there are several issues of upper rate programming that relate specifically to CRT patients.

Most patients with "regular" pacemakers have either sinus node dysfunction that will prevent them from reaching the upper tracking rate, or atrioventricular conduction system disease that will prevent intrinsic ventricular activation during rapid atrial rates. In contrast, most CRT patients have normal sinus and atrioventricular conduction system functions, and thus may develop, especially during exercise, rapid atrial rates that are above the programmed upper tracking rate. This may lead to Wenckebach function of the pacemaker with pacemaker atrioventricular delay becoming longer than the intrinsic atrioventricular conduction, resulting in intrinsic conduction with ventricular inhibition and loss of ventricular resynchronization [8]. Therefore, in CRT patients, it is of paramount importance to maintain programmed maximal tracking rate above the highest achievable sinus rhythm to ensure complete biventricular capture at higher atrial rates as well. Device diagnostics may help to ensure maintenance of appropriate upper rate (see section on Verifying Effective Biventricular Pacing in this chapter).

Output programming, left ventricular pacing thresholds, and battery longevity

The natural evolution of right ventricular (RV) pacing threshold over time has been recognized for many years. Following an initial rise, thresholds tend to fall to a steady level approximately two months after implantation. The initial rise in thresholds is blunted with steroid eluting leads. Most contemporary RV pacing leads maintain a steady pacing threshold which is usually below 1 V amplitude at 0.5 ms pulse width, and many patients can be safely paced with outputs of 2 V [9].

As opposed to RV pacing, LV pacing threshold characteristics have been less well studied. We recently looked at the evolution of LV pacing thresholds over one year in 61 patients following CRT system implantation. The average LV voltage thresholds were twice as high as the RV thresholds (energy thresholds were four times as high) and demonstrated a slow increase over time (Fig. 9.2) [10]. LV thresholds in our series were similar [11] or somewhat higher [12]

than those found in previous series. There is limited information on LV thresholds beyond the first year of follow-up, but there are longer term data that have demonstrated relatively stable mean thresholds below 2 V up to three years post implant [13]. There are certainly a subset of patients with LV thresholds above 2.5 V necessitating high output programming at or above 5 V that will likely result in premature battery depletion. In one series of patients thresholds above 2.5 V were seen at three months following implantation in 25% of patients [14]. Figure 9.3 illustrates a typical case of early end-of-life (EOL) due to a need for high output programming in a first-generation CRT pacemaker.

Although data are scarce regarding battery longevity in CRT devices, it is conceivable that LV energy thresholds four times as high as RV combined with 100% ventricular pacing will significantly affect battery longevity. This problem was even more common with first-generation CRT devices which had a common output programming for both ventricles that was determined by the higher threshold of the two ventricles, usually the left. Contemporary dual chamber ICDs, even without CRT, often have longevity that hardly reaches four years. Most CRT-D devices are expected to have even shorter longevity that exaggerrates the "mismatch between patient longevity and device longevity" [15].

As safety is not the main issue in determining LV pacing outputs we tend to program our LV pacing amplitudes to values of 1.5–2 times the pacing threshold in order to prolong battery life. We also try to find the configuration with the lowest pacing thresholds, as detailed below.

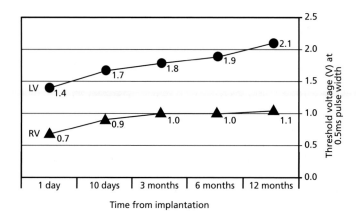

Figure 9.2 Evolution of LV pacing thresholds vs. RV pacing thresholds in 61 patients with CRT systems with CS LV lead (87% steroid eluting leads) [14].

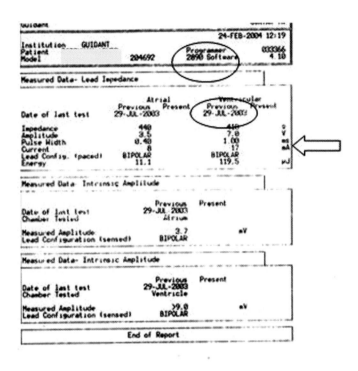

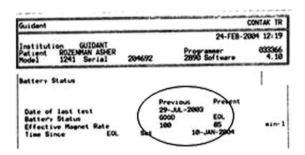

Figure 9.3 Short device longevity. Printout from a typical patient with a Contak TR (Guidant, Inc.) device programmed to pace at high output (7 V, arrow) due to high LV thresholds. The device reached end-of-life (EOL) two years after implantation, six months after the last checkup with no disclosed signs of impending elective replacement indicators (ERI) or EOL (ringed). Devices programmed in this way should be expected to drain early, and should be checked more frequently.

When pacing at high output cannot be avoided, frequent follow-up visits should be scheduled in anticipation of early pulse-generator battery depletion that may develop rapidly (Fig. 9.3).

Better lead design, better implantation techniques and capture verification algorithms [16] would contribute to resolving the problem of battery longevity of future CRT devices.

Anodal stimulation – an ECG curiosity or a clinically important phenomenon?

Myocardial pacing involves an electrical circuit being created between the cathode and the anode.

The cathode, located at the tip of the electrode, is by design smaller than the anode (either an electrically active collar proximal to the cathode in bipolar pacing configuration, or the pulse generator "can" in unipolar pacing configuration). The smaller surface area of the cathode results in higher current density. Therefore, under normal circumstances, the myocardial tissue adjoining the cathode is directly captured by the stimulus. High output pacing may result in current densities that are sufficiently strong to also capture myocardial tissue underlying the anode. This proarrhythmic condition [17] is termed "anodal stimulation." CRT devices, especially those with a unipolar LV lead, tend to use the RV ring or coil as an anode for LV pacing. When testing and programming LV output values one should be aware of the common phenomenon of anodal stimulation of the right ventricle which usually occurs with high output pacing when the RV ring or coil serves as the anode for LV pacing [18–20]. This phenomenon is more common with "true" rather than with "integrated" bipolar RV leads (using distal coil as anode), probably due to the smaller anodal surface area and thus higher current density of the former.

Anodal stimulation (also termed "triple site" pacing when it occurs during biventricular pacing) can be diagnosed when a sudden change in QRS morphology appears while decreasing the LV pacing output. This change is a manifestation of the loss of anodal capture while LV cathodal and RV cathodal capture continues. This change may be subtle, and may be better recognized with a 12-lead ECG than with a single channel monitor (Fig. 9.4A). The change is more easily recognizable in pacing only the left ventricle at decreasing amplitudes. In this case the QRS demonstrates a clear change in width and morphology (Fig. 9.4B).

Anodal capture has several clinical implications. As it is responsible for a sudden change in QRS morphology during threshold testing, loss of anodal capture may be misinterpreted as loss of LV capture during threshold testing, resulting in overestimation of LV threshold and excessive output programming. This phenomenon is more common with first-generation devices when thresholds are tested while pacing both ventricles and capture loss is determined by a change in the QRS morphology.

Anodal capture may also have some hemodynamic effects. In cases where LV only pacing is selected over biventricular pacing for hemodynamic reasons, RV anodal capture may be overlooked and has been shown to result in inconsistent hemodynamic improvement [20]. In serial evaluations of clinical or hemodynamic parameters (e.g by echo), it is very important to verify that values were taken consistently with the same mode of pacing (either with or without anodal capture). There are also hemodynamic differences between dual site and "triple site" pacing but their clinical significance is not established [18]. It also remains to be clarified whether anodal capture is arrhythmogenic in CRT patients.

(A)   (B)

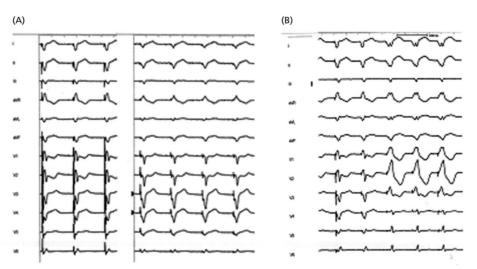

Figure 9.4 Anodal capture. (A) Biventricular pacing (LV tip to RV coil) in a patient with CRT device using 7.5 V (left) and 2 V (right). Left panel demonstrates ECG with anodal capture ("triple site pacing") and the right panel shows ECG with biventricular capture without anodal capture. The change in morphology may erroneously be misinterpreted as loss of LV capture and may result in programming excessive output energies. (B) Pacing the same patient – testing LV threshold (pacing LV only), using a configuration of LV tip to RV coil at decreasing outputs. With the decrease in output there is an abrupt change after the second beat in QRS width and morphology when anodal capture is lost but cathodal capture maintained.

Physicians who take care of CRT patients should be aware of the phenomenon of RV anodal capture in order to prevent threshold misinterpretation and to ensure consistent pacing over time with the same configuration to maintain hemodynamic benefit.

Unique programming issues in first-generation cardiac resynchronization therapy devices having a common ventricular channel

One of the unique features of first-generation CRT devices is that despite having separate ports for LV and RV leads, signals from both leads are processed through a common ventricular channel, and a common pacing output is split into the two ventricular leads. Given the long conduction times between the RV and LV lead tips in these patients (most of whom have a significant interventricular conduction delay that may exceed the ventricular blanking period), intrinsically conducted beats in these devices often result in double sensing and double counting of each beat on the ventricular channel (Fig. 9.5). Similarly, paced beats that capture only one of the ventricles are conducted slowly to the lead of the contralateral ventricle and are sensed there shortly after the pacing artifact (Fig. 9.6).

The phenomenon of double counting of intrinsically conducted beats could result in registration of

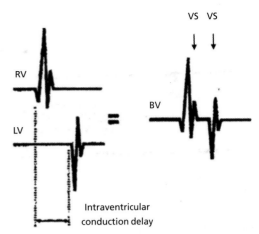

Figure 9.5 Double counting of an intrinsic beat in CRT systems with a common ventricular channel. Signals from both RV and LV leads, widely separated due to the conduction delay that exceeds the ventricular blanking period are combined to create two separate signals on the common ventricular channel (BV). Reproduced with permission of Guidant, Inc.

"high rate episodes" whenever there are several successive intrinsic beats (as discussed below under Use of Ventricular High Rate Episode Counter to Detect Double Counting in CRT Systems with a Common Ventricular Channel). Situations of intrinsic

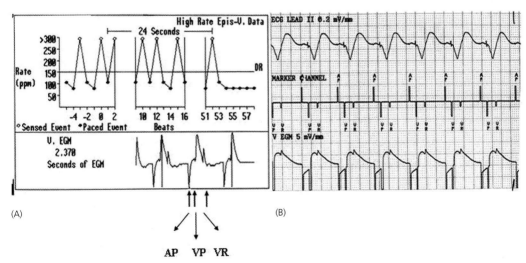

Figure 9.6 (A) The "high rate episode" is composed of alternating paced and sensed events in the ventricles (paced events are included in rate calculation of high rate episodes). The intervals as well as the captured EGM are consistent with atrial pacing (AP), ventricular pacing with capture at one ventricle (VP) with sensing of the evoked QRS by the contralateral ventricular lead (VR). This picture is typical of loss of capture in one ventricle (usually the left ventricle), which is confirmed by the real-time ECG (B). Increasing the output on the ventricular channel or repositioning of the CS lead is needed.

Table 9.1 Causes and prevention of intrinsic conduction and of consequent double counting

Cause of intrinsic conduction	Actions to consider
Intrinsic atrial/sinus rate above maximal tracking rate (MTR)	Ensure MTR above maximal achievable intrinsic rate at rest and during exercise
Intrinsic conduction time shorter than programmed atrioventricular delay	Ensure short atrioventricular delay at all circumstances (rest/exercise/sensed/paced)
Intrinsic P falls within PVARP due to long PVARP and long intrinsic PR	Ensure short PVARP Program tracking preference ON[b]
PVARP extended by double sensing on ventricular channel[a]	Cancel PVARP extension on PVC[a]
Atrial tachyarrhythmias with intact atrioventricular conduction	Increase maximal tracking rate, increase pacing rate during mode switch, atrioventricular nodal blockers, atrioventricular nodal ablation, program special features such as aggressive ventricular rate regularization and biventricular trigger[b]
Unilateral ventricular non-capture resulting in late sensing of V with subsequent PVARP[a]	Ensure consistent capture on both ventricles
Frequent ventricular premature contractions	Suppression by medications, program biventricular trigger[b]
Ventricular tachycardia	Suppress with medical/ablative treatment, change VF cutoff to prevent double counting as VF[a]

[a]Applies mainly to first-generation devices with a common ventricular channel.
[b]Applicable in advanced (non-first-generation) devices only.

conduction are listed in Table 9.1 and illustrated in Figs 9.7–9.9. In the case of the first-generation CRT-ICD demonstrated in Fig. 9.8, the phenomenon of double counting during intrinsic ventricular activation in a patient with atrial fibrillation leads to false ventricular fibrillation (VF) detection which may cause repeated inappropriate shocks and possible catastrophic consequences.

Double counting during ventricular tachycardia may also result in inappropriate VF therapies. Inap-propriate VF detection due to double counting was observed in one series in 17 out of 77 patients (22%) implanted with first generation CRT-ICD. Of these, 15 (88%) experienced inappropriate ICD therapy [21].

When a conducted beat occurs, either a premature ventricular beat (PVC) or one due to unilateral capture, loss of synchrony may be perpetuated by a peculiar mechanism. The second sensed component of the QRS (regarded by the device as PVC as it is not

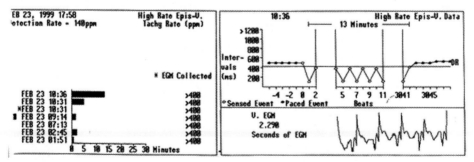

Figure 9.7 Interrogation of a first-generation pacemaker with a single channel sensing from both ventricles, in a patient with recent deterioration of his CHF status. There are prolonged "ventricular high rate episodes" in the common ventricular channel (left). A closer look at one of the episodes demonstrates initial tracking near the upper rate (that had been programmed to 120 bpm). As soon as the rate reaches the upper rate, intrinsic conduction takes over for 13 min as evidenced by the stored EGM. Since conducted QRS complexes are very wide they are being double sensed and are therefore counted as high rates. In first-generation devices ventricular high rates were often the clue to intrinsic conduction with loss of resynchronization.

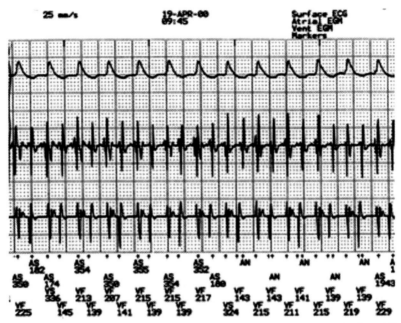

Figure 9.8 Example of double ventricular counting by a first-generation CRT-D during an episode of atrial fibrillation with rapid spontaneous ventricular response leading to false VF detection.

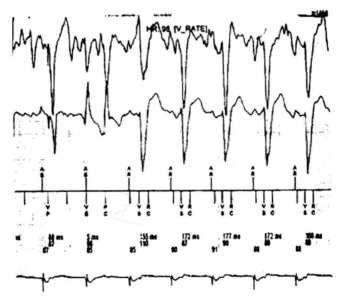

Figure 9.9 Mechanism of perpetuation of loss of synchrony due to extended PVARP in a device with a single channel for both ventricular leads. Having automatic PVC response programmed ON (as well as any other situation of long PVARP) may result in prolonged loss of biventricular synchronization. The first beat in the figure is a normally tracked sinus beat with capture of both ventricles. Following this, two PVCs (marked VS and PC) trigger an extension of PVARP due to "PVC response" algorithm.

The next sinus P wave falls into the extended PVARP (AR) and therefore is not tracked to the ventricles, resulting in atrioventricular nodal conduction manifested by wide QRS and double sensing. The second sensing that comes from the LV lead is again interpreted as a PVC (RC), PVARP extended again, next sinus beat is sensed within PVARP, and the mechanism is perpetuated for a very long time. PVC response should be turned off in biventricular pacemakers. Reproduced with permission of Medtronic, Inc.

preceded by a P wave) initiates another post-ventricular atrial refractory period (PVARP) that may sometimes be extended due to a post-PVC PVARP extension feature designed to prevent pacemaker-mediated tachycardia. As a result, the next sensed P wave may again fall into the PVARP, preventing ventricular tracking. In patients without atrioventricular block, intrinsic conduction to the ventricles will occur. The intrinsically conducted beat again has slow intramyocardial propagation, resulting in delayed sensing by the electrode located in the chamber ipsilateral to the patient's bundle branch block (LV electrode in patients with LBBB). Double counting occurs again, initiating a new PVARP that will again entrap the next spontaneous P wave, and so forth, in a self-perpetuating loop. The result is complete loss of biventricular pacing, and thus of CRT effect. This phenomenon is illustrated in Fig. 9.9, and is favored by long PR intervals and long PVARP, especially when the "PVC response" is programmed on for PVARP. The same mechanism is responsible for the phenomenon of perpetuation of intrinsic conduction when the upper rate is reached, and synchronization does not recover until the rate falls to a much lower rate than the upper tracking rate.

Figure 9.7 demonstrates an upper rate response that resulted in a 13 min loss of biventricular pacing. This occurred because once the upper tracking rate is reached (120 bpm in this example) in a patient with intact atrioventricular conduction system, intrinsic activation occurs, creating an extended PVARP. Under these circumstances the total atrial refractory period (TARP) may reach a much larger value which is explained by PR interval + time between two sensed components of the QRS + extended PVARP. This could reach lengths as great as 800 ms (250 + 150 + 400), thus delaying return to P-synchronous behavior until the sinus rate falls below 75 bpm. A similar, albeit less common, phenomenon may occur in patients with contemporary CRT devices who have a long intrinsic PR, long PVARP, and relatively rapid atrial rates. These will be discussed below.

Clinicians should keep in mind that one of the most important programming issues in first-generation CRT devices is prevention of intrinsic conduction and double counting with its consequences as previously described. Table 9.1 lists situations prone to double counting, and measures for prevention of intrinsic conduction are accordingly suggested.

Maintaining consistent biventricular capture and preventing intrinsic conduction

As benefits of CRT depend on the consistent capture of either both ventricles, or at least the left ventricle, capture should be maintained under all circumstances and under different physiologic conditions. Avoidance of intrinsic conduction is one of the most important steps in ensuring continuous biventricular pacing.

Methods to manage intrinsic conduction in the CRT patient include appropriate upper rate and atrioventricular delay programming, avoidance of unilateral loss of capture, short PVARP, avoidance of post-PVC PVARP extension, maintenance of higher pacing rates during mode switch, and the use of various pharmacological and ablative measures to suppress atrioventricular conduction (Table 9.1).

Unique programming features of cardiac resynchronization therapy devices
Special algorithms to maintain biventricular capture

The following features appear under different names in devices of various companies.

- Rate regularization, also termed "conducted AF response" is intended to maintain biventricular pacing during atrial fibrillation with irregular ventricular response. It is programmed to reduce RR variability and to preserve CRT delivery at a rate that slightly exceeds the rate of the intrinsic ventricular response, calculated on the basis of several preceding RR intervals. In cases when spontaneous conduction prevails during atrial fibrillation, aggressive programming of rate regularization may assist in maintaining biventricular pacing. The aggressiveness of regularization is programmable and may be adjusted based on diagnostic information from counters of percentage of paced beats during atrial fibrillation. Notably, rate regularization may be beneficial not only due to its effect on maintaining biventricular capture, but also due to the fact that ventricular cycle-length irregularity per se may severely affect both quality of life as well as myocardial function [22]. The use of rate regularization may be associated with some increase of the paced rate above the programmed lower rate or the programmed fallback lower rate. Figure 9.10 illustrates this feature and its effect in increasing the rate and in maintaining nearly 100% pacing.

- Biventricular trigger, also termed "ventricular sense response," has similarities to the VVT pac-

ing mode, and is designed to promote synchronization by pacing both ventricles immediately after an event (either a conducted beat or a PVC) is sensed by the RV lead. The biventricular trigger/ventricular sense response acts to enhance biventricular pacing during conducted atrial

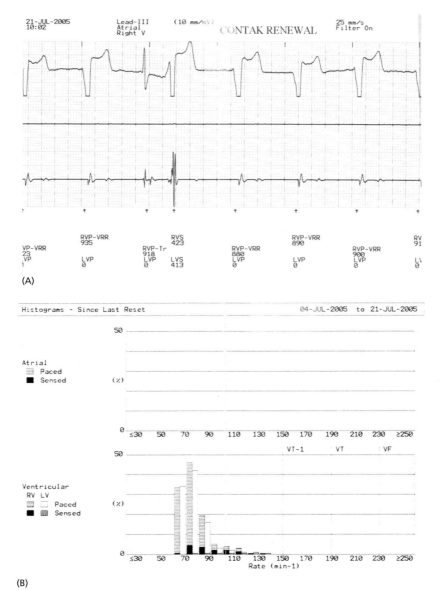

(A)

(B)

Figure 9.10 The effect of CRT maintenance mechanisms during AF in a patient with a Renewal 4 device programmed VVIR 60. (A) Real time telemetry. The first, fourth, fifth, and sixth beats are all paced at a rate higher than the lower rate due to ventricular rate regularization (designated VRR). The second beat is a conducted beat which immediately triggered pacing due to biventricular trigger (thus marked Tr). The third beat is a ventricular premature contraction (VPC) that was too early to activate biventricular trigger. As a result of the two mechanisms (VRR + TR) all beats in this tracing maintain biventricular capture. Indeed, the histogram of the patient at the same session (B) verifies high percentage pacing in both ventricles across all rates of AF.

fibrillation as well as when multiple PVCs disrupt normal synchronization. In patients with atrial fibrillation it should be used along with rate regularization to increase the percentage of paced ventricular beats (Fig. 9.10).

- Tracking preference, also termed "atrial tracking recovery," is designed to prevent the common occurrence where the sinus P wave falls repeatedly into the PVARP of the preceding beat due to a combination of relatively rapid rates (below maximal tracking rate (MTR)), long intrinsic atrioventricular conduction, long PVARP, and often initiated by a PVC. This may create prolonged episodes when CRT is not delivered secondary to intrinsic conduction causing ventricular pacing inhibition. As a potential solution to this problem, the device will automatically shorten the next PVARP when several successive beats occur in which RV sensing is preceded by a P wave that falls into the PVARP. The number of these beats differs according to the device and algorithm. This algorithm is illustrated in Fig. 9.11. The feature is optional, and should be programmed "on" when diagnostics demonstrate frequent sensed ventricular events suspected to have occurred as a result of a long TARP phenomenon.

Multiple programmable left ventricular pacing configurations – a tool or a toy?

Whereas conventional pacing systems have only two options for pacing configurations (unipolar and bipolar), some CRT systems have multiple programmable LV pacing configurations that use either the tip or the ring of the LV electrode as the cathode and the LV tip/ring, RV ring/coil, or the pulse generator "can" as the anode. Table 9.2 lists all available configurations in some of the currently available devices. Although there is no known consistent advantage of any one configuration over the others, in an individual patient this flexibility may help to overcome high LV pacing thresholds and avoid phrenic nerve stimulation.

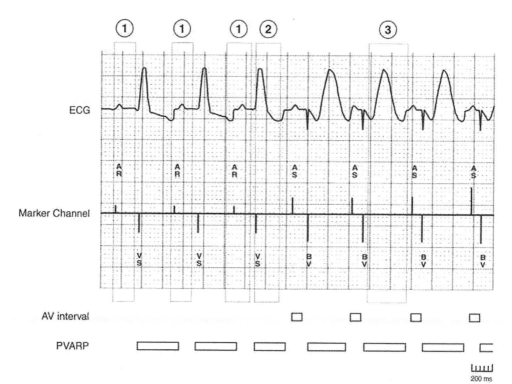

Figure 9.11 Atrial tracking recovery. After eight atrial events (1) occurring during PVARP (creating an AR–VS sequence) PVARP is shortened, thus the next atrial event is sensed (2) and subsequent beats are tracked again, with restitution of synchrony (3). Similar mechanisms exist in products of other manufacturers (e.g. tracking preference by Guidant). Reproduced with permission of Medtronic, Inc.

Table 9.2 Possible left ventricular pacing configurations according to device model[a]

	LV ring to RV coil	LV tip to RV coil	LV tip to LV ring	LV ring to LV tip	LV ring to RV ring	LV ring to can	LV tip to RV ring	LV tip to can
Guidant – H145			+	+	+	+	+	+
Guidant – H155	+	+	+	+				

[a]LV tip to LV ring was always the first configuration to be tested during implantation, and devices were initially programmed to this configuration.

We recently evaluated the utility of configuration changes in 43 patients with CRT or CRT-D systems with multiple programmable configurations, and compared them with 50 patients with systems lacking this feature [14]. Both patient groups had relatively frequent high LV pacing thresholds (30% and 50%, respectively, at some time during follow-up) and phrenic nerve stimulation (12% and 24%, respectively). However, while all cases with systems capable of programmable multiple LV pacing configurations could be solved by switching to another configuration, six patients (12%) that did not have extensive programmable configurations had to be re-operated or the LV lead abandoned due to loss of LV capture or intolerable phrenic nerve stimulation. Overall, we found this feature to be clinically useful in 42% of patients, helping to decrease pacing outputs and prevent phrenic nerve stimulation. Reducing pacing outputs by using the lowest capture threshold configuration may also contribute to increased battery longevity.

We recommend testing multiple LV pacing configurations when available in order to program the one with lowest myocardial capture threshold, and to avoid phrenic nerve stimulation.

Cardiac resynchronization therapy timing cycles and blanking periods

The fact that there is an additional lead for sensing and pacing the left ventricle adds to the complexity of timing cycles. Initially, first-generation CRT devices used inputs from both ventricular leads on a common channel. This approach created multiple problems as discussed above. Since the introduction of second-generation devices, each ventricle has been sensed separately. However, some devices ignore LV signals altogether thus following timing cycles based on RV signals only, similar to "regular" pacemakers, while in others LV sensing still has a limited role. The rationale behind this design is that

it was felt that ignoring signals originating from the left ventricle may at times create desynchronization or proarrhythmia and therefore developed special features that allow inhibition of LV pacing within a certain interval after an LV sensing event.

There are two features related to sensed LV events:

- Left ventricular protection period (LVPP) – prevents delivery of LV pacing shortly after an event has been sensed on the LV lead. This feature is designed to prevent potentially arrhythmogenic paced events during the LV vulnerable period (e.g. following a ventricular premature beat). Notably, when LVPP is programmed long it may compromise upper tracking rate, thus resulting in loss of biventricular pacing and resynchronization. Inappropriately long LVPP should be considered whenever a patient demonstrates pseudo-Wenckebach pacemaker behavior at rates lower than the programmed upper tracking rate. The importance of this feature in arrhythmia prevention remains to be established.
- Left ventricular refractory period limits the operation of LVPP during the initial period following an LV event by causing the device to ignore the very early sensed event.

Implantable cardioverter defibrillator programming issues in CRT-D patients

General principles of ICD programming are beyond the scope of this book. We will review only ICD programming issues that relate to CRT-D patients.

Shock energy programming and defibrillation thresholds

Numerous studies that looked at defibrillation thresholds (DFTs) describe low ejection fraction and advanced New York Heart Association (NYHA) class as predictors of high DFTs [23, 24]. Although information on DFTs in patients with CRT-D is limited, it is conceivable that the incidence of high DFTs in this population will be higher than in the general ICD population, and may encompass a significant proportion of CRT-D recipients. Although the issue of whether DFT testing should be performed is far from being resolved [23, 25], we feel that at least one induction during implantation is mandatory, in order to verify appropriate detection and conversion in this high-risk population. However, testing may be deferred according to the physician's discretion in patients whose risk of VF induction and conversion during implantation is prohibitive. These include patients with chronic atrial fibrillation in whom anticoagulation has been stopped in preparation for device implantation, and those with uncompensated and clinically significant heart failure. In these patients, DFT testing should be considered at a later stage when anticoagulation has been re-implemented, or heart failure symptoms better controlled.

Whether routine periodic evaluation of DFTs (or at least VF induction) should be performed is even more controversial than DFT testing during implantation, and many centers no longer perform routine VF induction [26].

Due to the expected high DFTs we tend to program maximal defibrillation energy in all CRT-D patients. When a patient is expected a priori to have high DFTs (such as with right-sided implantation or prior history of high DFTs) or in cases when DFT testing during implantation is considered unsafe (as detailed above) it is acceptable to implant high-energy devices.

Preliminary data suggest that the use of coronary sinus (CS) defibrillation leads may reduce DFTs. Anecdotal personal communications report off label use of ICD leads placed in the CS for pacing, sensing, and defibrillation. If substantiated by prospective studies, these data may pave the road for future use of this technology in resistant cases of high DFTs [27].

Anti-tachycardia pacing – right, left or both

Certain CRT-D devices enable anti-tachycardia pacing to be delivered from either the RV, LV lead, or both. Others devices use RV only anti-tachycardia pacing. Biventricular anti-tachycardia pacing seemed to perform better than RV pacing in the first InSync ICD trial [28] and this observation is supported by modeling of ventricular tachycardia wavefronts [29]. Ongoing studies are evaluating the efficacy of RV, LV, or biventricular anti-tachycardia pacing.

Rate smoothing – a useful tool or a double edge sword?

This feature is available in various models of CRT-D devices under different names (rate smoothing or rate stabilization). The relevancy of its perceived antiarrhythmic effect for CRT patients is attributed to the prevention of arrhythmogenic long–short sequences. The role of rate smoothing in long QT patients has already been shown and is based on a firm understanding of the sequence that leads to torsades de pointes in these cases [30]. It has been suggested that LV epicardial stimulation, as occurs with trans-CS LV pacing, prolongs the QT interval, and increases transmural dispersion of repolarization, which may contribute to arrhythmogenesis [31]. Therefore, it seems reasonable to expect that rate smoothing/rate stabilization may have an arrhythmia prevention effect in CRT patients. However, this hypothesis needs to be substantiated by clinical studies. Unpublished data in a study launched a number of years ago demonstrated some reduction in VT occurrence in ICD patients when rate smoothing was "on" [32]. Conversely, we [33] and others [34, 35] have shown that rate smoothing may adversely affect VT detection. At this stage we do not routinely use rate smoothing/rate stabilization in our CRT patients unless specifically indicated.

Diagnostic features for the management of cardiac resynchronization therapy

Apart from pacing and resynchronization of the failing heart, CRT devices, like other modern pacing systems, have the capability to acquire a significant amount of information regarding physiologic parameters. These data combine information from spontaneous atrial and ventricular electrical events sensed by intracardiac electrodes with other data collected by dedicated sensors imbedded in the pulse generator [36]. Overall, an abundance of clinically relevant information becomes available to the clinician, which may be used to improve patient follow-up and guide therapeutic decisions. Trans-telephonic transmitters are able to communicate diagnostic data from the device to care providers through specialized call centers, and emerging wireless technologies facilitate interrogation and transmission for the patient and the care providers, as well as enabling continuous data transfer. The physician is able to access these data through any internet-enabled PC (see section on Remote Patient Monitoring below).

Data provided by cardiac resynchronization devices should be made available not only to physicians who implant and follow patients with pacemakers. The data can be made available to all caregivers involved who may in turn familiarize themselves with device printouts and take advantage of relevant data in order to improve patient management.

In the future, device diagnostics will probably also include direct hemodynamic measurements from within the heart [37, 38]. These should become part of an auto-feedback mechanism [39–41], allowing the device to continuously optimize pacing parameters according to changes in the patient's hemodynamic status. For instance, heart rate, inter- and intraventricular and atrioventricular intervals may be modified on a beat to beat basis according to the patient's activity level, cardiac output, and lung fluid content. Such auto-feedback mechanisms are definitely more appropriate than current "fixed" programming to accommodate the changing needs of heart failure patients.

Like contemporary implantable pacemakers and defibrillators, cardiac resynchronization devices provide data regarding percentages of sensing and pacing, lead impedance, battery status, atrial and ventricular arrhythmias, etc. As these are thoroughly discussed in other pacing and ICD texts, this chapter will focus only on diagnostic features that are unique to cardiac resynchronization devices, and are aimed mainly at heart failure management. The use of intrathoracic impedance as an indicator for lung fluid content is discussed in Chapter 15 and heart rate variability (HRV) is discussed in Chapter 16. Examples of HRV monitoring are shown in Figs 9.12 and 9.13.

Verifying effective biventricular pacing

Effective CRT is obviously dependent on pacing the left ventricle the majority of the time. Spontaneous electrical events such as rapid atrial rates (either sinus tachycardia during exercise, or atrial arrhythmias) with rapid intrinsic ventricular response and frequent ventricular premature beats may reduce the amount of LV pacing and compromise effective CRT significantly. Several diagnostic features may be used to verify the adequacy of biventricular pacing delivery. These include counters of percentage of ventricular pacing, ventricular sensing episodes, and ventricular rate during atrial arrhythmias. For instance, the combination of atrial rates that are near or exceed the upper tracking rates and multiple ventricular sensed beats is typical of insufficient maximal tracking rate that should be increased. Potential programming measures to enhance biventricular pacing are suggested in the sections on

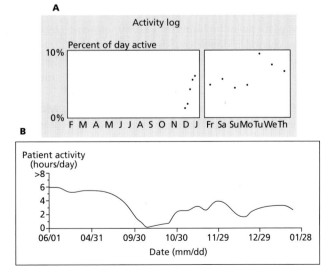

Figure 9.12 (A) Patient activity log representing weekly averages of percentage of day the patient was active for one year on the left, and average daily values for one week on the right. (B) A graph showing patient activity (expressed as hours active per day) for a one-year follow-up period. In September the patient was admitted to the hospital due to worsening heart failure. Reproduced with permission of Guidant, Inc.

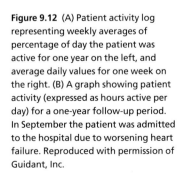

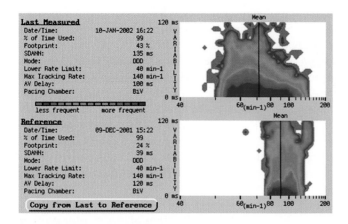

Figure 9.13 A heart rate variability (HRV) screen showing 24-h "footprint plot" (on top), compared with an older record (bottom). An obvious improvement in HRV indices over time is demonstrated by the increase in the percentage of the colored area of the plot from 24% in December to 43% in January. Note that in accordance with improvement in HRV, the lowest heart rate also decreased from 75 to 50 bpm. Reproduced with permission of Guidant, Inc.

Maintaining Consistent Biventricular Capture and Special Algorithms Aimed to Maintain Biventricular Capture in this chapter.

Use of ventricular high rate episode counter to detect double counting in cardiac resynchronization therapy systems with a common ventricular channel

While contemporary CRT devices have dedicated separate channels for the right and left ventricular leads, first-generation CRT systems have a common channel for both the right and left ventricular leads. These devices pose unique management challenges that may be tackled with the help of specific diagnostic tools. Please refer to previous discussion of this topic and underlying mechanisms under Unique Programming Issues in First-Generation Cardiac Resynchronization Therapy Devices.

One of the major problems with a common ventricular channel is double counting, which may be present during spontaneous non-paced ventricular events, as well as during paced ventricular events when loss of capture in one chamber occurs. Table 9.1 summarizes situations in which double counting may be encountered due to intrinsic conduction. Figures 9.6–9.9 illustrate various cases of double counting due to intrinsic conduction or unilateral non-capture. In Fig. 9.14 another unusual mechanism of double counting is illustrated where a patient had a coronary sinus lead positioned in a proximal location leading to non-capture of the left ventricle, and oversensing of left atrial events by the CS electrode leading to double ventricular counting.

One of the most valuable diagnostic tools to recognize the occurrence of double counting is the ventricular "high rate episode" counter. The typical event will have alternating beat to beat cycle lengths (Fig. 9.6A). The shorter cycle lengths represent double counting of the same beat and are equal to the time elapsing from the first chamber being activated or paced to the time that the beat is being sensed in the contralateral chamber. Therefore, the first signal of each pair may be a paced or a sensed signal (paced signal if non-capture underlies the double counting, sensed if any of the other mechanisms). The second signal is always a sensed signal coming from the chamber that is being activated later. An accompanying real-time ECG with markers (Fig. 9.6B) helps to verify the diagnosis by showing one QRS complex for each two ventricular markers. Diagnosing episodes of double counting should prompt the physician to solve the problem by either programming or repositioning of the LV lead (see previous section on Unique Programming Issues in First-Generation Cardiac Resynchronization Therapy Devices).

Monitoring patient physical activity level

Heart failure management is aimed at symptom reduction in order to enable patients to lead an active lifestyle. By monitoring a patient's activity levels the physician gains insight into the effects of medical and non-medical therapeutic measures. Patient activity, recorded by the device accelerometer function, is available in most devices, even when non-rate-adaptive pacing is programmed. The device registers

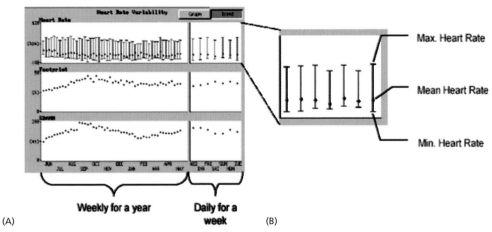

(A)

(B)

Figure 9.14 Graph showing heart rate variability trends over time. The left panel shows weekly means of lowest and highest heart rates (top panel), "footprint" values (middle panel), and standard deviation of normal to normal heartbeats (SDANN) values (bottom panel) for one year, while the right panel demonstrates mean daily values for one week. For each parameter lowest, highest, and average values can be retrieved. Reproduced with permission of Guidant, Inc.

the percentage of the day the patient's accelerometer indicated motion above the fixed threshold (for instance number of steps per minute walking, or heart rate above a pre-specified value). An activity log registers percentage of time the patient was active for every day of the last week, as well as average weekly data for one year (Fig. 9.14A). Alternatively, a graph shows evolution of patient activity expressed as average hours active per day over the follow-up period (Fig. 9.14B). Care providers may use patient activity data to detect early signs of heart failure worsening, as well as for monitoring response to treatment both for the individual patient, for study purposes, and to verify compliance to exercise regimens.

In a recent study [42] a measure of mean daily physical activity defined as more than 70 steps per minute walking showed gradual significant improvement over the first three months following CRT device implantation, which correlated with improvement in NYHA heart failure functional class and 6-minute walking distance.

Heart failure management reports

Most CRT devices will report some or all of the diagnostic parameters in a structured condensed heart failure report showing trends of atrial and ventricular arrhythmias, average day and night heart rates, atrial and ventricular pacing percentages, patient activ-

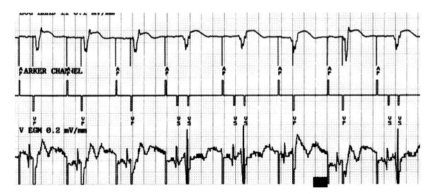

Figure 9.15 An example of double ventricular counting caused by a proximally located coronary sinus lead sensing left atrial activation on the ventricular channel of a first-generation CRT device.

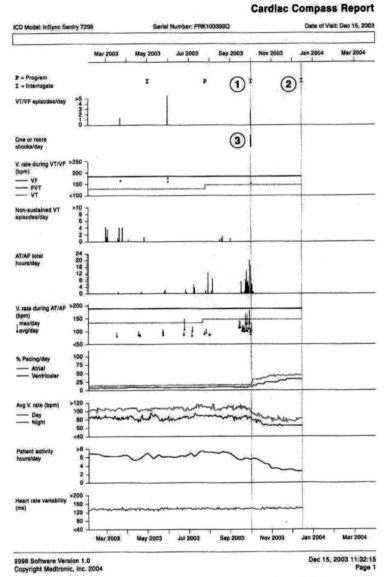

Figure 9.16 A condensed heart failure diagnostic report showing (from top to bottom) trends of VT/VF episodes per day, ventricular rates during VT/VF, number of non-sustained VT episodes per day, duration of atrial arrhythmias by hours per day, ventricular rates during atrial arrhythmias, percentage of atrial and ventricular pacing, average day and night ventricular rates, number of hours per day that the patient was active, and heart rate variability values over a follow-up period of six months. Reproduced with permission of Medtronic, Inc. Key: (1) last session indicator; (2) current session indicator; (3) high-voltage therapy indicator.

ity levels, heart rate variability, and in some newer devices also data regarding fluctuations in lung fluid content. In most cases care providers are able to specify the level of resolution for the sampling of data. For instance, sampling activity data may take place every 16 or every 60 min depending on physician's preferences. The type of data storage may also be specified in most cases, with "fixed storage" starting when setup is confirmed, and continuing until device memory storage is full, allowing the data to be viewed from initial setup for a fixed amount of time, or "continuous storage" that will overwrite new data on older records, allowing the clinician to view data for the recording duration immediately prior to data retrieval. Figure 9.16 shows an example of a condensed heart failure diagnostic report for a follow-up period of six months. In Fig. 9.17 a condensed heart failure report demonstrates clinical deterioration of the patient due to new onset of atrial fibrillation.

Remote patient management

In addition to in-clinic interrogation, CRT diagnos-

tic reports may also be transmitted electronically via the internet to care providers. This feature is currently available from several device manufacturers.

For home remote monitoring, two general technological approaches are currently in use. In one of them the patient initiates a session by putting a transmitter over the device that interrogates and transmits information through a home monitor

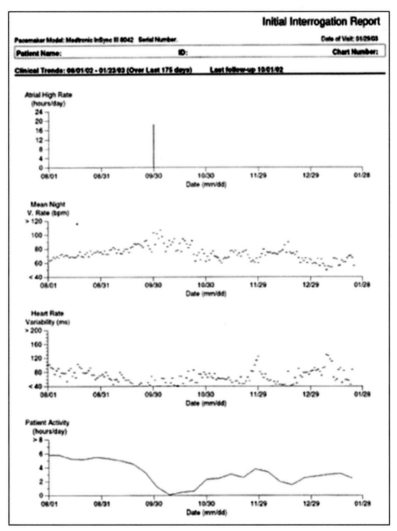

Figure 9.17 A heart failure diagnostic report showing signs of clinical deterioration due to new onset of atrial fibrillation. On the top panel the occurrence of an atrial high rate episode is noted on 30 September. This is accompanied by an increase in mean ventricular rate (second panel from top), and a decrease in patient activity (bottom panel). The patient was admitted to hospital and therapy for atrial fibrillation was initiated with gradual reduction of ventricular rates, and a concomitant improvement in patient activity. Note that the report also shows a decrease in HRV indices that accompanies the development of atrial fibrillation (third panel from top). However, this information should probably be disregarded since HRV can only be calculated from sinus beats. Reproduced with permission of Medtronic, Inc.

plugged into a phone line to a central secured computer. The other approach uses wireless technology in which the data is wirelessly transmitted by an internal antenna in the implantable device to a communicator unit that in turn transmits the information immediately to a central monitoring facility, accessible to physicians and other authorized users via the internet. The advantage of the latter approach is its ability to operate automatically and continuously or according to a schedule determined by the physician (as long as the patient is not very far from the base unit). It does not have to be actively triggered by the patient, and some systems may immediately transmit any real-time data including ongoing or recent arrhythmic events even before the patient is aware of them.

Using both methods, real-time EGM as well as data including device settings, battery status, lead impedance, signal amplitudes, atrial and ventricular arrhythmias, arrhythmia therapies and diagnostic information such as average heart rates, pacing percentages, patient activity, and heart rate variability are transmitted to a server facility. Call centers monitor transmitted data and forward them as scheduled (routine or on-demand interrogation) on a regular or on an urgent basis to care providers. These centers may also serve as trans-telephonic patient and physician support (Fig. 9.18).

Customized rules can be implemented to define different levels of alert situations indicating the degree of urgency with which physicians and patients need to be contacted. Care providers are able to access patient and device data from any internet-enabled PC. External sensors like weight scales and blood pressure cuffs and ability to answer symptom-related questions using the home communicator screen may also be added to the system, to transmit additional diagnostic information that is not available from the device. Remote home monitoring systems are especially important for patients living in remote areas, where access to a dedicated device outpatient clinic is limited. However, they may also prove to be very helpful in patients with congestive heart failure (CHF), where early detection of trends of impending decompensation may trigger steps to prevent further deterioration and hospitalization.

References

1 Janosik DL, Ellenbogen KA. Basic physiology of cardiac pacing and pacemaker syndrome. In: Ellenbogen KA, Kay GN, Wilkoff BL. eds. *Clinical Cardiac Pacing and Defibrillation*, 2nd edn. WB Saunders, Philadelphia, 2000: 333–382.
2 Delfaut P, Saksena S, Prakash A, Krol RB. Long-term outcome of patients with drug-refractory atrial flutter and fibrillation after single- and dual-site right atrial pacing

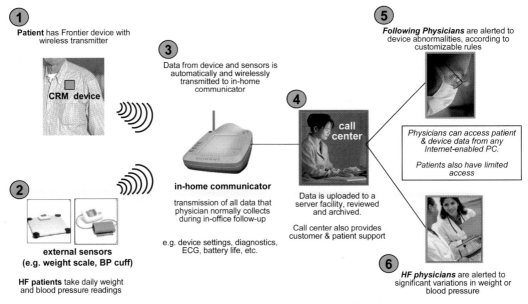

Figure 9.18 A wireless patient management system. Reproduced with permission of Guidant, Inc.

for arrhythmia prevention. *J Am Coll Cardiol* 1998; **32**: 1900–1908.

3 Bernheim A, Ammann P, Sticherling C *et al.* Right atrial pacing impairs cardiac function during resynchronization therapy: acute effects of DDD pacing compared to VDD pacing. *J Am Coll Cardiol* 2005; **45**: 1482–1487.

4 Young JB, Abraham WT, Smith AL *et al.* Combined cardiac resynchronization and implantable cardioversion defibrillation in advanced chronic heart failure: the MIRACLE ICD Trial. *JAMA* 2003; **289**: 2685–2694.

5 Bristow MR, Saxon LA, Boehmer J *et al.* Cardiac-resynchronization therapy with or without an implantable defibrillator in advanced chronic heart failure. *N Engl J Med* 2004; **350**: 2140–2150.

6 Abraham WT, Fisher WG, Smith AL *et al.* Cardiac resynchronization in chronic heart failure. *N Engl J Med* 2002; **346**: 1845–1853.

7 Cleland JG, Daubert JC, Erdmann E *et al.* The effect of cardiac resynchronization on morbidity and mortality in heart failure. *N Engl J Med* 2005; **352**: 1539–1549.

8 Barold SS, Herweg B. Upper rate response of biventricular pacing devices. *J Interv Card Electrophysiol* 2005; **12**: 129–136.

9 Mond HG. Engineering and clinical aspects of pacing leads. In: Ellenbogen KA, Kay GN, Wilkoff B, eds. *Clinical Cardiac Pacing and Defibrillation*, 2nd edn. WB Saunders, Philadelphia, 2000: 127–150.

10 Gurevitz O, Granit C, Carasso S *et al.* Evolution of left and right ventricular capture thresholds over time in patients receiving cardiac resynchronization therapy (abstract). *Heart Rhythm* 2005; **2**: S289.

11 Achtelik M, Bocchiardo M, Trappe HJ *et al.* Performance of a new steroid-eluting coronary sinus lead designed for left ventricular pacing. *Pacing Clin Electrophysiol* 2000; **23**: 1741–1743.

12 Tse HF, Yu C, Lee KL *et al.* Initial clinical experience with a new self-retaining left ventricular lead for permanent left ventricular pacing. *Pacing Clin Electrophysiol* 2000; **23**: 1738–1740.

13 Wheelan KR, Young JB, Abraham WT, Johnson WB, Witte LJ, Harsch MR. Left ventricular lead thresholds remain stable 36 months post implant in patients with heart failure. *Heart Rhythm* 2005; **2**: S169.

14 Gurevitz O, Tanami N, Luria D, Bar-Lev D, Eldar M, Glikson M. CRT systems with programmable multiple pacing configurations and a bipolar LV lead may help to maintain capture, conserve battery life and avoid phrenic nerve stimulation. *Europace* 2005; **7**: S158.

15 Hauser RG. The growing mismatch between patient longevity and the service life of ICDs. *J Am Coll Cardiol* 2005; **45**: 2022–2025.

16 Biffi M, Boriani G, Bertini M, Silvestri P, Martignani C, Branzi A. Pacing with capture verification in candidates

for resynchronisation therapy: a feasibility study. *Europace* 2005; **7**: 255–265.

17 Ellenbogen K, Kay N, Willkoff B. *Clinical Cardiac Pacing and Defibrillation*, 2nd edn. WB Saunders, Philadelphia, 2000.

18 Bulava A, Ansalone G, Ricci R *et al.* Triple-site pacing in patients with biventricular device-incidence of the phenomenon and cardiac resynchronization benefit. *J Interv Card Electrophysiol* 2004; **10**: 37–45.

19 van Gelder BM, Bracke FA, Pilmeyer A, Meijer A. Triple-site ventricular pacing in a biventricular pacing system. *Pacing Clin Electrophysiol* 2001; **24**: 1165–1167.

20 Thibault B, Roy D, Guerra PG *et al.* Anodal right ventricular capture during left ventricular stimulation in CRT-implantable cardioverter defibrillators. *Pacing Clin Electrophysiol* 2005; **28**: 613–619.

21 Chugh A, Scharf C, Hall B *et al.* Prevalence and management of inappropriate detection and therapies in patients with first-generation biventricular pacemaker-defibrillators. *Pacing Clin Electrophysiol* 2005; **28**: 44–50.

22 Melenovsky V, Hay I, Fetics BJ *et al.* Functional impact of rate irregularity in patients with heart failure and atrial fibrillation receiving cardiac resynchronization therapy. *Eur Heart J* 2005; **26**: 705–711.

23 Russo AM, Sauer W, Gerstenfeld EP *et al.* Defibrillation threshold testing: Is it really necessary at the time of implantable cardioverter-defibrillator insertion? *Heart Rhythm* 2005; **2**: 456–461.

24 Shukla HH, Flaker GC, Jayam V, Roberts D. High defibrillation thresholds in transvenous biphasic implantable defibrillators: clinical predictors and prognostic implications. *Pacing Clin Electrophysiol* 2003; **26**: 44–48.

25 Strickberger SA, Klein GJ. Is defibrillation testing required for defibrillator implantation? *J Am Coll Cardiol* 2004; **44**: 88–91.

26 Glikson M, Friedman P. Routine arrhythmia inductions for ICD follow-up: are they obsolete? *Pacing Clin Electrophysiol* 2001; **24**: 915–920.

27 Butter C, Meisel E, Tebbenjohanns J *et al.* Transvenous biventricular defibrillation halves energy requirements in patients. *Circulation* 2001; **104**: 2533–2538.

28 Kuhlkamp V. Initial experience with an implantable cardioverter-defibrillator incorporating cardiac resynchronization therapy. *J Am Coll Cardiol* 2002; **39**: 790–797.

29 Byrd IA, Rogers JM, Smith WM, Pollard AE. Comparison of conventional and biventricular antitachycardia pacing in a geometrically realistic model of the rabbit ventricle. *J Cardiovasc Electrophysiol* 2004; **15**: 1066–1077.

30 Viskin S, Glikson M, Fish R, Glick A, Copperman Y, Saxon LA. Rate smoothing with cardiac pacing for preventing torsade de pointes. *Am J Cardiol* 2000; **86**(suppl 1): K111–K115.

31 Fish JM, Di Diego JM, Nesterenko V, Antzelevitch C.

Epicardial activation of left ventricular wall prolongs QT interval and transmural dispersion of repolarization: implications for biventricular pacing. *Circulation* 2004; **109**: 2136–2142.

32 Fromer M, Wietholt D. Algorithm for the prevention of ventricular tachycardia onset: the Prevent Study. *Am J Cardiol* 1999; **83**: 45D–47D.

33 Glikson M, Beeman A, Luria DM, Hayes DL, Friedman PA. Impaired detection of ventricular tachyarrhythmias by a rate-smoothing algorithm in dual-chamber implantable defibrillators: Intradevice interactions. *J Cardiovasc Electrophysiol* 2002; **13**: 312–318.

34 Cooper JM, Sauer WH, Verdino RJ. Absent ventricular tachycardia detection in a biventricular implantable cardioverter-defibrillator due to intradevice interaction with a rate smoothing pacing algorithm. *Heart Rhythm* 2004; **1**: 728–731.

35 Shivkumar K, Feliciano Z, Boyle NG, Wiener I. Intradevice interaction in a dual chamber implantable cardioverter defibrillator preventing ventricular tachyarrhythmia detection. *J Cardiovasc Electrophysiol* 2000; **11**: 1285–1288.

36 Kadhiresan K, Carlson G. The role of implantable sensors for management of heart failure. *Stud Health Technol Inform* 2004; **108**: 219–227.

37 Adamson PB, Magalski A, Braunschweig F *et al.* Ongoing right ventricular hemodynamics in heart failure: clinical value of measurements derived from an implantable monitoring system. *J Am Coll Cardiol* 2003; **41**: 565–571.

38 Braunschweig F, Linde C, Eriksson MJ, Hofman-Bang C, Ryden L. Continuous haemodynamic monitoring during withdrawal of diuretics in patients with congestive heart failure. *Eur Heart J* 2002; **23**: 59–69.

39 Griesbach L, Gestrich B, Wojciechowski D *et al.* Clinical performance of automatic closed-loop stimulation systems. *Pacing Clin Electrophysiol* 2003; **26**: 1432–1437.

40 Occhetta E, Bortnik M, Audoglio R, Vassanelli C. Closed loop stimulation in prevention of vasovagal syncope. Inotropy Controlled Pacing in Vasovagal Syncope (IN-VASY): a multicentre randomized, single blind, controlled study. *Europace* 2004; **6**: 538–547.

41 Rom R, Erel J, Glikson M, Rosenblum K, Ginosar R. Adaptive cardiac resynchronization therapy device: A simulation report. *Pacing Clin Electrophysiol* (in press).

42 Braunschweig F, Mortensen PT, Gras D *et al.* Monitoring of physical activity and heart rate variability in patients with chronic heart failure using cardiac resynchronization devices. *Am J Cardiol* 2005; **95**: 1104–1107.

SECTION 4

Implantation

CHAPTER 10

Implantation techniques for cardiac resynchronization therapy

Michael O. Sweeney, MD

Implementation of cardiac resynchronization therapy

There are currently three approaches to achieving left ventricular (LV) pacing. The transvenous approach utilizes specially designed delivery sheaths and tools for cannulating the coronary sinus in order to permit delivery of pacing leads into the epicardial coronary venous circulation. LV pacing lead placement can also be achieved under direct visualization using a cardiac surgical approach. Finally, transvenous LV endocardial pacing via trans-septal puncture has been described in the rare circumstance where neither the transvenous epicardial nor surgical options are viable [1–3].

Approach to transvenous left ventricular lead placement

Early attempts at epicardial LV pacing via the coronary veins utilized standard endocardial pacing leads designed for right ventricular (RV) pacing or coronary sinus (CS) leads designed for left atrial pacing [4]. This approach was met with predictable difficulties, including inability to cannulate the coronary sinus and first or second order target veins, unacceptably high epicardial pacing thresholds, and a high incidence of lead dislodgement. Experienced implanters using currently available tools, techniques, and leads specifically designed for coronary veins can achieve optimal LV stimulation in >90% of cases. The techniques for transvenous delivery of cardiac resynchronization therapy (CRT) have been previously described [5]. Some technical aspects merit special mention in order to increase the probability of achieving an optimal LV stimulation site.

Preparing the patient for cardiac resynchronization therapy device implantation

The preparation of the patient for CRT implantation is superficially similar to conventional transvenous cardiac pacing and defibrillation. However, because candidates for CRT have advanced systolic heart failure, meticulous management of the procedural process is mandated to reduce the risk of complications.

Hydration and cardiovascular medications

The matter of optimal volume status for CRT implantation contains an inherent conflict. The patient must be able to lie comfortably flat for several hours. Therefore, there is a desire to optimize the patient's volume status with diuretics prior to the procedure. However, relative volume depletion in the preload dependent patient may increase risk for procedural hypotension. Such patients are often unpredictably sensitive to the venodilating effects of intravenous conscious sedation and even small volume blood loss. On the other hand, agitation due to air hunger in the supine volume overloaded patient may be misinterpreted as anxiety or pain. Excessive administration of sedation in this situation may precipitate acute respiratory failure and result in premature termination of the procedure.

Therefore, a practical balance must be achieved between these two competing needs. The patient's diuretic program should be adjusted to achieve a "dry" weight the evening prior to the procedure. During overnight fasting, intravenous fluids should be administered to replace insensible losses (i.e. dextrose 5% with saline at 75 mL/h). Electrolytes should be measured and replaced as needed coincident with pre-procedural maintenance hydration. In particular, every effort should be made to prevent hypokalemia or hyperkalemia, either of which may increase the risk of procedure-related arrhythmia. Most experts recommend that the serum potassium be targeted in the 4.0–5.0 mmol/L range during chronic heart failure management. It is reasonable to withhold some cardiovascular medications such as afterload reducing agents (angiotensin-converting enzyme (ACE) inhibitors, angiotensin receptor blockers, nitrates, hydralazine), and beta blockers on the morning of the procedure to reduce the risk of intraoperative hypotension related to intravenous conscious sedation.

Many patients with advanced heart failure have impaired renal function due to atherosclerotic disease, chronic underperfusion due to reduced cardiac output, or diabetes. The risk of contrast-induced nephrotoxicity increases progressively when the serum creatinine exceeds 1.6 mg/dL. In elderly heart failure patients or others with low muscle mass the serum creatinine levels often underestimate the glomerular filtration rate. Preoperative hydration may reduce the risk of contrast-induced nephrotoxicity. Serum creatinine greater than or equal to 2.5 mg/dL in men or greater than or equal to 2.0 mg/dL in women may identify patients at particularly high risk for contrast-induced nephrotoxicity. This risk may be reduced by pre-treatment with *n*-acetylcysteine (i.e. 600 mg twice daily, beginning the day prior to the procedure and continued for 2 days post procedure).

Anticoagulation

Ideally, chronic anticoagulation can be completely reversed pre-operatively and resumed in a leisurely manner post-operatively in order to reduce the risk of intra-operative bleeding and post-operative pocket hematoma. This is often possible in many low-risk patients who are receiving anticoagulation for stroke prophylaxis in the setting of reduced ejection fraction, paroxysmal atrial fibrillation, or permanent atrial fibrillation with no prior history of embolic stroke. In these situations, the incidence of embolic stroke in the absence of anticoagulation is extremely low.

However, in many patients chronic anticoagulation cannot be safely withheld for more than 24 h because of embolic risk (i.e. mechanical valve prostheses or history of embolic stroke). There are two approaches in this situation. The first is to discontinue coumadin several days in advance of the procedure and bridge anticoagulation with intravenous unfractionated heparin or subcutaneous low molecular weight heparin. Intravenous unfractionated heparin should be discontinued at least 5 h prior to the scheduled procedure, whereas the last dose of subcutaneous low molecular weight heparin should be given 24 h prior to the procedure, particularly in patients with impaired renal function. Either form of heparin is then typically resumed 12 h post-operatively along with coumadin until the International Normalized Ratio (INR) is in the appropriate target range. The disadvantages of this approach are the costs associated with the medication (particularly low molecular weight heparin) and the extended hospitalization and the significantly increased risk of a pocket hematoma due to anticoagulation overshoot.

An alternative approach is to perform CRT implantation with a therapeutic INR (range 2–3). This eliminates the need for interruption of anticoagulation and the use of post-operative unfractionated or low molecular weight heparin, which is associated with significant increased risk of pocket hematoma. For some implanters, this decision is influenced by the presence or absence of prior cardiac surgery. The risk of tamponade in the event of myocardial penetration or coronary venous laceration is remote due to the chronic adhesive pericarditis that follows pericardiotomy. This is an entirely different matter among patients with no prior history of cardiac surgery and in this situation it is prudent to include the subxyphoid space in the surgical preparation in case urgent pericardiocentesis is needed.

Most experienced implanters recognize that the bleeding risks of antiplatelet therapy are far greater than antithrombotic therapy with coumadin. Recommendations for discontinuation of antiplatelet therapy are similar to those for cardiac surgery. Aspirin can generally be safely continued, but thienopyridines (clopidogrel, ticlopidine) should be discontinued for at least 5 days, and preferably 7 days prior to the procedure. This recommendation is based on the excess bleeding among patients undergoing coronary artery bypass surgery for acute coronary syndromes after receiving thienopyridines [6].

Surgical approach
Right- versus left-sided approach

Many electrophysiologists are familiar with the right superior approach to CS cannulation via the internal jugular vein for placement of diagnostic electrophysiology catheters. A potential advantage to CRT implantation from the right-sided approach, besides this familiarity, is that the fluoroscopic tube does not interfere with the implanter when lateral views are used for CS cannulation, venography, and LV lead placement. There are two potential disadvantages to the right-sided approach. First, manipulation of the CS guiding sheaths and LV lead may be constrained by the two opposing 90-degree curves at the junction of the right subclavian vein and superior vena cava and the low right atrium and coronary sinus ostium. Secondly, right-sided pectoral implantable cardioverter defibrillator (ICD) implantation has been associated with higher defibrillation threshold energy requirements [7, 8]. For experienced implanters, the choice of approach is unlikely to be influenced by these considerations.

The left-sided approach has an anatomic advantage since the path of the CS guiding sheaths and LV lead pursues a gentle C-shaped curve from the left innominate vein to the superior vena cava (SVC), low right atrium (RA) and CS ostium. This reduces binding points that may impede sheath and lead manipulation. Lateral fluoroscopic views are awkward, however, because the fluoroscopic tube often interferes with the implanter's upper body and the image intensifier collides with the implanter's body/head. This is a relatively minor inconvenience that can be overcome by using shallow left anterior oblique views (i.e. 45 degrees) and cranial or caudal angulation.

Venous access

The technique of obtaining venous access should minimize the chance of lead damage, which is mainly due to mechanical stress at the sterno-clavicular joint due to poor implantation technique. Conventional pacemaker and ICD leads can be implanted using a cephalic vein cutdown with peel away sheaths and a retained guidewire [9]. This approach eliminates the possibility of sterno-clavicular "crush" and

should be recommended. Some implanters have reported good experience with a cephalic guidewire approach for three CRT pacing leads (but not ICD leads) [10]. However, it is often the case that the small-diameter cephalic vein cannot accommodate a right atrial pacing lead, an RV ICD lead, and the CS guiding sheath for LV leads delivery, or lead–lead interaction renders this approach unnecessarily difficult. In this situation, or when the cephalic vein is absent or cannot be navigated with a guidewire, an axillary vein puncture is recommended to reduce the risks of sterno-clavicular "crush" and pneumothorax associated with subclavian vein puncture [11, 12]. The axillary vein puncture should be done after the cephalic vein is cannulated but before the RA and RV leads are placed, using either the guidewire or contrast injection for visualization of the cephalic–axillary juncture.

"Planning" retrograde coronary venogram

Some implanters prefer to do a "planning" retrograde coronary venogram (see also below, Retrograde Coronary Venography) the day prior to CRT implantation. This is often done from the right internal jugular approach, similar to an electrophysiology procedure. The arguments in favor of this approach include spacing the contrast dye load over 2 days in order to reduce nephrotoxicity and a detailed examination of the coronary venous anatomy to better inform the surgical approach. This 2-day strategy is impractical in many centers and the additional costs of hospitalization cannot be justified. More recently, non-invasive visualization of the coronary sinus and its tributaries by fast CT has been proposed. Experience with this technique is considerably limited and the quality of images is still relatively low.

Some implanters prefer to place a temporary transvenous pacing wire from femoral approach in almost all patients, but particularly those patients with non-ischemic dilated cardiomyopathy and proximal left bundle branch block (LBBB) in order to prevent asystole caused by traumatic atrioventricular block which occurs in 1–2% of cases [13]. Placement of a temporary transvenous pacing wire can be easily combined with a planning retrograde coronary venogram. The Swartz SL-3 ablation sheath (St. Jude Medical) is ideally suited for this purpose (see below) [14]. A slight counterclockwise rotation of the tip of this sheath in the low right atrium usually permits engagement of the CS ostium in less than 1–2 min in most patients. After the retrograde CS venogram is performed, the sheath is withdrawn into the right atrium and rotated clockwise, and a temporary transvenous pacing wire is then advanced through the sheath and into the right ventricle. The tip of the sheath is preferentially positioned anteriorly and the temporary wire is placed in the RV inflow, so as not to interefere with subsequent RV lead placement and CS cannulation from the superior approach.

Approach to left ventricular lead placement using the coronary veins
Order of lead placement
The RV lead should be placed first in all circumstances, even if a temporary RV pacing wire is in place. The rationale, as noted above, is that repeated attempts to cannulate the CS may result in traumatic atrioventricular (AV) block due to bumping of the compact AV node or the proximal right bundle branch (see above). Many implanters prefer to place the right atrial lead second so that no further manipulations are needed after LV lead placement and CS guiding sheath removal. Coronary sinus cannulation and LV lead placement are therefore the last stage of the procedure.

Coronary sinus cannulation
Early attempts at LV pacing via the coronary veins were done with conventional endocardial pacing leads and unassisted CS cannulation. This was only possible with stylet-driven leads and required considerable technical prowess. The technique mandated selective bending of stylets to achieve a favorable shape of the tip of the lead to permit CS cannulation. Additional stylet shapes were necessary to permit engagement of the ostium of first and second order coronary venous branches. Some contemporary implanters continue to advocate this approach [10], though this often requires tedious and needlessly heroic stylet and lead manipulations. However, there is no obvious merit to this approach except to eliminate the use of CS guiding sheaths, which may reduce the chances of implant success, particularly in difficult anatomic situations.

Typically, the CS is cannulated with a pre-shaped sheath that serves as a workstation for retrograde coronary venography and LV lead placement. First-generation sheaths were straight or minimally curved and had two immediately obvious limitations relating to RA and CS anatomy. First, straight sheaths tended to track along the lateral RA wall. Consequently, the tip of the sheath often did not reach the CS ostium, or only with great difficulty, especially in patients with marked RA enlargement (such as is often encountered in permanent atrial fibrillation) (Fig. 10.1). Secondly, the tip of the straight sheath would often fall abruptly to the floor of the RA upon removal from the CS, dislodging the LV lead (see below).

Recognition of these limitations resulted in the development of CS sheaths with a variety of diameters and shapes intended to overcome unpredictable anatomic variation in right heart chamber dimensions and orientation due to remodeling. Most

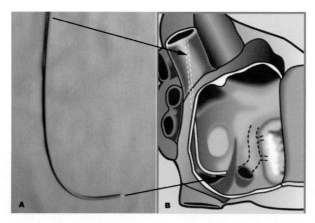

Figure 10.1 Coronary sinus sheath with minimal primary curve. Note tip of sheath is directed towards the floor of the right atrium, rather than the CS ostium. See text. Reproduced from www.bivtips.com with permission of Seth Worley, MD.

designs incorporate a J-shaped primary curve that directs the tip towards the CS ostium. Additionally, the heel of the curve rests on the floor of the RA and provides support during sheath removal from the CS, reducing LV lead dislodgement (Fig. 10.2). Some sheaths also incorporate an Amplatz-type secondary curve at the tip to facilitate CS cannulation or even sub-selection of proximal first-order coronary veins (see below).

Though such sheaths permit unassisted cannulation of the CS ostium in some cases, most implanters assist CS cannulation using a deflectable electrophysiology catheter, a coronary angiography catheter or a hydrophilic coated 0.038″ guidewire within the CS

guiding sheath. Increasingly elaborate technologies to assist with CS cannulation have been developed, including deflectable inner guides capable of contrast dye injection, ultrasound catheters and infrared imaging [15]. All of these are quite expensive and whether they are worth the cost is debatable, since coronary angiography catheters are quite cheap. A less expensive technique utilizes an Amplatz AL-3 coronary guide catheter, which has primary and secondary curves uniquely suited to CS cannulation.

The technique of CS cannulation using an Amplatz AL-3 coronary guide catheter within the CS sheath is as follows (Fig. 10.3). The sheath is advanced using a straight dilator over a wire to the

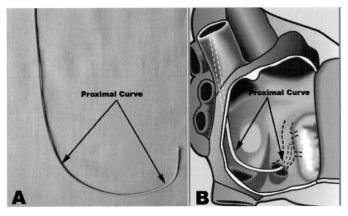

Figure 10.2 Coronary sinus sheath with large J-shaped primary curve. Note tip of sheath is directed towards the CS ostium. Reproduced from www.bivtips.com with permission of Seth Worley, MD.

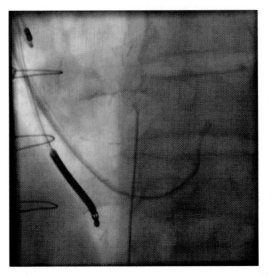
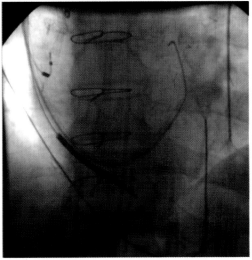

Figure 10.3 Coronary sinus cannulation using a coronary guide catheter (AL-3) and an over-the-wire technique. Note LV lead delivery sheath within main body of coronary sinus.

mid right atrium. When the dilator is removed, the distal segment of the sheath will begin to assume the primary curve and the tip will begin to point slightly upwards towards the tricuspid valve orifice. The guide catheter is then advanced over the guidewire until the tip and primary curve extend just beyond the sheath tip. Despite radiographic markers, the tip of the guide catheter is often difficult to see and visualization is improved by positioning the tip of the guidewire flush with the tip of the sheath. The tip of the guide catheter is then advanced and directed posteriorly by applying counterclockwise rotation. Localization of the CS ostium is greatly facilitated by stored fluoroscopic images if a planning venogram from either the superior or inferior approach was previously performed (see above). Engagement of the CS ostium results in a characteristic "rocking" motion of the guide catheter due to systolic movement of the AV groove that is transmitted as a tapping tactile sensation to the fingertips. The absence of ventricular ectopy, though cited by some implanters as useful, is an unreliable indicator of successful CS cannulation because catheter manipulation in the RV outflow tract may not result in ectopy and guidewire or catheter manipulation in the coronary sinus may elicit ectopy. Proper positioning of the guidewire or guide catheter in the CS is best demonstrated by lateral fluoroscopic views (30 or 45 degree left anterior oblique projection) or a small contrast injection. In any event, a similar technique for CS cannulation is applied with a deflectable electrophysiology catheter or any other inner guide.

Once the CS is cannulated a floppy tip guidewire is advanced into the main body CS. Depending upon the diameter of the guide sheath and the LV lead, it may be possible to leave this guidewire in place to facilitate re-cannulation in the event that sheath manipulations or LV lead placement result in dislodgement. The sheath is then advanced into CS using the guidewire and/or catheter as a railing system (Fig. 10.3). Often there is some resistance to sheath advancement due to binding at the CS ostium or within the main body of the CS. The latter typically occurs when the tip of the sheath is not coaxially aligned with the outer wall of the CS. Anatomic explanations for resistance to sheath advancement include the valve of Vieussens, present in ~80–90% of hearts, or an acute bend in the great

cardiac vein, found in ~50–60% of hearts [16]. The precise cause of resistance can be impossible to discern by fluoroscopic examination and is denoted by a tendency of the sheath to back out into the low RA during attempted advancement. The implanter must train their eye to monitor the main body CS and the RA, rather than just the tip of the sheath during advancement. There is a tendency amongst novice implanters to push harder when resistance is encountered, which inevitably results in complete displacement of the sheath into the RA. Forward resistance to sheath advancement can be overcome by advancing the guidewire and guide catheter deeper into the CS and applying clockwise or counterclockwise rotational torque to the sheath until advancement is possible, which often occurs as a sudden forward "jump." The guide catheter can then be removed. Some implanters prefer to leave the guidewire in place (above), but many smaller diameter sheath systems do not permit this. Even so, the retained CS guidewire often interferes with LV lead manipulation and has to be abandoned.

Retrograde coronary venography

Once the CS is successfully cannulated, retrograde venography is performed to delineate the coronary venous anatomy (Fig. 10.4). The importance of a complete and accurate coronary venogram to identify optimal target veins for LV stimulation cannot be overstated. This is done with a standard balloon occlusion catheter and hand injections of contrast dye. Underfilling the coronary venous system is a common mistake that may result in failure to identify potentially suitable targets for LV pacing lead placement. Care must be taken to achieve a good seal within the main body of the CS in order to obtain maximal opacification of the distal vasculature. This is not always possible when the CS is massively dilated. In this situation, intentional overinflation of the balloon may be needed to achieve a minimally acceptable seal and prevent torrential backwash of contrast dye. Occasionally the inflated balloon will occlude the ostium of a suitable branch vessel for LV lead placement, therefore occlusive venography at multiple levels within the main CS is advisable (Fig. 10.5). Moreover, it is advisable to take a long cine sequence which may allow a delayed visualization of the occluded site branches. Care must be taken to avoid trauma to the venous endothelium, which

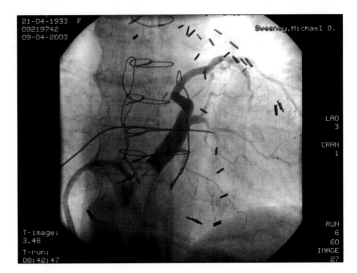

Figure 10.4 Retrograde coronary venogram via femoral approach. Note large lateral vein with three second-order branches, and a smaller posterolateral vein.

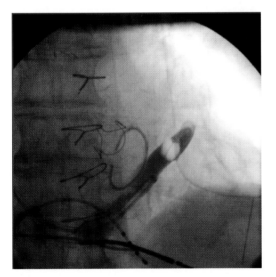

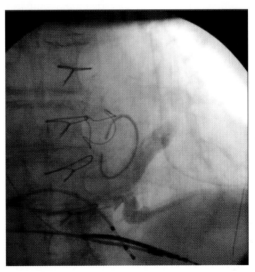

Figure 10.5 Retrograde coronary venogram via left superior approach. Left: Balloon is inflated in mid-CS. No target veins are visualized. Right: Sheath and balloon are withdrawn to proximal CS. Venography now reveals a large posterolateral vein. The ostium of this vein was occluded by the sheath on the first injection.

may result in dissection. The tip of the balloon catheter is quite stiff and in many implanters' experience is the most common cause of dissection (see Acute Complications of Left Ventricle Lead Placement in the Coronary Veins, below). Despite best efforts at retrograde venography, it is often the case that guidewires and leads unexpectedly traverse second-order branches not visualized by venography. It is important to remember that unlike coronary arteriography, where contrast dye is carried forward under high pressure, the flow of coronary venous blood is against contrast injection. Also, many smaller coronary veins are under low pressure and underfilled, or compressed during ventricular systole.

Selecting a target vein for optimal left ventricular stimulation

The optimal site for LV pacing is an unsettled and complex consideration. It is probably true that the optimal site varies between patients and is likely to be modified by venous anatomy, regional and global LV mechanical function, myocardial substrate, characterization of electrical delay, and other factors. In patients with abnormal ventricular conduction due to LBBB and systolic heart failure the stimulation site influences the response to LV pacing. The success of resynchronization is dependent on pacing from a site that causes a change in the sequence of ventricular activation that translates to an improvement in cardiac performance. Such systolic improvement and mechanical resynchronization does not require electrical synchrony [17] and explains the lack of correlation between change in QRS duration and clinical response to CRT [18]. Ideally, the pacing site or sites that produce the greatest hemodynamic effect would be selected.

However, current clinical evidence permits some generalizations regarding LV pacing site selection for optimal acute hemodynamic response. Multiple independent investigations comparing the acute and chronic effects of different pacing sites in similar dilated cardiomyopathy populations have reported concordant evidence that stimulation site is a primary determinant of CRT hemodynamic benefit.

Auricchio *et al.* [19, 20] showed a positive correlation between the magnitude of pulse pressure and LV +dP/dt increases and LV pacing site. The percentage increases in pulse pressure and LV +dP/dt averaged over all AV delays were significantly larger at mid-lateral free wall LV epicardial pacing sites compared with any other sample LV region. Furthermore, increases at the mid-anterior sites were smaller than at all other sites. These observations were extended in an analysis of 30 patients enrolled in the PATH-CHF II trial [21]. LV stimulation was delivered at the lateral free wall or mid-anterior wall. Free wall sites yielded significantly larger improvements in LV +dP/dt and pulse pressure than anterior sites. Furthermore, in a third of patients stimulation at anterior sites worsened acute LV hemodynamic performance, whereas free wall stimulation improved it, and the opposite pattern was never observed. This difference in acute hemodynamic response correlated with intrinsic conduction delays. This may be interpreted as evidence that stimulating a later activated LV region produces a larger response because it more effectively restores regional activation synchrony. Thus, the negative effect of anterior wall stimulation at all AV delays in some patients may be due to pre-excitation of an already relatively early-activated site thereby exaggerating intraventricular dyssynchrony [22].

Stimulation at the latest electrically activated (most delayed) region of the LV is associated with greatest hemodynamic response. This is usually on the posterior or posterolateral–basal wall as demonstrated by endocardial voltage mapping [23–25] and Doppler myocardial imaging [26, 27]. CRT with stimulation at a LV free wall site consistently improves short-term systolic function more than stimulation at an anterior site does. Lateral or posterolateral LV vein lead positions are associated with acute improvements in +dP/dt and pulse pressure [19, 21, 28], significant chronic improvements in functional capacity and ventricular function [29, 30] and possibly mortality compared to anterior vein sites in some [30] but not other studies [29]. However, within a specific coronary vein, the hemodynamic response to LV stimulation at different sites from apex to base is heterogeneous, suggesting that optimization of specific pacing sites within a target vein might be necessary for optimal CRT response [28].

It is likely, then, that inadequate LV lead positions contribute significantly to CRT non-response. In the MIRACLE study a lateral or posterolateral vein site was obtained in only 77% of patients, whereas the anterior interventricular vein or middle cardiac vein were used in 19.5% and 4.5% of patients, respectively. A similar situation was reported in the VENTAK CHF/CONTAK CD study where a lateral or posterolateral vein site was obtained in 67% of patients and an anterior interventricular vein site in the remaining 33% [31]. Furthermore, even among patients in whom the transvenous approach failed, necessitating surgical placement of LV leads, a lateral or posterolateral site was obtained in only 34%, whereas the remaining 66% were placed in the anterior or apical LV positions [31]. Thus, even in RCTs of CRT as many as 23–33% of patients receive LV stimulation from a sub-optimal site. It is conceivable that some of these patients were actually made worse by CRT due to LV pacing in the anterior vein, particularly those with relatively narrow QRSd (less than 150 ms) [21].

These differences in LV stimulation sites may partly account for the varied results and large individual difference observed among clinical studies.

Methods for identifying the best site during implantation are not yet of proven clinical benefit. Furthermore, even if optimal LV pacing sites could be identified a priori, access to such sites is potentially constrained by variations in coronary venous anatomy. The coronary venous circulation demonstrates considerably more variability than the parallel arterial circulation (Figs 10.6 and 10.7). Careful surveys of retrograde coronary venography have revealed that the anterior interventricular vein is present in 99% of patients and the middle cardiac vein is present in 100% [32, 33]. These veins are generally undesirable for resynchronization therapy because they do not reach the late activated portion of the LV free wall. Unfortunately, approximately 50% patients have only a single vein serving the LV free wall [34]. Anatomically, this is a lateral marginal vein in slightly more than 75% and a true posterior vein that ascends the free wall in approximately 50% of patients [33].

Selecting a left ventricular lead

Conventional endocardial pacing leads were poorly suited to LV pacing via the coronary veins. The electrodes, particularly the anodal ring of bipolar leads, prevented cornering of tortuous target vein take-offs. Even if the tip of such leads could be manipulated into the ostium of first-order target veins, the cross-sectional diameter of the lead body often exceeded the luminal diameter of the vein and prevented advancement. Ironically, the only relative merit of conventional pacing leads was the larger cross-sectional diameter that assisted with passive fixation within a target vein. This size trade-off between maneuverability and mechanical stability has not been resolved despite considerable advancements in LV lead design. The experienced implanter recognizes that a design advantage in one anatomic situation is almost invariably a disadvantage in another and therefore, the "ideal" LV lead suitable for use in all patients and anatomic situations does not exist.

The implanter must therefore be prepared to select a LV lead that best meets the constraining conditions of the individual patient. Several factors figure unpredictably in this choice, including coronary venous anatomy, phrenic nerve stimulation, and LV epicardial pacing thresholds.

The initial choice of a LV lead should be almost entirely informed by the coronary venogram. Decision-making should initially focus on the ostial take-off of the target vein, followed by an exami-

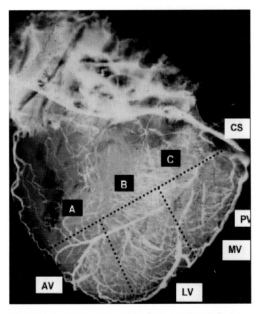

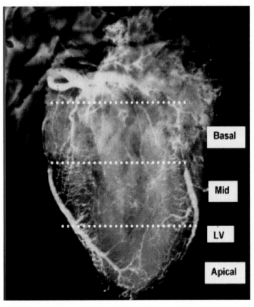

Figure 10.6 Coronary venogram from a cadaveric heart. The dotted lines indicate segmental divisions along the horizontal plane. A, anterior segment; B, lateral segment; C, posterior segment; AV, anterior interventricular vein; LV, lateral marginal vein; PV, posterior cardiac vein; MV, middle cardiac vein [50].

A

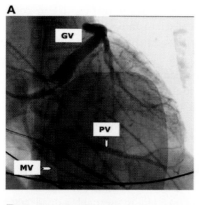

B

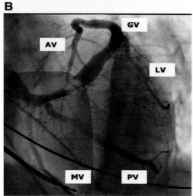

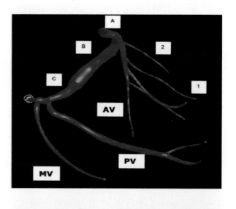

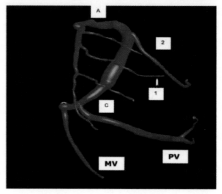

Figure 10.7 Left: Rotational venous angiogram, with still frames in anteroposterior (A) and left anterior oblique 30° (B). PV, posterior vein; MV, middle cardiac vein; GV, great cardiac vein; AV, anterior cardiac vein. Right: Three-dimensional reconstructed images of the coronary venous system. From Singh *et al.* [50].

nation of the main body of the target vein. Often times, these two considerations are in opposition – for example, a tight ostial take-off accompanied by a large diameter vein. In this situation, a smaller diameter, flexible tip lead would be optimal for navigating the take-off, possibly assisted by a guidewire. However, an undesirable characteristic of smaller diameter leads is that they tend to descend distally within larger target veins ("apex seekers") until a matched cross-sectional diameter is encountered and fixation by wedging occurs. In contrast, a larger diameter, stiffer lead is more likely to achieve proximal fixation, reducing the chance of phrenic nerve stimulation, but may not be able to navigate the ostial take-off of the target vein.

Currently available transvenous LV pacing leads may be either stylet driven or use over-the-wire (OTW) delivery similar to percutaneous coronary intervention (PCI) (Fig. 10.8). Lead diameter can be reduced in only three ways: reducing lumen size,

eliminating a conductor (unipolar), or reducing insulation (undesirable). Therefore, in general the smallest diameter leads are unipolar and are delivered exclusively over a PCI guidewire. Larger diameter leads may accommodate a conventional stylet or a PCI guidewire ("hybrids"). In some cases, fixation relies primarily on "wedging" the lead tip into a distal site within the target vein such that the outer diameter of the lead closely approximates the inner luminal diameter of the vein. Some other current LV lead designs incorporate one or more tines, which may assist with fixation by catching on a valve or promoting thrombosis, but are probably otherwise irrelevant. Finally, some other LV leads have a self-retaining cant at the tip that has two intended purposes. The cant unfolds within the target vein simultaneously compressing the distal segment of the lead against the outer wall of the vein, improving fixation, and forcing the tip electrode against the epicardium, improving electrical contact for pacing (Figs 10.8 and

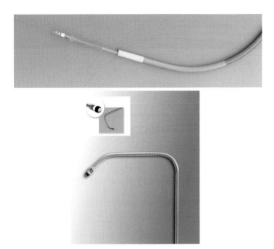

Figure 10.8 Examples of purely OTW LV lead (top) and hybrid stylet or OTW LV lead (bottom).

10.9). More recently, enhancements to lead design have been directed at combining the maneuverability of smaller diameter leads with the mechanical stability of large leads. This is achieved by incorporating reversible, self-retaining S- or pigtail-shaped curves at the lead tip, which increase the "effective" diameter of smaller leads for mechanical stability without degrading maneuverability (Fig. 10.10).

Selecting the target vein

Prior to attempting placement of an LV lead in the target vein, the ostium and proximal segment should be carefully examined in at least two fluoroscopic views (anteroposterior and left anterior oblique). The apparent origin of the target vein can be quite misleading, particularly if it arises on the posterior wall of the CS, which is not easily visualized by any fluoroscopic view. The investment of additional contrast injections prior to attempted sub-selection of the target vein may avoid the selection of an inappropriate lead design for the anatomic situation and an excessively time consuming and futile effort. Some implanters recommend systemic anticoagulation with intravenous unfractionated heparin after CS cannulation but before attempted target vein sub-selection. The rationale for this recommendation is based on the common observation that extensive clots are often found on the tips and bodies of LV leads when they are removed and exchanged during attempted placement, raising the possibility that acute coronary vein thrombosis may prevent successful LV lead placement. Systemic anticoagulation is then reversed with intravenous protamine at the conclusion of the procedure, analogous to coronary arteriography or PCI.

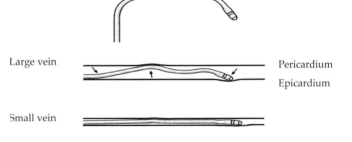

Figure 10.9 Use of self-retaining cant to achieve mechanical stability and epicardial contact for optimal pacing performance.

Large vein

Small vein

Pericardium

Epicardium

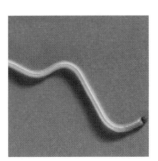

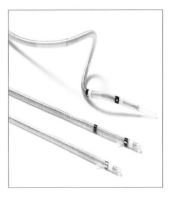

Figure 10.10 Examples of LV leads incorporating reversible, self-retaining S- or pigtail-shaped curves at the tip, which increase the "effective" diameter of smaller leads for mechanical stability without degrading maneuverability.

The approach to cannulating the ostium of the target vein is influenced by the take-off anatomy and the lead choice, which are interdependent.

Stylet-driven coronary sinus leads
If a stylet-driven lead is chosen, a 30–60 degree bend is applied to the distal tip of the stylet (Fig. 10.11). This results in a similar but less severe angle at the tip of the LV lead that assists with target vein ostial cannulation. If the tip of the LV lead has a pre-formed cant, then slight withdrawal of the stylet will achieve the same goal in some cases. The lead is then slowly rotated clockwise and counterclockwise while simultaneously advancing or retracting until the target vein ostium is encountered. Once the tip has engaged the target vein several techniques facilitate advancement. Occasionally, slight withdrawal of the stylet and forward pushing of the lead body will permit the tip to jump forward into the target vein (Fig. 10.12). Repeated pushing of the lead body and pulling of the stylet may be needed in some situations. Lead advancement is often facilitated by clockwise rotation from the left superior approach. Whereas counterclockwise rotation is necessary to cannulate the CS, clockwise rotation is necessary to exit the CS and descend a coronary vein on the posterior LV wall. It is helpful to apply torque and hold the lead body securely with the fingertips while allowing cardiac motion to transmit the torque to the tip. This need not be done under fluoroscopic observation as it may take several minutes. A large amount of torque may need to be applied in order to transmit to the tip for two reasons: the leads are long and they typically bind at several points (venous entry, within sheath proximally and distally, at ostium of target vein, and within target vein body), and the counterclockwise torque required to enter the CS from the low RA must be overcome.

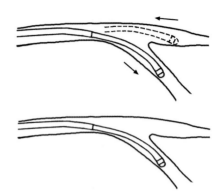

Figure 10.12 Manipulation of a stylet-driven lead to achieve target vein cannulation.

Guidewire-driven coronary sinus leads
The approach with OTW leads is entirely different. Occasionally the PCI guidewire can be manipulated into the target vein with minimal effort (Fig. 10.13). In some situations, the lead is then simply advanced over the guidewire although this is not guaranteed (Fig. 10.14) (see below). When the unassisted PCI guidewire cannot be easily manipulated into the

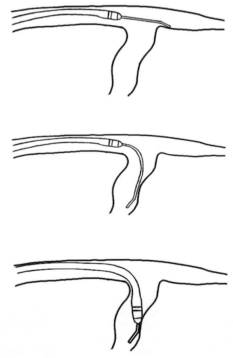

Figure 10.13 Use of guidewire to achieve target vein cannulation.

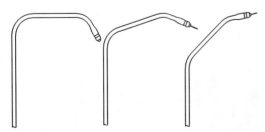

Figure 10.11 Use of stylets and guidewires to create lead tip angulation to assist with target vein ostial cannulation.

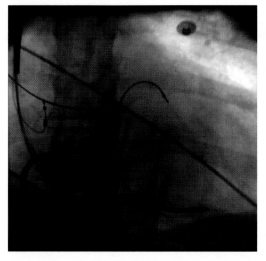
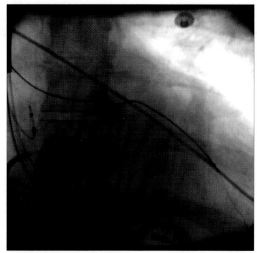

Figure 10.14 A pure OTW lead is advanced over a PCI guidewire into a lateral coronary vein.

target vein, a guide catheter is employed (Fig. 10.15). Coronary and non-coronary angiography catheters may be used for this purpose and the choice of catheter depends on the target vein ostial anatomy [35]. In general, the four French Judkins right coronary catheter (JR-4), an internal mammary artery (IMA) catheter, or Bern or Berenstein angiography catheters are effective for this purpose. Selective injections of contrast can help localize the target vein ostium and facilitate cannulation. Once the tip of the guide catheter has engaged the target vein ostium, the PCI guidewire is advanced as distally as possible

into the vein and the guide catheter is withdrawn completely. This must be done under continuous fluoroscopic observation to be certain that the PCI guidewire is not inadvertently withdrawn from the target vein, or worse, the main body CS. Thereafter, the lead is advanced over the PCI guidewire and into the target vein.

Inability to advance the lead despite tip engagement of the target vein ostium is frustratingly common. The most common scenario is that axial push on the lead results in prolapse of the tip out of the ostium of the target vein and into the main body

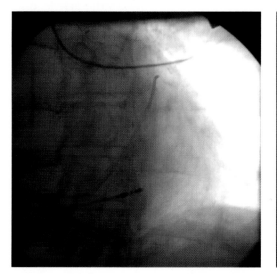
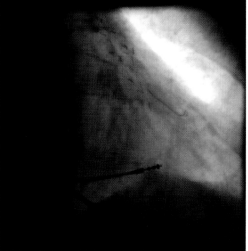

Figure 10.15 Selective cannulation of a high lateral coronary vein with a 5 French LIMA catheter (left). Placement of PCI guidewire into the target vein using the LIMA catheter.

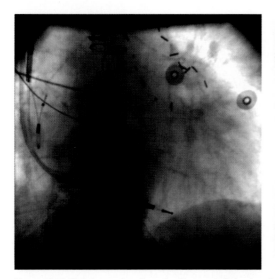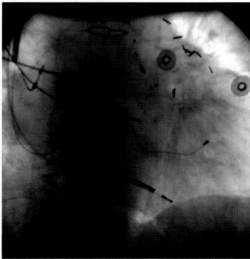

Figure 10.16 Tightly angulated proximal segment ("shepherd's crook") of a lateral vein (left). Straightening of the angulated segment with a PCI guidewire permitting successful LV lead placement.

CS. This is particularly common with first-order venous branches that have a "shepherd's crook" take-off (Fig. 10.16). Several techniques increase the probability of success in this situation. Occasionally, advancing the PCI wire deep into the target vein or a tertiary branch arising from the target vein will provide enough distal support to permit sufficient axial push to be applied to the lead tip so that guidewire tracking advancement occurs. The use of a stiffer PCI guidewire is sometimes useful in this regard. Additionally, advancing the CS sheath to a nearly adjacent position to the target ostium will provide enough support within the main body CS that backwards prolapse is prevented. If both of these techniques are unsuccessful, then the use of a "buddy" wire may be considered. This is a technique well known to interventional cardiologists, in which a separate PCI guidewire is advanced into the target vein to achieve straightening of the tortuous segment. A second PCI guidewire is then placed adjacent to the "buddy" wire and the LV lead is advanced through the now straightened proximal vein segment. If all of these approaches fail, then sub-selection of the target vein with telescoping sheaths may be necessary (see below). An important caveat when performing this technique is represented by the diameter of the inner lumen of the guiding catheter. Indeed, guiding catheters from different manufacturers may present different inner lumen diameters which may impede simultaneous introduction of guidewire and pacing lead.

Positioning the left ventricular lead within the target vein

Once the lead tip has successfully negotiated the proximal portion of the target vein, further advancement is usually desirable to prevent dislodgement. Similar difficulties with lead advancement may occur and can be addressed with techniques described above. A particular virtue of stylet-driven leads in this situation is that the support of the stylet permits considerable axial pressure and rotational torque to be applied to the lead, facilitating advancement, particularly when there is residual binding of the lead body at the ostium of the target vein.

The design of the terminal portion of the lead may influence the ability to advance within the target vein. Leads that incorporate a self-retaining cant are often difficult to advance with a stylet alone because of a "snowplow" effect. In this situation a hybrid approach using a PCI guidewire alternating with a stiff stylet is often necessary. The "snowplow" effect can be overcome by exchanging the stylet for a PCI guidewire which, when advanced distally in the vein, has the effect of straightening the cant and "lifting" the tip off the epicardial surface. Lead advancement then occurs with the "push–pull" guidewire technique described above. Simultaneous to and fro advancement of the lead and retraction of the guidewire permits the lead to creep forward like an "inchworm." This technique works equally well with purely OTW leads but axial push is dramatically limited due to the lack of a supporting structure (i.e. stylet).

The choice of PCI guidewire is probably not as important as a mastering a few crucial guidewire techniques. A half-loop at the guidewire tip greatly facilitates advancement within the vein. Some guidewires have pre-formed J-tips and a hydrophilic coating to facilitate movement with the target vessel. Alternately, a half-loop can be manually created by gently pulling the guidewire tip over the barrel of an 18-gauge needle. Occasionally, a half-loop can be formed by holding forward pressure on the guidewire with the tip partially lodged in a tertiary branch. The guidewire is then withdrawn into the target vein and advanced as desired. Rarely, the guidewire tip will become ensnared just distal to the LV lead tip and cannot be easily withdrawn. Overaggressive traction may result in severing of the guidewire tip with distal embolization (Fig. 10.17). The safest approach is to remove the LV lead and ensnared guidewire from the body and disengage the guidewire under direct vision.

Acute electrical testing of the left ventricular lead

Once the LV lead is in a mechanically stable position acute electrical testing is performed in the usual manner. The experienced implanter develops pragmatic expectations regarding LV stimulation thresholds, which are typically, but not always higher than endocardial stimulation thresholds in the right heart. All other considerations being equal (i.e. mechanical stability, absence of phrenic stimulation, optimal site), a stimulation threshold less than maximum programmed voltage output of the pulse generator is accepted because the alternative may only be a separate cardiac surgical procedure for LV lead placement.

Testing for phrenic nerve stimulation is critical and should be performed at maximum permissible voltage and pulse duration (typically, 10 V/up to 2.0 ms). This should be accompanied by fluoroscopic observation of the left hemidiaphragm and also a hand positioned on the chest wall, because occasionally direct chest wall stimulation occurs when the RV or LV is massively enlarged. This produces a faint "tapping" that is palpable and distinctly different from phrenic stimulation. Some implanters advocate rejecting any vein in which phrenic nerve stimulation is encountered on the apparent premise that no site will eliminate the problem.

Experienced implanters recognize that potentially ideal target veins can be salvaged by careful manipulation of the lead to a different site (see below). A final important consideration pertains to LV lead implantation under general anesthesia. In this situation, muscle relaxants should be temporarily reversed to perform testing for phrenic stimulation.

Coronary sinus sheath removal

Sheath removal is often the most stressful point in the procedure, particularly if LV lead placement was challenging and required exhaustive ancillary techniques. Many factors may threaten LV lead dislodgement during sheath removal, including poor technique. As noted above, the sheath itself may provide critical support for the lead that is necessary for mechanical stability within the target vein. As the sheath is withdrawn the lead may begin to back out from the target vein and into the main body CS. Recognition and readvancement of the sheath can temporarily prevent dislodgement while an alternative strategy is developed. A related scenario is that there is retained torque within the body of the LV lead related to manipulations during positioning. This torque is temporarily "hidden" by the support-

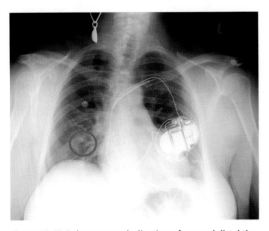

Figure 10.17 Pulmonary embolization of severed distal tip of PCI guidewire during LV lead placement.

ing structure of the sheath, which when removed, permits the lead to uncoil and spring backwards out of the target vein. Finally, complete dislodgement may occur when the sheath tip drops abruptly to the floor of the right atrium after exiting the CS ostium, dragging the LV lead body with it. This complication is partially mitigated by sheath design, specifically use of sheaths with a J-shaped primary curve, as previously discussed (Fig. 10.18).

Several techniques simultaneously applied greatly reduce the probability of LV lead dislodgement during sheath removal. Regardless of whether a stylet only, hybrid, or OTW only LV lead is used, some sort of supporting wire is needed during sheath removal. A PCI guidewire provides insufficient support for this purpose. The use of a curved stylet is advocated for stylet driven leads, whereas a "finishing wire" is recommended for purely OTW LV leads (Figs 10.19 and 10.20). Once the supporting stylet or finishing wire is in place and LV lead tip position is confirmed, the sheath is slowly withdrawn under continuous fluoroscopic observation. The critical moment is when the sheath reaches the ostium of the CS. There is a natural inclination to push the lead forward when the sheath begins to fall into the right atrium and this usually has disastrous consequences. A redundancy forms in the body of the lead, which falls to the floor of the right atrium and drags the LV lead body out. This is avoided by applying backwards traction to the LV lead as the sheath exits the CS, which prevents formation of a redundancy and paradoxically stabilizes the lead.

Sheath cutting should not be performed until the sheath tip is clearly within the right atrium and LV lead stability is assured. This requires practice and patience. The lead body (and guidewire, if retained) is "collected" in the cutting tool. The cutting tool is held in the dominant hand, which is firmly pressed against the patient's chest wall. The sheath is then pulled back over and against the cutting tool using the nondominant hand. This should be done in one continuous, smooth motion. Stopping and starting is often problematic because it is difficult to reestablish a clean cutting plane. Under no circumstances should the cutting tool be advanced. This will create a lead redundance beyond the sheath tip and risk dislodgement into the low right atrium. Once the sheath is removed, lead slack and tip position should be verified. This is best done in the lateral view. The anterior–posterior view often gives the mistaken impression that there is too much slack in the LV lead. The lateral view should reveal that the body of the lead traverses the floor of the right atrium. LV pacing thresholds should be redetermined even in the absence of gross movement of the LV lead tip, since "microdislodgement" not visible by fluoroscopy may have occurred.

Repositioning the LV lead after sheath removal is a challenging task, particularly when the support provided by the sheath was necessary to achieve implantation success. It is sometimes possible to carefully advance a PCI guidwire to the tip of the LV lead without the sheath in place, but great care must be taken to avoid a redundancy at the low RA–CS ostial junction that could result in prolapse dislodgement. Once the PCI guidewire is beyond the tip of the LV within the target vein, an exchange for a curved stylet or finishing wire can be made to facilitate

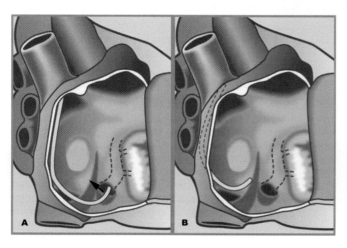

Figure 10.18 Importance of J-shaped curve in CS sheath to prevent lead dislodgement during sheath removal. As sheath is withdrawn from the CS, the tip elevates toward the SVC rather than falling to the floor of the RA and dislodging the LV lead. Reproduced from www.bivtips.com with permission of Seth Worley, MD.

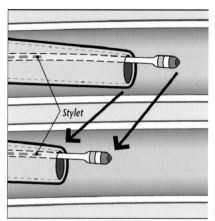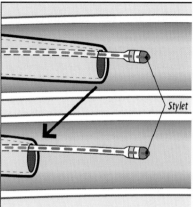

Figure 10.19 Importance of guidewire position during CS sheath removal. A gently curved stabilizing stylet should be advanced all the way to the tip of the lead prior to attempted sheath removal. When the stylet is not advanced to the tip of the lead, friction between the sheath and the lead will slide the lead back over the stylet as the sheath is withdrawn even when the position of the stylet is fixed. Left, top: The stylet is not advanced to the tip of the pacing lead. The tip sheath is in contact with pacing lead. Left, bottom: The sheath has been withdrawn. Contact between the tip of the sheath and the lead body pulled the pacing lead back along the stylet. Right, top: The tip of the sheath is in contact with the lead. The stylet is at the tip of the lead. Right, bottom: The sheath has been withdrawn. The tip of the lead remains in position. As long as the stylet does not move the lead will remain in position. Reproduced from www.bivtips.com with permission of Seth Worley, MD.

fine movement adjustments of the lead. Either the stylet or finishing wire is then removed using the approach described above.

Techniques for overcoming factors limiting successful transvenous left ventricular lead placement

Complex and unpredictable anatomic and technical considerations may preclude successful delivery of the LV lead to an optimal pacing site.

Inability to localize or cannulate the coronary sinus ostium

It is difficult to estimate the true percentage of cases in which the coronary sinus cannot be cannulated because this is clearly influenced by operator experience. It is probably in the range of 1–5%. Besides

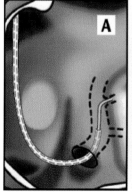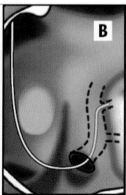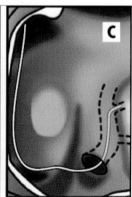

Figure 10.20 Importance of adjusting slack in LV lead during sheath removal. Left: Lead is within sheath. Middle: When the sheath is removed without advancing additional lead, tension may displace the tip of the lead from the target vein. Right: Additional slack has been added to ensure that the tip of the lead is not dislodged when the patient changes position. Reproduced from www.bivtips. com with permission of Seth Worley, MD.

operator inexperience, several anatomic situations may render localization of the CS ostium problematic. These include an unusually high or low position of the CS ostium, or very rarely, absence of the CS orifice. Some implanters advocate bolus contrast injections to visualize the CS ostium. The presence of myocardial staining with visible trabeculations indicates that the CS sheath (and guide catheter) is in the RV whereas the absence of trabecular staining indicates an atrial position. It is often difficult, however, to achieve adequate opacification of the RA with small volume (10–20 mL) hand injections due to swirling of blood within the enlarged RA and torrential competitive flow out of the CS. In this situation, equipment for performing a power injection may be particularly useful.

Cannulation of the CS ostium can be facilitated by a working knowledge of the right heart anatomy. The CS ostium is bounded inferiorly by the thebesian valve and on the atrial side by the eustachian ridge (Fig. 10.21). The thebesian valve is usually thin and crescent shaped in about one-third of hearts but multiple variations have been described, including fibrous bands, strands, filigree network, and large redundant "fishnets" continuous with a Chiari network [16]. In one autopsy study, large membrane-like thebesian valves almost completely occluded the CS ostium in 25% of specimens [36].

These structures tend to impede forward progress of the CS sheath and coronary guide catheter (or deflectable catheter) when approached from the atrial side (Fig. 10.22). On the other hand, these structures (in particular, the eustachian ridge) tend to direct the CS sheath and guide catheters into the ostium when approached from the ventricular side (Fig. 10.22). Therefore, in difficult cases it is useful to advance the tip of the CS sheath and guide catheters into the RV, then rotate counterclockwise during gradual withdrawal so as to encounter the CS ostium (Figs 10.23–10.26). If this approach fails, an adaptation of the inferior approach described for complex electrophysiology procedures is often successful in localizing the CS ostium (see above, Fig. 10.5). Alternately, intracardiac ultrasound can be used to assist localization of the CS ostium.

Having localized the CS ostium, it is sometimes very difficult to advance the guide catheter or sheath due to kinking at the neck of the CS. This is most commonly encountered with a "goose neck" proximal CS which is often associated with massive cardiomegaly. This can result in sheath kinking that prevents LV lead passage. This problem has been virtually eliminated by braided sheath designs (see above, discussion of sheaths). Rarely, a combined inferior and superior approach is needed to overcome sheath kinking in the proximal CS. A deflectable electrophysiology catheter is placed in the CS ostium from the inferior approach and downward pressure is applied to "straighten" the "goose neck" segment. This may permit advancement of the CS sheath and guide catheters from the superior approach.

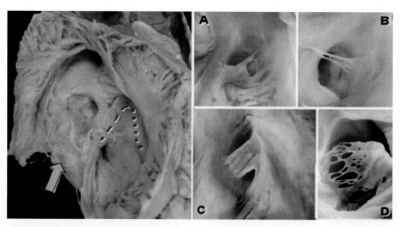

Figure 10.21 Anatomy of the coronary sinus ostium. Left: The CS ostium is bounded by the eustachian ridge and the thebesian valve. Right: Examples of variations in thebesian valve morphology. (A) Crescent with fenestrations, (B) fine strand, (C) broad fibrous band, and (D) aneurysmal fenestrated valve almost covering the os. From Ho *et al.* [16].

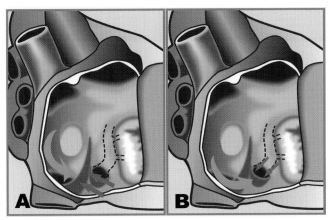

Figure 10.22 Left: Both the eustachian ridge and thebesian valve (small arrows) block entrance to the CS OS as it is approached from the atrium along the inferior posterior wall (large arrow). Right: Both the eustachian ridge and thebesian valve (small arrows) direct the tip of the guide into the CS OS as it is approached from the posterior superior tricuspid annulus (large arrow). Reproduced from www.bivtips.com with permission of Seth Worley, MD.

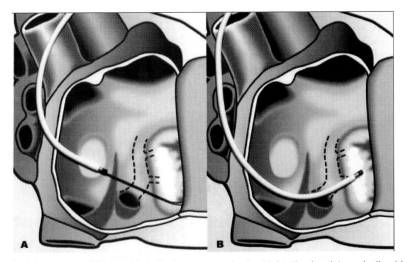

Figure 10.23 Left: Advancement of LV sheath into the RV over a guidewire. Right: The sheath is gradually withdrawn and rotated counterclockwise to enter the CS ostium. Reproduced from www.bivtips.com with permission of Seth Worley, MD.

Coronary venous anatomy: absent or inaccessible target veins

Despite rapid evolution of implantation techniques including guiding sheaths and catheters and OTW delivery systems, a suitable pacing site on the LV free wall cannot be achieved in 20–30% of patients. In many patients this is simply because of absence of coronary veins reaching the LV free wall. In some instances target veins are present but too small for cannulation with existing lead systems, or paradoxically too large to achieve mechanical fixation with reduced diameter LV leads that rely primarily on "wedging" the lead tip into a distal site within the target vein for fixation such that the outer diameter of the lead closely approximates the inner luminal diameter of the vein. A fairly common observation is that potentially ideal target veins serving the posterobasal LV wall are of insufficient caliber to accommodate any available LV lead. In this situation, coronary venoplasty can achieve sufficient cross-sectional diameter to permit successful LV lead placement [37]. This approach is also useful when the target vein cannot be navigated from the antegrade approach due to ostial kinking, proximal segment tortuosity, etc. Careful inspection of the coronary venogram may often reveal collateralization of

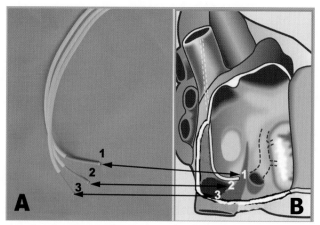

Figure 10.24 Using the eustachian ridge and thebesian valve to direct a CS cannulation from the ventricular approach. Left: Three positions of a guide with progressive application of torque are superimposed. A, initial counterclockwise torque at the hub of the guide directs the tip of the guide back; B, with additional counterclockwise torque the guide tip can no longer move back. The torque thus directs the tip of the guide down and to the left. C, as more counterclockwise torque is added, the tip of the guide continues to move down and to the left. In B and C the proximal section of the guide lifts off the surface (out of the plane of the illustration). Right: Drawing of the area of the CS OS demonstrates the relative position of the tip of the guide as torque is applied assuming an initial position on the posterior superior tricuspid annulus. If the tip of the guide is above the CS on the tricuspid annulus when torque is applied it will be directed posterior inferior toward the right atrium into the CS. However, if the guide is at or below the CS as torque is applied, the tip will move inferiorly away from the CS. For counterclockwise torque to be effective in finding the OS, the initial tip position must be superior and on the RV side of the OS. As an aside, clockwise torque will direct the tip of the guide anterior away from the OS. Reproduced from www.bivtips.com with permission of Seth Worley, MD.

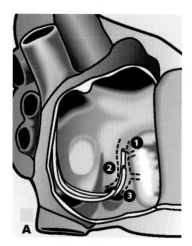

Figure 10.25 Effect of counterclockwise torque on CS sheath tip position. Position 1: 45–90 degrees of counterclockwise torque. Position 2: 90–120 degrees of counterclockwise torque. Position 3: 120–180 degrees of counterclockwise torque. Note that without advancing or withdrawing the sheath/guide combination, progressive counterclockwise torque directs the tip inferior and toward the right atrium. Reproduced from www.bivtips.com with permission of Seth Worley, MD.

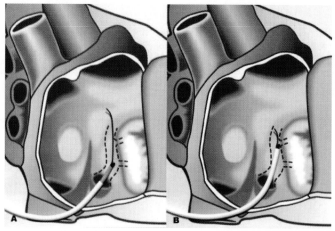

Figure 10.26 Advancement of CS sheath over inner guide and guidewire.

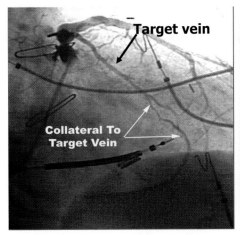

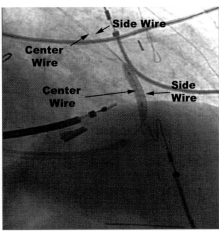

Figure 10.27 Target lateral vein has sharply angulated take-off that could not be navigated by any technique. Careful inspection of the coronary venogram often reveals collateralization of the distal target vein from a lower posterolateral coronary vein. However, the collateral anastomosis was quite small and prevented lead advancement. Venoplasty of the narrowed collateral segment permitted retrograde access to the target vein for successful LV lead. Reproduced with permission of Seth Worley, MD.

the distal target vein from another coronary vein. However, the collateral anastomosis may be quite small, and coronary venoplasty can be exploited to gain retrograde access to the target vein for successful LV lead placement (Fig.10.27).

Prior cardiac surgery may impose further limitations on coronary venous anatomy. Rarely, mitral valve surgery may result in impassable strictures in the main body CS, presumably related to encroachment of the sewing ring. Similarly, adhesive bands that form after pericardiotomy may create coronary venous strictures. Both of these situations can be overcome with venoplasty [37]. However, great technical skill is required. Finally, secondary and tertiary coronary venous branches are often surgically ligated or clipped during arterial anastomosis, preventing advancement of LV pacing leads. This can be immediately recognized by coronary venography and cannot be overcome by any technique.

In all of these situations where the coronary venous approach fails due to insuperable anatomic constraints, surgical placement of epicardial LV pacing leads or endocardial LV stimulation are final options.

Coronary venous tortuosity

Another commonly encountered difficulty in transvenous LV lead placement is tortuosity of the target vessel take-off or main segment (Figs 10.28 and 10.29). These anatomic constraints can be extremely difficult to overcome and often require the use of multiple LV lead designs and delivery systems not specifically designed for this application. Large-diameter stylet driven leads are likely to fail in this

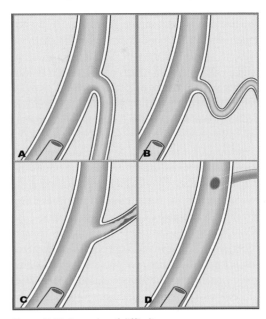

Figure 10.28 Examples of difficult coronary venous anatomy. (A) Acutely angulated take-off. (B) Tortuous proximal segment. (C) Partial occlusion. (D) Posterior take-off. Reproduced from www.bivtips.com with permission of Seth Worley, MD.

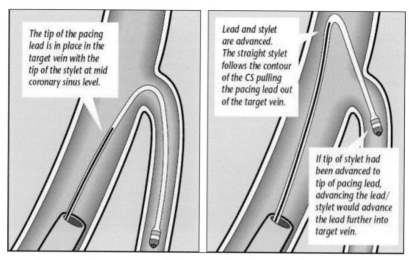

The tip of the pacing lead is in place in the target vein with the tip of the stylet at mid coronary sinus level.

Lead and stylet are advanced. The straight stylet follows the contour of the CS pulling the pacing lead out of the target vein.

If tip of stylet had been advanced to tip of pacing lead, advancing the lead/stylet would advance the lead further into target vein.

Figure 10.29 Importance of stylet position. When straight stylet is not advanced to the tip of the LV lead, the stylet follows the contour of the CS and pulls the LV lead out of the target vein. When a gently curved stylet is advanced to the tip of the LV lead, coaxial pressure advances the lead into the target vein. Reproduced from www.bivtips.com with permission of Seth Worley, MD.

situation and most implanters reflexively select the smallest diameters OTW lead upon inspection of the coronary venogram.

One approach utilizes coronary, renal or other angiography catheters to selectively cannulate the small and tortuous target vein (see above, Fig. 10.15). Advancement of a PCI guidewire will often straighten the tortuous segment of the vein, permitting nagivation with an OTW LV lead. Occasionally, the OTW lead cannot be advanced through the proximal segment despite a straight path of the guidewire. The likely explanation in this situation is that the guidewire has not truly straightened the tortuous segment of the target vein. This is more likely when the target vein has a relatively large diameter. In these conditions, the very small-diameter guidewire may pursue a straight course through the vessel lumen without exerting any effective straightening pressure on the wall of the vein. Occasionally, this can be overcome by using a stiffer guidewire. However, more often, significant resistance to lead advancement persists despite a stiffer guidewire and a "buddy wire technique" is required. This refers to one or more guidewire placed alongside the first which may sufficiently straighten the vein to permit lead advancement [38]. After successful placement of the LV lead but before sheath removal, the "buddy wires" are removed.

Despite these techniques, proximal segment tortuousity may persist and prevent advancement of even the smallest diameter OTW leads. An alternative technique that many experienced implanters have adopted as the first line approach to this situation is the use of telescoping sheaths. Sub-selection of the target vein with an inner guiding sheath permits straightening of the tortuous proximal segment and direct delivery of the LV lead. This approach often eliminates the use of a guidewire altogether and permits delivery of large-diameter stylet driven leads if desired, which would otherwise likely fail in this situation.

Telescoping sheaths may require the use of a larger diameter (i.e. 9 French) CS sheath. The target vein is typically cannulated with a stiff PCI guidewire as described above. A smaller diameter straight CS sheath is then advanced over the guidewire into the proximal segment of the target vein. Often the PCI guidewire does not provide enough support for advancement of the inner straight sheath into the target vein. This can be overcome either by using multiple PCI guidewires, or preferably, a floppy tipped 0.035″ guidewire. Occasionally the inner straight sheath cannot be advanced into the target vein using any guidewire technique. In this situation, an angiography catheter can be placed within the inner sheath (triple catheter/sheath approach) (Fig. 10.30). An angiography catheter that closely approximates the shape of the tortuous proximal segment of the target vein should be chosen. A "shepherd's crook" renal angiography catheter is particularly well suited to this requirement. The tip of the angiography catheter is manipulated into the target vein using puffs of contrast if needed. A floppy-tipped 0.035″ guidewire is then placed for distal support. The inner straight sheath can then be advanced over the stiff angiography catheter, definitively straightening the tortuous proximal segment. The floppy-tipped guidewire and angiography catheter are then removed, and the LV lead of choice is delivered directly through the inner straight sheath (Fig. 10.30). The inner straight sheath is then cut away using techniques previously described.

Some comments are necessary to reduce complications and increase success of the telescoping sheath technique. First, the patient should be prepped for urgent pericardiocentesis and thoracotomy (which is generally recommended for CRT implantation). Second, excessive force should not be applied to any guidewire or sheath within the coronary veins. Pressure on the vessel wall may causes tension and reduces the normal distensibility of the vein, increasing the probability of perforation. Resistance to advancement of the inner sheath (within or without an inner guide catheter for support) should sponsor a contrast injection to assess the mechanical situation. Third, the inner sheath should have a relatively soft tip segment. Lastly, the telescoping sheath technique should not be applied to small-diameter veins (i.e. <3–3.5 mm).

The telescoping sheath technique may be not ideally suited to lateral coronary veins that arise beyond the proximal third of the main body CS. Inability to apply forward axial pressure typically results in failure of this approach, despite the extra support of a 0.035″ guidewire or an angiography guide catheter. Additionally, straight LV sheaths are typically not long enough to reach the proximal segments of lateral veins that arise beyond the proximal third of the CS.

Therefore, the telescoping sheath technique is most useful for posterolateral veins that arise within 1–3 cm of the CS ostium. This approach is particularly helpful in the situation where the middle cardiac vein and posterolateral vein share a common ostium within the proximal neck of the CS. This anatomical arrangement poses a unique problem for LV lead placement using a single sheath. In order to permit cannulation of the target vein ostium with the LV lead or guidewire, the sheath must be withdrawn to within 1 cm or less of the CS ostium. This commonly results in abrupt dislodgement of the sheath to the floor of the right atrium, pulling the LV lead and guidewire along with it. Occasionally using a stylet-driven lead and intentionally withdrawing the LV sheath from the CS in a controlled manner can defeat this. The lead is advanced to the mid-portion of the CS and the sheath and lead are simultaneously withdrawn

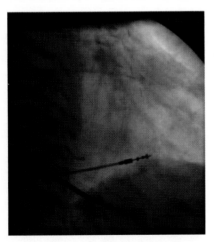 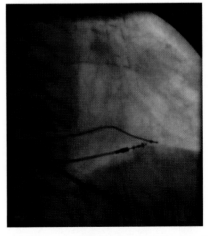

Figure 10.30 "Triple catheter/sheath" for straightening tortuous proximal coronary veins. Left: 5 French "shepherd's crook" renal angiography catheter has engaged the ostium of a posterolateral vein. Right: Inner straight sheath is advanced over the angiography catheter, which was supported distally by a 0.035 gauge floppy-tip guidewire (not shown). Guidewire and angiography catheter are removed and LV lead is delivered directly through the inner straight sheath.

while rotating the lead tip into the ostium of the target vein. Attention must be paid to the point when the sheath exits the CS ostium so as to avoid the creation of a redundancy in the LV lead body that could result in prolapse onto the right atrial floor.

Alternatively, a variation of the telescoping sheath approach is often successful in the "common ostium" situation (Figs 10.31–10.33). An inner guide catheter with a 45–60 degree tip angle (i.e. Bern or Berenstein) is advanced through the inner

straight sheath (triple catheter/sheath approach) to the mid CS. The outer LV sheath is withdrawn over the inner straight sheath until it has exited the CS ostium. The inner straight sheath and inner guide catheter are then simultaneously withdrawn while rotating the guide catheter tip until the ostium of the target vein is engaged. A floppy-tipped 0.035″ guidewire is advanced into the target vein, followed by the inner guide catheter and the inner straight sheath. The outer LV sheath is essentially irrelevant at this point and can be withdrawn to

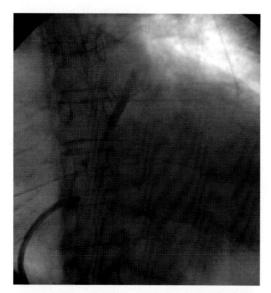
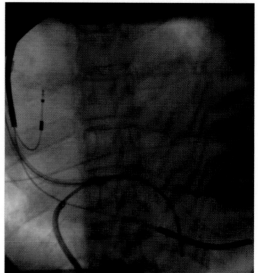

Figure 10.31 Same technique as Fig. 10.30. See text for details.

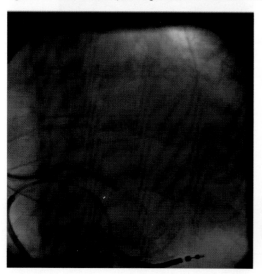
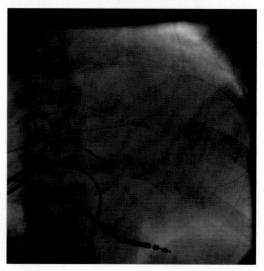

Figure 10.32 Continuation of technique in Fig. 10.31. See text for details.

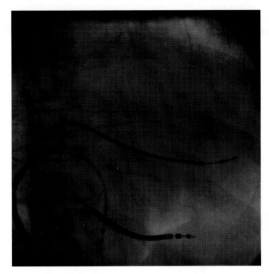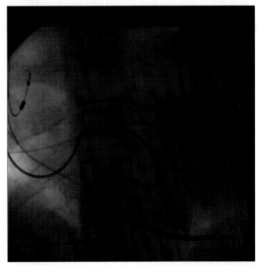

Figure 10.33 Continuation of Figs 10.30–10.32. Final LV lead placement in posterolateral vein via an inner straight sheath. See text for details.

the mid right atrium. The inner guide catheter and guidewire are removed and the LV lead is delivered directly into the target vein through the inner straight sheath. The inner straight sheath and outer sheath are removed in the usual manner. Though these posterolateral veins present unique challenges to LV lead placement, they often yield mechanically stable positions because of the relatively straight course pursued from the low right atrium through the proximal coronary sinus to the lateral LV wall.

Inner guide catheters specifically packaged for coronary venous application are available. Some of these guide catheters have a deflectable tip to enhance sub-selection of target veins. These inner guide catheters serve a similar role to the coronary and renal angiographic catheters adapted for this role as described previously. Their primary purpose is to assist with delivery of a guidewire to the target vein. More recently, inner sheaths of sufficient diameter to deliver LV leads directly have been developed. These have several different distal segment shapes (hockey stick, multipurpose, hook) intended to match patterns of coronary venous take-off anatomy (Figs 10.34 and 10.35). Such inner sheaths are particularly useful for low-lying posterior and posterolateral veins, but typically do not provide sufficient reach for use with mid and high lateral veins.

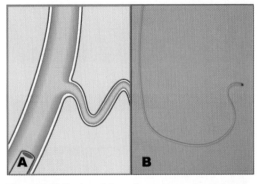

Figure 10.34 Hockey stick pre-formed inner sheath for sub-selecting and straightening tortuous proximal target veins.

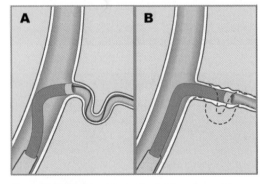

Figure 10.35 Use of guidewire to direct pre-formed inner sheath through the tortuous proximal segment of the target vein, permitting direct delivery of the LV lead. Reproduced from www.bivtips.com with permission of Seth Worley, MD.

Preventing and overcoming high left ventricular stimulation thresholds and phrenic nerve stimulation

The principal limitation of the transvenous approach is that the selection of sites for pacing is entirely dictated by navigable coronary venous anatomy. A commonly encountered problem is that an apparently suitable target vein delivers the lead to a site where ventricular capture can be achieved at only very high output voltages or not at all, rendering potentially optimal target veins unsuitable for use. This presumably relates to the presence of scar on the epicardial surface of the heart underlying the target vein or inadequate contact with the epicardial surface and cannot be anticipated by fluoroscopic examination a priori. Occasionally mapping of the proximal segment of such veins will yield sites with suitable capture thresholds. Upsizing of the LV lead, or use of a lead with a self-retaining "S" shape or cant may be required to achieve mechanical stability depending on the characteristics of the original lead selected (Figs 10.36–10.38). Similarly, before abandoning such veins a sub-selective venogram should be performed because potentially useful

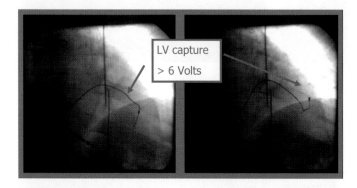

Figure 10.36 LV capture could not be demonstrated at any distal location using a 4 French OTW LV lead in the lateral vein.

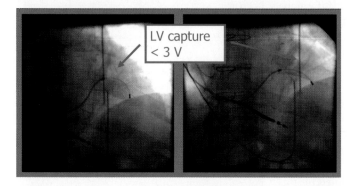

Figure 10.37 Same patient as Fig. 10.36. A larger diameter LV lead was wedged more proximally within the same vein, yielding a capture threshold <3 V.

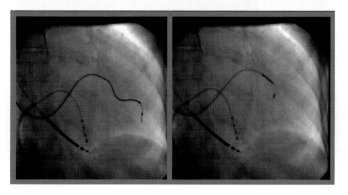

Figure 10.38 Left: Continuous phrenic nerve stimulation at the only mechanically stable position obtained with a reversible fixation LV lead. Right: Elimination of phrenic stimulation at a more proximal position in the same lateral vein using a canted LV lead design.

tertiary branches are often not visualized during main body CS injection due to low flow and systolic compression. Such tertiary branches may serve a region of myocardium with an acceptable pacing threshold. Depending upon the size of the tertiary branch, downsizing of the LV lead to a purely OTW design may be necessary if not originally utilized. If this is not successful, surgical placement of LV leads permits more detailed mapping of viable sites in the anatomic region of interest.

A second common problem is that the target vein delivers the lead to a site that results in phrenic nerve stimulation and diaphragmatic pacing. Careful examination of cadaver hearts demonstrates that the phrenic nerve passes over the lateral coronary veins in ~80% of specimens and over the anterior interventricular vein in the remaining ~20% [39]. This presents a high probability of anatomic conflict between the optimal site for LV stimulation and unacceptable phrenic nerve stimulation. Phrenic stimulation can be difficult to demonstrate during implantation when the patient is supine and sedated but may be immediately evident when the patient is later active and changes body positions, even in the absence of lead dislodgement. It is important to recognize that once phrenic nerve stimulation is observed acutely (during implantation), it is almost invariably encountered during follow-up despite manipulation of output voltages and therefore alternative site LV pacing is sought (Figs 10.39 and 10.40). As with high

LV capture thresholds, phrenic nerve stimulation can often be overcome by repositioning the LV lead more proximally within the target vein. Occasionally, if there is a significant differential in the capture thresholds for phrenic nerve stimulation versus LV capture, this can be overcome by manipulation of LV voltage output in devices that permit separate RV and LV outputs. More recently, some LV leads have ≥2 electrodes that permit selection of specific LV sites for dual cathodal biventricular stimulation, biventricular stimulation with true bipolar LV stimulation, or true bipolar LV-only univentricular stimulation. It has not been convincingly demonstrated that true bipolar LV stimulation reliably overcomes phrenic stimulation compared with dual cathodal or unipolar LV pacing. On the other hand, selecting alternate LV electrodes for dual cathodal biventricular stimulation may occasionally overcome phrenic stimulation by altering the LV–RV pacing vector. This can be achieved non-invasively using some pulse generators and is referred to as "electronic repositioning." In either case, the problem of phrenic nerve stimulation is more reliably addressed by LV lead repositioning at implant. If phrenic stimulation during attempted transvenous LV pacing cannot be overcome by any means, surgical placement of LV leads should be considered. Phrenic stimulation can occur with surgically placed epicardial leads if careful visualization of the course of the nerve sheath is not performed prior to fixation. Chronic development of phrenic

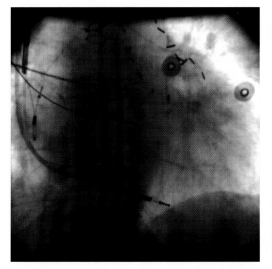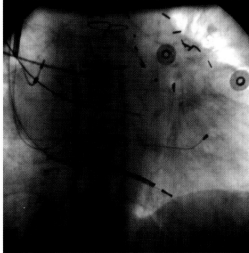

Figure 10.39 Continuous phrenic nerve stimulation at all points in a lateral vein.

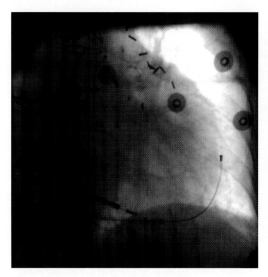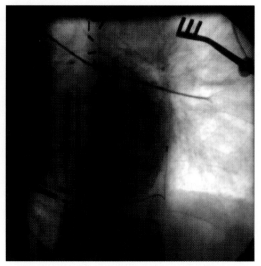

Figure 10.40 Same patient as Fig. 10.39. Elimination of phrenic stimulation by using a posterolateral vein that ascended the LV free wall.

nerve stimulation results in permanent loss of CRT in about 1–2% of patients [40].

Loss of cardiac resynchronization therapy due to differential left ventricular capture threshold rise

There are relatively limited data on long-term pacing thresholds with transvenous or thoracotomy leads for LV pacing. Loss of ventricular capture occurred in 10% of patients in the VENTAK CHF/CONTAK CD study and was the second most common cause of interrupted CRT [40]. Three-quarters of these cases were due to gross dislodgement of the LV lead, whereas 23% were due to chronic pacing threshold elevation that was overcome by increasing voltage output in the majority of cases. The reasons for chronic increase in tranvenous LV pacing thresholds are not well characterized. Possible explanations include "microdislodgement" not evidenced by radiographic examination or exit block that occurs as a consequence of inadequate mechanical stability. Hansky [41] has pointed out that an important technique-related factor to post-operative increase in pacing thresholds is an unstable, but not grossly dislodged, lead position. This is based on speculation that repetitive chronic endothelial injuries due to "rocking" of the lead tip may result in progressive fibrotic reorganization of the adjacent vessel wall (Fig. 10.41). It is also pos-

sible that late rises in previously acceptable transvenous LV thresholds relate to implantation technique. Aggressive lead manipulations, repeated lead exchanges, or guidewire maneuvers may traumatize the endothelium of the target vein, resulting in a fibrotic reaction, thrombosis or dissection, all of which may degrade the pacing threshold.

A comparison of thoracotomy and transvenous lead system performance in 87 patients who received CRT-D systems between 1998 and 2001 reported no significant differences in chronic thresh-

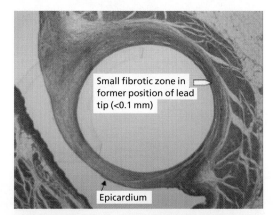

Figure 10.41 Lateral coronary vein (magnification 2.5 × 10) at former lead tip. Explanted heart for heart transplantation eight months after LV lead implantation. From Hansky *et al.* [41].

olds with either approach, which on average were between 1.5 and 2.0 V up to 30 months post implant [42]. Similarly, there were no chronic threshold differences between transvenous lead designs (OTW versus pre-formed shape). An interim progress report of the InSync Registry Post-Approval Study [43] in 903 patients showed similar range and stability of LV thresholds (mean 1.88 ± 1.44 V) with two different pre-formed transvenous lead designs at six months that were retained at 36 months. In this same report, epicardial voltage thresholds were similarly stable, but slightly higher (2.42 ± 0.74 V) at 12 months, though data were available on a much smaller number of patients.

A particularly difficult problem with chronic epicardial leads is exit block, which in some instances results in voltage thresholds that exceed pulse generator output and results in permanent loss of CRT. Though this is infrequent, it is a devastating problem for the patient, since the epicardial approach is usually taken only when the transvenous approach fails. Several factors contribute to this problem relating to lead design and surgical technique. The epicardial pacing lead which most commonly shows poor long-term performance is a fixed helix mechanism without steroid, and chronic doubling of the implant threshold is common. Furthermore, this situation is made worse by multiple applications of the helix and incautious use of suturing which increase local tissue trauma and the subsequent inflammatory response.

Loss of cardiac resynchronization therapy due to lead dislodgement

Acute dislodgement of RA and RV electrodes is uncommon, particularly with active fixation leads, although this is not a specific issue of CRT implantation. The incidence of LV lead dislodgement is considerably higher and has a reported incidence of 5–10% in larger studies [13, 44, 45]. This relates to implanter experience and other technical factors such as the lack of fixation mechanisms and stresses placed on the proximal portion of the lead at the junction of the right atrium and CS ostium. Lead dislodgements are readily identified by change in QRS duration and morphology in ECG as well as by chest radiography but usually suspected on the basis of device interrogation that discloses a significant decline in local signal amplitude and/or change in pacing capture threshold. Typically, RA

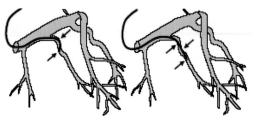

Supported at two points: **Unstable position**   Supported at three points: **Stable position**

Figure 10.42 Support at multiple (>2–3) positions increases mechanical stability. From Hansky *et al.* [41].

leads dislodge onto the floor of the RA and RV leads dislodge towards the inflow of the RV. LV leads typically dislodge into the main body of the CS, and less commonly into the RA.

Several techniques reduce the chances of LV lead dislodgement. Probably of most importance is an optimal match between the diameter of the LV lead and the luminal diameter of the target vein. Support at multiple (>2–3) positions increases mechanical stability (Fig. 10.42). Larger leads with pre-formed shapes should be advanced sufficiently within the target vein to completely unfold (Fig. 10.43). In the case of the smallest diameter purely OTW leads, it is useful to position the tip in a tertiary branch to achieve support at more than one position and increase mechanical stability. In extreme situations,

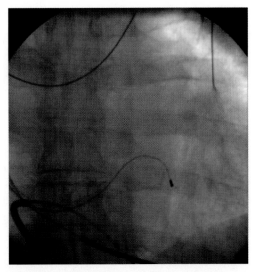

Figures 10.43 Larger leads with pre-formed shapes should be advanced sufficiently within the target vein to completely unfold. In this position, subtle lead tip instability was observed during systolic contraction, despite apparent gross mechanical stability of the lead body.

bare metal stents have been deployed in the coronary vein adjacent to the LV lead to achieve mechanical stability at a desired site (Seth Worley, personal communication). This approach should be considered with great caution as stent struts may damage lead insulation over time but also chronic CS thrombosis or stenosis may result. Alternatively, 4 French lumenless, catheter-delivered fixed helix activation fixation pacing leads designed for endocardial use have been used for coronary venous pacing (Bert Hansky, personal communication). Many obvious questions regarding safety, long-term performance, and approach to removal will arise. Only the most experienced implanters should attempt such exotic approaches to coronary venous pacing.

Approach to avoiding or correcting a sub-optimal left ventricular lead position

Ideally, a sub-optimal LV lead position should be identified and rejected at the time of implantation. The most common mistake of the uninformed or uncommitted implanter is to place the LV lead in the anterior vein and "see how the patient does." If a patient is not responding to CRT and the LV lead is in the anterior vein, an attempt to reposition the LV lead (or a different lead) in a lateral vein should be made. If this is not possible due to limitations in coronary venous anatomy or other insuperable technical obstacles (see below), the patient should

be referred for surgical placement of the LV lead in an optimal location.

Cardiac surgical approach to left ventricular lead placement

The approach to surgical implantation of epicardial LV leads depends on whether the reason is planned cardiothoracic surgery (i.e. coronary revascularization, valve repair/replacement) or because of failed transvenous approach for any reason (Figs 10.44 and 10.45). This technique is extensively discussed in Chapter 11.

Acute complications of left ventricular lead placement in the coronary veins

Endothelial flaps at the coronary sinus or coronary sinus dissection are by far the most common complications (~6–8%) for the novice implanter and relate largely to poor technique. The three most common causes of CS dissection are stiff guidewires used to support the CS sheath, deflectable electrophysiology catheters for CS cannulation, and balloon catheters for retrograde coronary venography. The tips of electrophysiology and balloon catheters, in particular, are quite rigid, and overaggressive or careless manipulation may shear the endothelial surface of the main body CS. In one prospective randomized study of coronary venogram techniques, CS dissections were observed only during balloon occlusion

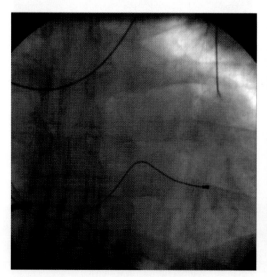
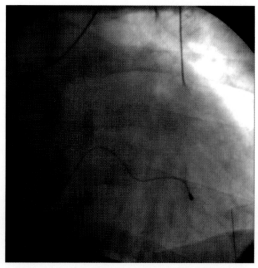

Figure 10.44 Same patient as Fig. 10.43. In the case of the smallest diameter purely OTW leads, it is useful to position the tip in a tertiary branch to achieve support at more than one position and increase mechanical stability. Note fully deployed self-retaining cant when lead is advanced deeper into the target vein.

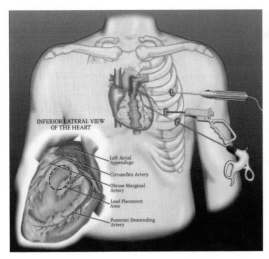
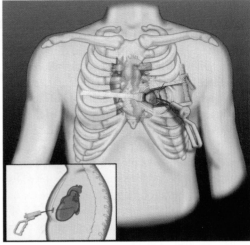

Figure 10.45 Surgical approach to minimally invasive placement of epicardial LV pacing leads via "port hole" approach (left) or limited left lateral thoracotomy (right).

venography and never during direct catheter venography [46], suggesting that balloon inflation was the cause of endothelial disruption. This is easily recognized during coronary venography as staining of the CS wall, which may track retrogradely to the ostium and into the pericardial space. However, pericardial tamponade virtually never occurs, probably because a true perforation or rupture of the vessel wall does not accompany endothelial dissection. Nonetheless, a CS dissection may force premature termination of the procedure if the implanter cannot be certain that advancement of the LV lead or delivery system is not within a false lumen created by the dissection or if the advancing dissection flap occludes the ostium of the target vein. When a dissection is noted after advancement of the CS sheath, particularly if the dissection is proximal to the tip of the sheath and the ostium of the target vein, LV lead placement can usually be safely carried out in the usual manner. A CS dissection that forces premature termination of the procedure does not preclude future attempts at coronary venous pacing. It is advisable to wait 60–90 days before re-attempting CS cannulation. Angiographic follow-up studies of CS dissection indicate that the intimal flap heals completely within at least 2–3 months and is not accompanied by any residual structural damage or venous remodeling [47].

Intimal dissection of the target vein is a rare event that is influenced by LV lead design. Leads with an exposed metal ring at the tip, such as "side wire" de-

signs, or conventional unipolar endocardial pacing leads, are more likely to disrupt the venous endothelium. Misadventure with guidewires in OTW lead designs may also result in venous intimal damage. Target vein dissection may result in premature procedural termination for the reasons cited above, as well as acute thrombotic occlusion. A non-threatening complication is hematoma in the wall of the target vein. This also may contribute to venous thrombosis but is usually not clinically evident. However, coronary vein hematomas due to failed transvenous lead placement are frequently seen at the time of cardiac surgery for "bail out" epicardial LV lead placement.

A much more feared acute complication is coronary venous laceration or perforation. This almost invariably occurs as a result of PCI guidewire manipulation during LV lead positioning. The factors that cause this complication are unknown; however, perforation tends to occur during lead/guidewire manipulations at the distal terminus of the target vein, where the lead tip diameter is equal to or slightly exceeding the luminal diameter of the vein. As a result, excessive outward pressure may be exerted on the vessel wall that reduces the usual distensibility of the vein and facilitates penetration by the advancing guidewire. A rigid and straight guidewire and operator inexperience are the most frequent cause of vein perforation. Coronary venous perforation is recognizable by sudden free movement of the guidewire within the pericardial space. Though coronary venous pressure and intrapericardial pressure are similarly low, a pressure gradient may exist, resulting in pericardial fluid accumulation and tamponade. The management of this complication may be quite difficult. Obviously, pericardiocentesis is mandated in the event of tampondade. Coronary venous bleeders are characteristically slow to cease bleeding, despite low pressure, because of the lack of elastic recoil, unlike arterial injuries. Compression of the culprit vessel by clot formation in the pericardial space is the most likely explanation for coronary venous perforations to cease bleeding. Therefore, removal of blood from the pericardial space may actually hamper hemostasis at the venous bleeding site. In this circumstance, continued accumulation of blood in the pericardial space, even when tamponade is controlled, should sponsor cardiac surgery for definitive evacuation and oversewing of the culprit vessel.

Transvenous extraction of chronic left ventricular pacing leads

Few physicians who have implanted coronary venous LV pacing leads have experience with chronic extraction and the published experience is even less. Therefore, specific comments regarding techniques, success and failure rates, mitigating conditions in either success or failure, and complication rates cannot be made. Many experienced implanters have enduring anxiety about the eventual necessity of removing some chronically implanted coronary venous leads for conventional (lead disruption, infection) and unconventional (exit block, desire for alternate site stimulation, multisite stimulation, etc.) indications. These concerns relate almost entirely to the perceived fragility of the coronary venous system, but should also include consideration that certain aspects of lead design might render chronic extraction more difficult.

Concerns about disruptions of coronary veins during chronic extraction are warranted. The coronary veins are extremely forgiving in their native state due primarily to distensibility. The body of a LV lead that closely approximates the luminal dimensions of the vein eliminates such distensibility. Furthermore, it can be anticipated that the majority of coronary veins likely thrombose after LV lead placement and this might increase binding along the length of the lead. It is also uncertain whether

the use of surgical dissection sheaths (i.e. laser, electrocautery) can be tolerated in the human coronary sinus, reflecting upon the small but catastrophic incidence of laceration of the much larger superior vena cava seen during conventional RA and RV endocardial pacing and ICD lead extraction. Certainly, the experience with the use of laser sheaths in the ovine coronary venous system has not been reassuring, where a 30% incidence of great cardiac vein laceration was reported [48].

It is also unclear whether locking stylets can be safely used for LV lead extraction. One report described a high incidence of lumen loss in OTW LV leads encountered at extraction [41]. This lumen loss may be mechanical (due to crush) or due to thrombosis, since some OTW LV leads do not incorporate a one-way diaphragm at the tip to prevent blood ingress. In either case, the lack of a central lumen for locking stylets would mandate direct (unassisted) traction and presumably increase the probability of incomplete or failed extraction, similar to the experience with conventional transvenous endocardial pacing and ICD leads. Some LV leads incorporate one or more tines to assist with fixation and it is unknown how this may impact extraction. Similarly, some LV leads utilize reversible self-retaining "S" shapes that can only be straightened by a guidewire. Lumen loss due to "crush" or thrombosis that prevented guidewire advancement would necessitate extraction of such leads with the distal portion in the expanded state, potentially increasing resistance to traction. Finally, "side-wire" type leads may pose an increased risk of venous injury during extraction due to the exposed metal ring at the tip.

The published experience is somewhat optimistic despite these considerations. Hansky et al. [41] reported no complications associated with extraction of 10 chronic transvenous LV leads (implant duration three months to two years) with or without locking stylets. As anticipated, the lumen of OTW leads was frequently occluded by thrombus. The most common binding points were the CS ostium and the distal CS (Hansky B, personal communication) [49]. Burke et al. recently reported experience with a laser sheath in 4/10 chronic LV leads (implant duration 5–59 months). Laser energy was applied without complication at the CS ostium and within anterolateral and posterolateral branch vessels. Notably, immediate post-extraction venograms demonstrated that 50% of coronary veins from which chronic LV leads were extracted were thrombosed and unusable for further use [49]. Alternate coronary veins for optimal LV stimulation may not be usable, mandating direct surgical lead placement (Figs 10.46–10.48).

Final comments

The education of the expert LV lead implanter is marked by a series of plateaus. The first of these is developing skill and confidence at CS cannulation. Subsequent skill achievements evolve in a naturally progressive order beginning with a sound familiar-

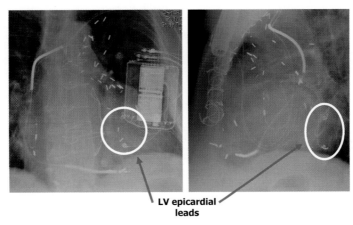

LV epicardial leads

Figure 10.46 Chest radiographs of surgically placed epicardial LV pacing leads. Note LV free wall position of leads approximates obtuse marginal artery location in circumflex territory, where epicardial mapping identified viable sites for LV pacing.

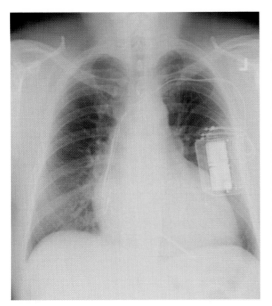
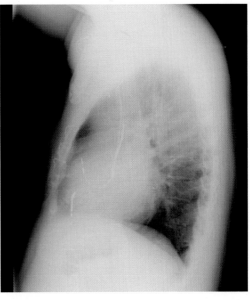

Figure 10.47 CRT "responder." The patient was a 48-year-old male with non-ischemic dilated cardiomyopathy and LBBB, in whom a CRT-D was implanted on 7 January 2000. Note position of LV lead in lateral vein. Note spatial separation of RV and LV leads in lateral view. The patient had an immediate and sustained clinical response to CRT.

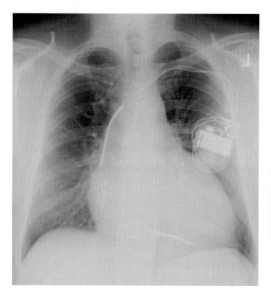

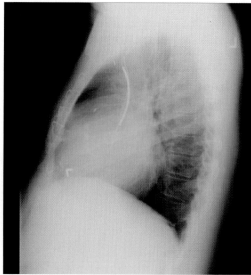

Figure 10.48 Same patient as in Fig. 10.47. Fifty months after CRT-D implant the patient had an abrupt clinical deterioration at which time it was discovered that LV capture could no longer be achieved at maximum device output, despite no evidence of lead dislodgement or conductor discontinuity. The presumptive diagnosis was exit block. The LV lead was extracted; however, the lateral vein could not be reaccessed presumably due to thrombus. A new LV lead was implanted in the anterior interventricular vein.

ity with the basic tools and techniques for routine anatomic situations. During this phase, the implanter comes to appreciate that successful LV lead placement requires a "tool box" approach and that no single LV lead design or delivery system is optimal for every patient. Along with this comes awareness that the advantages to any lead design in specific anatomic situations are likely to be disadvantages

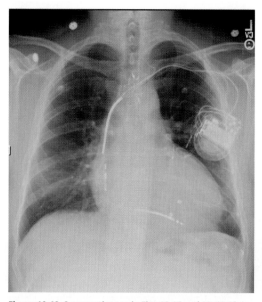

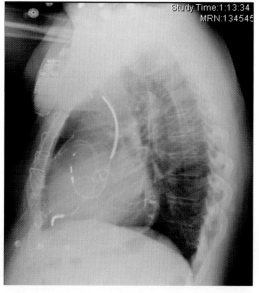

Figure 10.49 Same patient as in Figs 10.47 and 10.48. The patient's heart failure status continued to deteriorate after LV lead revision. Five months later two epicardial LV leads were placed on the posterobasal LV, in close proximity to the original transvenous LV lead site. The patient had an immediate and sustained response to CRT with this stimulation site configuration.

in others. Only when these concepts are mastered can the implanter begin to develop the insight and imagination needed to create innovative solutions to complex and unpredictable obstacles to LV lead placement. Finally, the experienced implanter recognizes that the difference between success and failure is often simply the willingness to labor a difficult task.

References

1 Garrigue S, Jais P, Espil G et al. Comparison of chronic biventricular pacing between epicardial and endocardial left ventricular stimulation using doppler tissue imaging in patients with heart failure. Am J Cardiol 2001; **88**: 858–862.

2 Jais P, Takahashi A, Garrigue S et al. Mid-term follow-up of endocardial biventricular pacing. Pacing Clin Electrophysiol 2000; **23**: 1744–1747.

3 Leclercq C, Hager FX, Macia JC, Mariottini CJ, Pasquie JL, Grolleau R. Left ventricular lead insertion using a modified transseptal catheterization technique: A totally endocardial approach for permanent biventricular pacing in end-stage heart failure. Pacing Clin Electrophysiol 1999; **22**: 1570–1575.

4 Daubert CJ, Ritter P, LeBreton H et al. Permanent left ventricular pacing with transvenous leads inserted into the coronary veins. Pacing Clin Electrophysiol 1998; **21**: 239–345.

5 Leon A, Delurgio DB, Mera F. Practical approach to implanting left ventricular pacing leads for cardiac resynchronization. J Cardiovasc Electrophysiol 2005; **16**: 100–105.

6 Yusuf S, Zhao F, Mehta SR et al. for the Clopidogrel in Unstable Angina to Prevent Recurrent Events Trial Investigators. Effects of clopidogrel in addition to aspirin in patients with acute coronary syndromes without ST-segment elevation. N Engl J Med 2003; **345**: 494–502.

7 Epstein AE, Kay GN, Plumb VJ, Voshage-Stahl L, Hull ML. Elevated defibrillation threshold when right-sided venous access is used for nonthoracotomy implantable defibrillator lead implantation. The Endotak Investigators. J Cardiovasc Electrophysiol 1995; **6**: 979–986.

8 Kirk MM, Shorofsky SR, Gold MR. Right sided active pectoral pulse generators do not reduce defibrillation thresholds. Pacing Clin Electrophysiol 1999; **22**: 747. Abstract.

9 Ong LS, Barold SS, Lederman M, Falkoff M, Heinle RA. Cephalic vein guide wire technique for implantation of permanent pacemakers. Am Heart J 1987; **114**: 753–756.

10 Romeyer-Bouchard C, Da Costa A, Abdellaoui L et al. Simplified cardiac resynchronization implantation technique involving right access and a triple-guide/single in-

troducer approach. Heart Rhythm 2005; **2**: 714–719.

11 Magney JE, Flynn DM, Parsons JA et al. Anatomical mechanisms explaining damage to pacemaker leads, defibrillator leads, and failure of central venous catheters adjacent to the sternoclavicular joint. Pacing Clin Electrophysiol 1993; **16**: 373–376.

12 Magney JE, Staplin DH, Flynn DM, Hunter DW. A new approach to percutaneous subclavian venipuncture to avoid lead fracture or central venous catheter occlusion. Pacing Clin Electrophysiol 1993; **16**: 2133–2142.

13 Abraham WT, Fisher WG, Smith AL et al., for the MIRACLE Study Group. Cardiac resynchronization in chronic heart failure. N Engl J Med 2002; **346**: 1845–1853.

14 Pepper CB, Davidson N, Ross DL. Use of a long preshaped sheath to faciliate cannulation of the coronary sinus at electrophysiologic study. J Cardiovasc Electrophysiol 2001; **12**: 1335–1337.

15 Nazarian S, Knight BP, Dickfeld TL et al. Direct visualization of coronary sinus ostium and branches with a flexible steerable fiberoptic infrared endoscope. Heart Rhythm 2005; **2**: 844–888.

16 Ho SY, Sanchez-Quintana D, Becker AE. A review of the coronary venous system: a road less traveled. Heart Rhythm 2004; **1**: 107–112.

17 Leclercq C, Faris O, Runin R et al. Systolic improvement and mechanical resynchronization does not require electrical synchrony in the dilated failing heart with left bundle-branch block. Circulation 2002; **106**: 1760–1763.

18 Kass DA. Predicting cardiac resynchronization response by QRS duration: the long and short of it. J Am Coll Cardiol 2003; **42**: 2125–2127.

19 Auricchio A, Klein H, Tockman B et al. Transvenous biventricular pacing for heart failure: can the obstacles be overcome? Am J Cardiol 1999; **83**: 136D–142D.

20 Auricchio A, Stellbrink C, Sack S et al. The Pacing Therapies for Congestive Heart Failure (PATH-CHF) study: rationale, design, and endpoints of a prospective randomized multicenter study. Am J Cardiol 1999; **83**: 130D–135D.

21 Butter C, Auricchio A, Stellbrink C et al. for the Pacing Therapy for Chronic Heart Failure II Study Group. Effect of resynchronization therapy stimulation site on the systolic function of heart failure patients. Circulation 2001; **104**: 3026–3029.

22 Fauchier L, Marie O, Casset-Senon D, Babuty D, Cosnay P, Fauchier JP. Interventricular and intraventricular dyssynchrony in idiopathic dilated cardiomyopathy: a prognostic study with fourier phase analysis of radionuclide angioscintigraphy. J Am Coll Cardiol 2002; **40**: 2031–2033.

23 Vassallo JA, Cassidy DM, Machlinski FE et al. Endocardial activation of left bundle branch block. Circulation 1984; **69**: 914.

24 Auricchio A, Fantoni C, Regoli F et al. Characterization

of left ventricular activation in patients with heart failure and left bundle branch block. *Circulation* 2004; **109**: 1133–1139.

25 Rodriguez LM, Timmermans C, Nabar A, Beatty G, Wellens HJ. Variable patterns of septal activation in patients with left bundle branch block. *J Cardiovasc Electrophysiol* 2003; **14**: 135–141.

26 Ansalone A, Giannantoni P, Ricci R *et al*. Doppler myocardial imaging in patients with heart failure receiving biventricular pacing treatment. *Am Heart J* 2001; **142**: 881–896.

27 Ansalone G, Giannantoni P, Ricci R, Trambaiolo P, Fedele F, Santini M. Doppler myocardial imaging to evaluate the effectiveness of pacing sites in patients receiving biventricular pacing. *J Am Coll Cardiol* 2002; **39**: 489–499.

28 Gold MR, Auriccchio A, Hummel JD *et al*. Comparison of stimulation sites within left ventricular veins on the acute hemodynamic effects of cardiac resynchronization therapy. *Heart Rhythm* 2005; **2**: 376–381.

29 Rossillo A, Verma A, Saad EB *et al*. Impact of coronary sinus lead position on biventricular pacing: mortality and echocardiographic evaluation during long term followup. *J Cardiovasc Electrophysiol* 2004; **15**: 1120–1125.

30 Koos R, Sinha A, Markus L *et al*. Comparison of left ventricular lead placement via the coronary venous approach versus lateral thoracotomy in patients receiving cardiac resynchronization therapy. *Am J Cardiol* 2004; **94**: 59–63.

31 Higgins SL, Hummel JD, Niazi IK *et al*. Cardiac resynchronization therapy for the treatment of heart failure and intraventricular conduction delay and malignant ventricular tachyarrhythmia. *J Am Coll Cardiol* 2003; **42**: 1454–1459.

32 Gilard M, Mansourati J, Etienne Y *et al*. Angiographic anatomy of the coronary sinus and its tributaries. *Pacing Clin Electrophysiol* 1998; **21**: 2280–2284.

33 Meisel E, Pfeiffer D, Engelmann L *et al*. Investigation of coronary venous anatomy by retrograde venography in patients with malignant ventricular tachycardia. *Circulation* 2001; **104**: 442–447.

34 Gerber TC, Sheedy PF, Bell MR *et al*. Evaluation of the coronary venous system using electron beam computed tomography. *Int J Cardiovasc Imaging* 2001; **17**: 65–75.

35 Debruyne P, Geelen P, Janssens L, Brugada P. Useful tip to improve electrode positioning in markedly angulated coronary sinus tributaries. *J Cardiovasc Electrophysiol* 2003; **14**: 415–416.

36 Hellerstein HK, Orbison JL. Anatomic variations of the orifice of the human coronary sinus. *Circulation* 1951; **3**: 514–523.

37 Hansky B, Lamp B, Minami K *et al*. Coronary vein balloon angioplasty for left ventricular pacemaker lead implantation. *J Am Coll Cardiol* 2002; **40**: 2144–2149.

38 Chierchia G-B, Geelen P, Rivero-Ayerza M, Brugada P. Double wire technique to catheterize sharply angulated coronary sinus branches in cardiac resynchronization therapy. *Pacing Clin Electrophysiol* 2005; **28**: 168–170.

39 Sanchez-Quintana D, Cabrera JA, Climent V, Farre J, Weiglein A, Ho SW. How close are the phrenic nerves to cardiac structures? Implications for cardiac interventionalists. *J Cardiovasc Electrophysiol* 2005; **16**: 309–313.

40 Knight BP, Desai A, Coman J, Faddis M, Yong P. Long-term retention of cardiac resynchronization therapy. *J Am Coll Cardiol* 2004; **44**: 72–77.

41 Hansky B, Schulte-Eistrup S, Vogt J *et al*. Lead selection and implantation technique for biventricular pacing. *Eur Heart J Suppl* 2004; **6**(suppl D): D112–116.

42 Daoud E, Kalbfleisch FJ, Hummel JD *et al*. Implantation techniques and chronic lead parameters of biventricular pacing dual-chamber defibrillators. *J Cardiovasc Electrophysiol* 2002; **13**: 964–970.

43 Storm C, Harsch M, DeBus B. InSync Registry: Post Market Study: Progress Report No. 7. Medtronic, Inc., 2005.

44 Bristow MR, Saxon LA, Boehmer J *et al*., the Comparison of Medical Therapy P, and Defibrillation in Heart Failure (COMPANION) Investigators. Cardiac-resynchronization therapy with or without an implantable defibrillator in advanced chronic heart failure. *N Engl J Med* 2004; **350**: 2140–2150.

45 Young JB, Abraham WT, Smith AL *et al*., Multicenter InSync ICD Randomized Clinical Evaluation (MIRACLE ICD) Trial Investigators. Combined cardiac resynchronization and implantable cardioversion defibrillation in advanced chronic heart failure: the MIRACLE ICD Trial. *JAMA* 2003; **289**: 2685–2394.

46 De Martino G, Messano L, Santamaria M *et al*. A randomized evaluation of different approaches to coronary sinus venography during biventricular pacemaker implants. *Europace* 2005; **7**: 73–76.

47 de Cock CC, van Campen CM, Visser CA. Major dissection of the coronary sinus and its tributaries during lead implantation for biventricular stimulation: angiographic follow-up. *Europace* 2004; **6**: 43–47.

48 Tacker WA, Vanvleet JF, Shoenlein WE, Janas W, Ayers GM, Byrd CL. Post mortem changes after lead extraction from the ovine coronary sinus and great cardiac vein. *Pacing Clin Electrophysiol* 1998; **21**: 292–298.

49 Burke DC, Morton J, Lin AC *et al*. Implications and outcome of permanent coronary sinus lead extraction and reimplantation. *J Cardiovasc Electrophysiol* 2005; **16**: 830–837.

50 Singh JP, Houser S, Heist EK, Ruskin JN. The coronary venous anatomy: A segmental approach to aid cardiac resynchronization therapy. *J Am Coll Cardiol* 2005; **46**: 68–74.

CHAPTER 11

Anatomy of the coronary sinus

Samuel J. Asirvatham, MD

Introduction

It is several centuries since the basic anatomy of the venous system for the heart, including the coronary sinus, was first described, but it is only in the last two decades that there has been a tremendous and sustained interest in the anatomy of these veins [1]. Although the main reason for this recent interest has been the advent of biventricular pacing, electrophysiologists have increasingly used coronary venous access to ablate epicardial cardiac arrhythmias. Even more recently the cardiac venous system has been proposed for the deployment of devices to aid cardiac function and decrease valvular regurgitation [2–5].

The aim of this chapter is to describe the gross and histological anatomy of the coronary veins with the biventricular device implanter in mind. Although basic structural descriptions will be presented, focus will be on details of anatomy and electrophysiology that should aid the novice implanter. For those who are more experienced, we provide a

brief description of anatomical variation, anomalies, and pathology related to the implant complications that will hopefully yield greater success in coronary venous manipulation. A brief description of the neighboring anatomy of the venous system including the arteries, phrenic nerve, and autonomic nerve will also be given since an understanding of these associated structures is critical when the coronary venous system is instrumented.

Gross anatomy

Most of the left ventricle and portions of the right ventricle and intraventricular septum are drained by the coronary venous system (Fig. 11.1). The anterior wall of the left ventricle and intraventricular septum is drained by branches of the anterior intraventricular vein [3, 6–8]. These drain back to the mitral annulus and are joined by branches of the lateral venous system (Fig. 11.2). Anterolateral, lateral, and posterolateral veins are frequently found. On the annulus, the vein is named the great cardiac

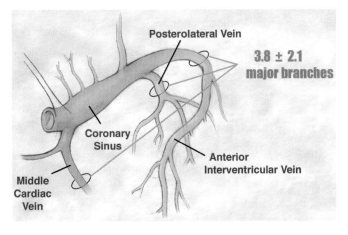

Figure 11.1 Diagram of the coronary sinus showing the three principal tributaries. Note the ostium of the posterolateral vein demarcates the coronary sinus from the great cardiac vein. In a series of 600 autopsied heart specimens, an average of 3.8 ± 2.1 major branches were noted. Reproduced from [52] with permission. © Mayo Foundation for Medical Education and Research.

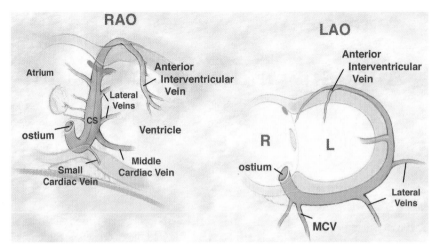

Figure 11.2 Diagrammatic representation of the positioning of the coronary sinus in the right anterior oblique and left anterior oblique projections. Note the numerous atrial tributaries and two lateral veins shown in the diagram. Also note the small cardiac vein that is in proximity to the posterior fat pad and rightward in the left anterior oblique projection. Reproduced from [52] with permission. © Mayo Foundation for Medical Education and Research.

vein. Where the great cardiac vein is joined by the main posterior lateral vein, the coronary sinus itself is formed. The coronary sinus in turn often receives posterior venous supply in the form of a posterior vein and the middle cardiac vein. Throughout its course, the atrial musculature is drained into the venous system via various atrial veins. The most consistent atrial vein is one formed at the junction of the great cardiac vein and posterolateral vein and is called the vein of Marshall [9]. The vein of Marshall is a remnant of the left superior vena cava. The length of the coronary sinus itself is variable (3–5.5 cm) as would be expected with an arbitrary definition dependent on the site of drainage of the posterolateral vein (see below) [10]. The diameter of the coronary sinus is also highly variable and is dependent on the loading conditions on the heart, presence and extent of atrial myocardium within the coronary vein (see below), and the presence of cardiac disease or prior cardiac surgery. Distinctly aneurysmal coronary sinus and great cardiac veins have been reported as well as diverticular enlargement of the primary and secondary branches of the coronary system.

The orientations of the coronary sinus and its tributaries are defined by the blood flow through this venous system. Thus, the most distal end is the coronary sinus ostium in the right atrium. The proximal end of the main coronary sinus is described as the beginning or distal most part of the great cardiac vein. This transition from coronary sinus to great cardiac vein is usually stated to be at the site of the valve of Vieussens. Also located at this site is the main posterolateral vein as well as the ostium of the vein or ligament of Marshall (Figs 11.3 and 11.4). These anatomic definitions often overlap because of the variability in finding the valve of Vieussens or the ligament of Marshall, making it difficult at times to find the exact length of the coronary sinus.

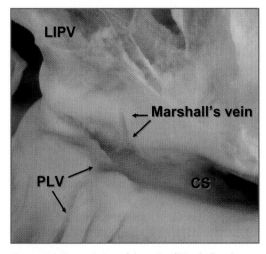

Figure 11.3 External view of the vein of Marshall and posterolateral vein.

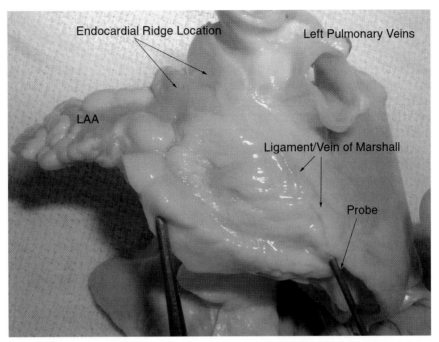

Figure 11.4 Course of the vein of Marshall anterior to the pulmonary veins and posterior to the left atrial appendage; a probe passes into a patent vein of Marshall.

The average length of the coronary sinus as defined above is 40–45 mm with an average diameter of 10 mm. It is at times slightly "atrialized" with up to 10 mm atrial to the atrioventricular sulcus and thus not precisely on the annulus. It thus courses along the left atrial myocardium. This fact is known to electrophysiologists because of the large near-field atrial signal noted on catheters placed within the coronary sinus. This is again understandable from the developmental anatomy because both the posteroinferior left atrium and coronary sinus arise from the left horn of the sinus venosus. More proximally the tributaries of the coronary vein are closer to the left ventricle and more truly in the atrioventricular sulcus.

The coronary sinus lies in relation to the posterior mitral annulus and drains through the posteroseptal portion of the right atrium on the interatrial septum into the right atrium. Atrial myocardium is present to various extents into the coronary veins. Typically described is the extension of the myocardium up to the portion of great cardiac vein that is the junction of the posterolateral vein [11–13]. Occasionally myocardial sleeves can extend beyond this portion and even into the atrial and ventricular

branches. This myocardial sleeve is always continuous in its entirety with the right atrial myocardium at the ostium and at variable portions and to a variable extent with the left atrial myocardium through interdigitations. These myocardial sleeves are not usually continuous with ventricular myocardium. If such a continuation is formed, this constitutes an atrial–ventricular bypass tract referred to an epicardial pathway [14–17].

Various valves can be found in the cardiac venous system (Fig. 11.5) [18–22]. Most frequently present is the thebesian valve found at the ostium of the coronary sinus (Fig. 11.6). Vieussens' valve is also frequently seen at the ostium of the primary posterolateral vein opposite to the opening of the vein of Marshall (Fig. 11.7). Valves may be found in other ventricular and atrial veins. Rarely seen, but most common of the non-Vieussens' variety, is a valve at the ostium of the middle cardiac vein.

The right ventricular venous drainage and portions of the interventricular septum are primarily through the thebesian [23] venous network directly into the right ventricle. The most proximal of the branches of the coronary venous system is the small cardiac vein which drains the posterior and postero-

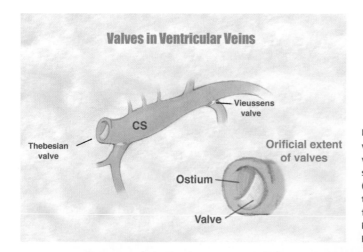

Figure 11.5 Valves in the coronary venous system. Typically found are veins of the ostium of the coronary sinus, ostium of the posterolateral vein (Vieussens' valve) and the ostium of the middle cardiac vein. Reproduced from [52] with permission. © Mayo Foundation for Medical Education and Research.

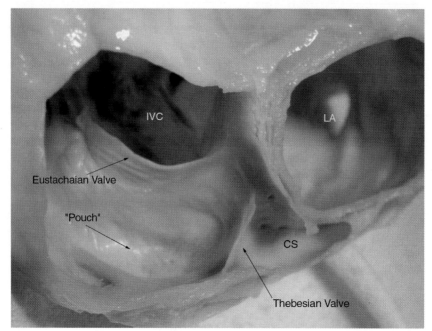

Figure 11.6 A prominent thebesian valve shown at the ostium of the coronary sinus. Note a subeustachian pouch that is bordered by the thebesian, eustachian, and tricuspid valves.

lateral portions of the right ventricle and right atrium opening into the coronary sinus at its ostium in the right atrium.

Embryology of the coronary sinus

The primordial atrium and sinus venosus originate from a single cardiac tube that separates in the third week of life. The right horn of this sinus venosus is absorbed by the right atrium to become the smooth portion of the superior vena cava and the area between the cava extending to the coronary sinus os [24]. The left horn of the sinus venosus progressively disappears until the tenth week (Fig. 11.8). Of the remnants of the left common cardinal vein, only the vein of Marshall (see below) or its ligamentous remnants survive. The remainder of the left horn of the sinus venosus becomes the coronary sinus. It is because of this development that the proximal end of the coronary sinus is marked by the vein of Marshall tributary [25].

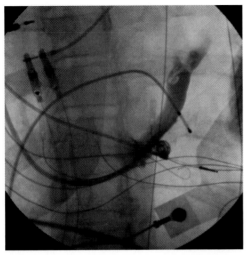 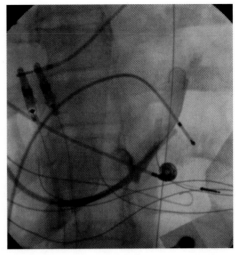

Figure 11.7 Coronary sinus angiogram showing a prominent Vieussens' valve at the ostium of the posterolateral vein. Reproduced from [52] with permission. © Mayo Foundation for Medical Education and Research.

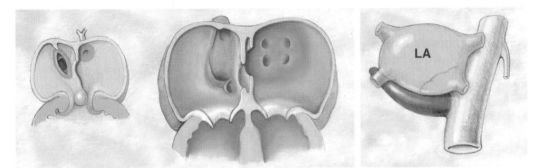

Figure 11.8 Venous and primordial atrial tissue contribute to the formation of the right atrium, left atrium, as well as the coronary sinus itself. The left venous horn remains as the vein of Marshall and the coronary sinus. See text for details.

The coronary sinus ostium

The coronary sinus ostium typically measures 5–15 mm in diameter. The ostium is almost always located on the posterior interatrial septum anterior to the eustachian ridge and valve and posterior to the tricuspid annulus [8, 10, 20–22]. It is frequently guarded by the thebesian valve (Fig. 11.9) The valve typically covers about a third of the ostium but may sometimes nearly completely occlude the ostium. When near circumferential valves are found, multiple fenestrations are usually seen. When the circumference is only partially covered, it is usually the superior and posterior surfaces that are covered. Thus, entering the coronary sinus from an inferior and ventricular starting point avoids valvular contact. Rarely the valve covers the inferior hemi-circumference making it necessary to enter the coronary sinus

from a superior route dragging the catheter sheath supero-inferiorly on the interatrial septum anterior to the eustachian ridge.

Traversing the floor of the coronary sinus ostium in about a third of normal hearts are extensions of the pectinate muscles that course from the lateral wall across the sub-eustachian isthmus and into the proximal coronary veins where they form part of the atrial myocardial sleeve described above. In some patients, a sub-eustachian aneurysm or pouch is noted. These patients have minimal myocardial sleeves entering into the coronary sinus and well-formed thebesian valves at the coronary sinus ostium. The atrial myocardial sleeves that course from the roof of the coronary sinus across the ostium in the tendon of Todaro cephalad towards the atrio-ventriacular (AV) node constitute part of the slow pathway input to the AV node.

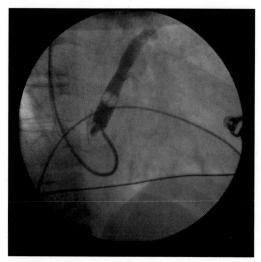

Figure 11.9 Coronary angiogram showing an abrupt narrowing at the ostium of the coronary sinus. Reproduced from [52] with permission. © Mayo Foundation for Medical Education and Research.

Atrial venous drainage

The atrial veins have been used when pacing the left atrium has been required. The total number of atrial venous branches are highly variable, but typically the largest branch occurs opposite to the posterolateral vein coursing between the anterior surface of the left-sided pulmonary veins and the posterior surface of the route of the left atrial appendage. This is the embryological remnant of the left superior vena cava and is patent to a variable extent. When completely patent, it is called a persistent left superior vena cava draining into the coronary sinus; when patent in its atrial myocardial course it is called the vein of Marshall; and when partially or completely obliterated it is referred to as the oblique vein of Marshall [9, 26, 27]. A pericardial fold is raised by the structure epicardially and an endocardial invagination is seen consistently between the left pulmonary veins and the left atrial appendage (echocardiographic "Q-tip" or endocardial ridge). Typically three or four atrial veins are seen between the vein of Marshall and the ostium of the coronary sinus and two to three atrial veins are seen anterior to the vein of Marshall.

Ventricular veins

The anterior intraventricular vein

The anterior intraventricular vein courses from the ventricular apex to the annulus just lateral to the anterior ventricular septum. Various tributaries drain the anterior wall of the left ventricle and parts of the anterior wall of the right ventricle. In the right anterior oblique projection, this vein is seen just behind the sternum and is the most anterior vein seen in this view. The largest tributary of the anterior intraventricular vein arises proximally and drains a large portion of the anterolateral wall of the left ventricle. Frequent anastomoses with the lateral venous system are seen through this vein. In about 30% of hearts, the proximal branch (apical) of the anterior intraventricular vein interdigitates and is continuous with similar branches of the posterior and middle cardiac veins [8, 10, 25, 28–30]. Thus, a guidewire advanced apically into the anterior intraventricular vein in these patients will enter the middle cardiac venous system and through this vein reenter the coronary sinus and right atrium. The course of the anterior intraventricular vein is similar to the left anterior descending coronary artery and the primary anterolateral tributary to the anterior ventricular vein is analogous to the first diagonal branch of the left anterior descending coronary artery (Fig. 11.10). More laterally, that is over the anterolateral wall of the left ventricle, the vein (anterior intraventricular vein) is leftward of the corresponding coronary artery and more septally (rightward) the vein crosses anterior to the coronary artery and is found to its right [16, 31, 32]. In approximately 20% of patients the left phrenic nerve will form an anterior relation to the anterolateral branch of the anterior intraventricular vein. A fat pad of various thicknesses is found consistently over the mid portion of the anterior intraventricular vein. The anterolateral tributary and distal tributaries are often superficial and not covered by fat. Because of the absence of fat over the anterolateral tributary, when the phrenic nerve forms an immediate relation to this vein, phrenic nerve stimulation with unipolar or wide bipolar stimulation from this site can be expected.

Lateral cardiac veins

Typically three distinct veins are seen draining the lateral wall of the left ventricle [8, 10, 25, 28–30]. The posterolateral vein is most consistent and often the largest and occurs directly opposite to the vein of Marshall. A smaller straight lateral vein and one

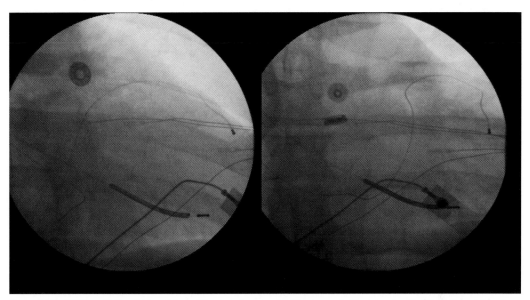

Figure 11.10 Right and left anterior oblique fluoroscopic views showing access to the lateral wall of the left ventricle via the anterior interventricular vein.

or more anterior lateral veins can be seen. When the anterior lateral veins are large, draining into the great cardiac vein, the anterolateral tributary of the anterior interventricular vein is often small or absent (Fig. 11.11). Occasionally atrial myocardium can be seen just distal to the posterolateral vein and almost never seen in the great cardiac vein at sites adjacent to the lateral and anterolateral tributaries. The great cardiac vein itself is the accompanying vein of the circumflex coronary artery and is usually superficial to the artery. The lateral tributaries accompany and frequently cross over the obtuse marginal branches of the circumflex artery. Less common in comparison to the anterior intraventricular vein are continuous anastomoses via the apex to the middle cardiac venous distribution. Frequently seen, however, are large multiple anastomoses between the various lateral veins, the posterior cardiac vein and the anterolateral tributary of the anterior intraventricular vein. Intimal sleeves of adipose tissue are seen in the lateral tributaries of the great cardiac vein. The phrenic nerve typically courses lateral to the left atrial appendage, crossing superficial to the great cardiac vein forming variable relations with the lateral vein, posterior branches of the anterolateral vein and anterior branches of the posterolateral cardiac vein. It should be noted that because of the thickness of the ventricular myocardium at this

site, fairly large secondary tributaries of these lateral veins can be seen going intramyocardially. A pacing lead placed in one of the secondary tributaries will avoid stimulation of the phrenic nerve.

Posterior ventricular vein

The posterior ventricular vein arises just distal to the middle cardiac vein and is often confused by implanters with the middle cardiac vein. In about a quarter of patients, the middle cardiac vein and the posterior vein share a common cloacal ostium [8, 10, 25, 28–30]. In even fewer patients the posterior vein arises as a proximal tributary of the middle cardiac vein. The vein, regardless of the nature of its origin, courses directly to the lateral wall and accompanies the posterolateral branches of the right coronary artery. This is the only normally occurring tributary of the venous system whose main body runs parallel or nearly parallel to the annulus and its tributaries coursing from apex to base or vice versa. Because of this course, it is frequently mistaken to be a branch of the middle cardiac vein. This vein, regardless of origin, can be consistently used to place a pacing lead to the lateral wall of the left ventricle even when the posterolateral and lateral veins are absent, tortuous or otherwise not amenable to implant. The distal branches of the posterior ventricular vein interdigitate with tributaries of the

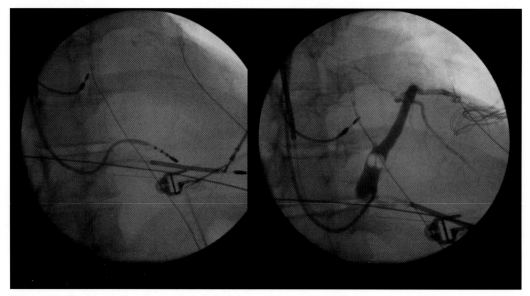

Figure 11.11 The venous tributaries, particularly the left posterior and posterolateral veins are rather constant in their presence. In this example, coronary angiography does not reveal a posterolateral vein. However, probing with a deflectable catheter easily cannulates this vein, probably occluded by the balloon, and the delivery sheath is tracked over the catheter into this tributary. Reproduced from [52] with permission. © Mayo Foundation for Medical Education and Research.

lateral venous system and are frequently related to the phrenic nerve at these sites. Because the ostium of this vein is very close to the ostium of the middle cardiac vein, selective cannulation of this vein can be difficult. Thus attempting to enter the vein from the right atrium directly will cause sub-selection of the middle cardiac vein and when sheaths are placed into the coronary sinus, the ostia of both the posterior vein and middle cardiac vein are covered, rendering these veins inaccessible. Understanding the anatomy of this vein allows its cannulation by placing the sub-selecting catheter or lead into the main body of the coronary sinus, withdrawing the sheath back to the right atrium and with clockwise torque engaging, upon withdrawal of the lead or catheter, the ostium of the posterior ventricular vein (Fig. 11.12) [32–35].

Middle cardiac vein

The middle cardiac vein is the largest proximal tributary to the coronary sinus (Figs 11.13 and 11.14). The ostium is located between the orifice of the small cardiac vein and the left posterior vein [3, 32, 36]. These two latter veins may arise as tributaries of the middle cardiac vein. The middle cardiac vein courses from apex to base on the posterior interventricular groove where it is accompanied by the posterior descending artery and covered by fat. Tributaries that drain the posterior and posterolateral left ventricle as well as rightward tributaries that drain part of the posterior right ventricle, drain into the middle cardiac vein along its course in the posterior interventricular sulcus. Cardiac autonomic fibers, particularly vagal afferents and some sympathetic efferents are found in the posterior crux near to the junction of the middle cardiac vein with the coronary sinus.

Rarely the middle cardiac vein may arise as a separate ostium where its orifice can be found superior to the main orifice of the coronary sinus. Even rarer is a direct opening of the middle cardiac vein apical to the septal attachment of the tricuspid valve. Distal tributaries of the middle cardiac vein have numerous anastomoses near the apex with the apical tributaries of the anterior intraventricular vein and the lateral cardiac veins. The phrenic nerve typically does not have an anatomic relation (right or left phrenic nerves) with the middle cardiac vein. However, pacing leads placed apically in the distal middle cardiac vein may directly capture the left hemidiaphragm.

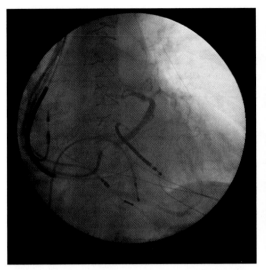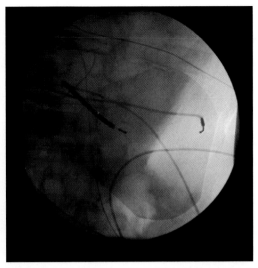

Figure 11.12 Extensive collateralization between the main tributaries of the coronary sinus with placement of a lead to the lateral wall of the left ventricle through one of these tributaries. Reproduced from [52] with permission. © Mayo Foundation for Medical Education and Research.

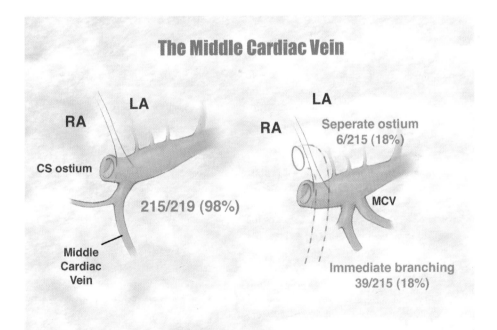

Figure 11.13 Variations in the presence of the middle cardiac vein include a separate ostium and immediate branching of the middle cardiac vein. When there is immediate branching of the middle cardiac vein, a separate left posterior vein is not seen.

Venous drainage of the lateral left ventricular wall

Intraoperative hemodynamic studies suggest that left ventricular stimulation with a pacing electrode located in the mid portion of the left ventricular free wall results in the greatest benefit. Fortunately, the venous drainage of the lateral wall tends to be extensive with interdigitating branches of all the main tributaries of the coronary sinus and great cardiac

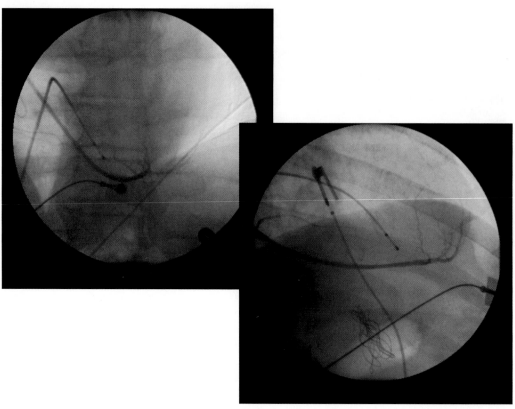

Figure 11.14 Angiographic subselection of the middle cardiac vein showing numerous lateral branches, some large enough to place a lead. Top right anterior oblique, bottom left anterior oblique views. Reproduced from [52] with permission. © Mayo Foundation for Medical Education and Research.

vein. The most direct anatomic drainage of this site is via the lateral high posterior, high posterolateral, or anterolateral veins (Figs 11.15–11.17). At times cannulation of these veins can be difficult as typically the ostium and proximal tributary is at near right angles to the access of the great cardiac vein. Furthermore, the main posterolateral vein is frequently guarded by a valve (Vieussens' valve) making sub-selection of this tributary challenging. In addition, because of the direct opposition of the vein of Marshall, guide wires and catheters may curl into this sometimes large atrial branch and then prolapse into the distal coronary venous circulation, not allowing cannulation of a lateral vein. While several techniques have been described to aid cannulation of the lateral veins, it should be kept in mind that alternate venous drainage to this site exists. Most notably, lateral branches of the anterior interventricular vein and, in almost all hearts, the left posterior vein will either

directly drain this site or anastomose with branches of the lateral venous circulation.

Histological anatomy

Like most veins the coronary veins have an intimal and adventitial layer. Venular smooth muscle that is electrophysiologically active is found throughout the course of the coronary venous tree. In addition to this, atrial syncytial myocardium is found ostially and extends up to the region of the posterolateral vein/vein of Marshall. The venous valves, including the thebesian and Vieussens' valves, do not have atrial myocardium.

The coronary sinus wall is largely composed of striated muscle sheaths with a structure similar to that of the atrial myocardium [15, 37–39]. This muscular sheath surrounds the venous tissue and is in fact an extension of the right atrial myocardium.

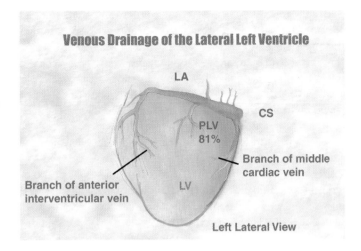

Figure 11.15 The lateral wall of the left ventricle is often a target site for left ventricular pacing. This myocardial site can be arrived at via the posterolateral vein, lateral branches of the middle cardiac vein or lateral branches of the anterior interventricular vein in the majority of patients. Reproduced from [52] with permission. © Mayo Foundation for Medical Education and Research.

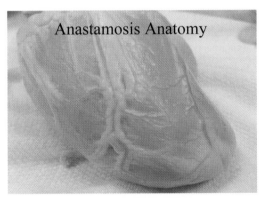

Figure 11.16 Autopsied specimen showing extensive anastomoses in the lateral wall of the left ventricle.

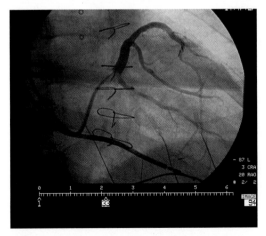

Figure 11.17 Angiogram showing anastomoses of the principal tributaries of the coronary sinus. Reproduced from [52] with permission. © Mayo Foundation for Medical Education and Research.

It represents the intermingling of derivatives of the left and right horns of the sinus venosus. Its electrophysiological significance is that it is one of the three main electrical connections between the right and left atrium (in addition to Bachmann's bundle and the fossa ovalis). The left atrial musculature surrounds the venous tissue of the coronary sinus and the right atrial sleeve. Of the venous tributaries, the middle cardiac vein and the small cardiac vein are the most likely to carry right and left atrial muscular sheaths along their course.

Electrophysiology of the coronary sinus

The coronary sinus is an electrophysiologically active structure. In many ways the coronary sinus represents a third atrium [12]. Like the right and left atrium, an admixture embryologically of venous and cardiac musculature derivatives exists. In the tributaries and distal circulation, the coronary venous circulation is much like the systemic veins. More proximally in the great cardiac vein and the coronary sinus there is a presence of both myocardium as well as venular structures. The venular smooth muscle is by itself electrically active capable of spontaneous depolarization and slow conduction from one site to another [40–42]. In addition, the atrial myocardial sleeves show typical syncytial cardiac muscle conduction and automaticity and form one of the normal electrical connections between the right and left atrium. For electrophysiologists, these electrical connections are important in the pathogenesis of various arrhythmias including atrial fibrillation, coronary sinus tachycardias, atypical AV node reentry and interatrial flutters [17, 43–45]. For implantation of a left ventricular lead, it should be noted that leads placed in the proximal tributaries may give rise to both inappropriate atrial sensing and capture of the right atrium through the musculature of the coronary sinus.

Early experiments showed that the coronary sinus is capable of automaticity and represents one of the main secondary sites of impulse initiation when the sinus node fails [37, 39, 46–48]. There is a close relationship between the leftward margins/extensions of the atrioventricular node and the coronary sinus orifice. The anatomical basis for this electrophysiological activity includes the lining of atrial muscle from the coronary sinus ostium to the junction of the great cardiac vein, or the smooth venular muscle of the vein itself. Despite the anatomical proximity of the AV node, the action potentials recorded from cells at the ostium of the coronary sinus are different from the action potentials typically seen from the AV nodal tissue. This inherent automaticity coupled with the complex anatomy of encircling right atrial and left atrial myocardial sleeves with venular smooth muscle is the basis for the complex

arrhythmogenicity of the coronary sinus. Arrhythmias related to enhanced automaticity, triggered activity, and complex reentrant mechanisms have all been described.

Anomalies and variation in coronary sinus anatomy

The prevalence of coronary sinus anomalies is difficult to ascertain as they are of little pathophysiological significance. Described anomalies include absence of the coronary sinus, atresia of whole or part or a tributary of the coronary sinus and hypoplasia of the coronary sinus (Fig. 11.18) These anomalies are often associated with a persistent left superior vena cava. Coronary sinus diverticula are malformations typically associated with the main tributaries of the coronary sinus and great cardiac vein and have been associated with epicardial accessory pathways [10, 20, 22, 49–51].

Persistent left superior vena cava
One to two per cent of normal hearts show persistence of the left superior vena cava as it courses between the left upper pulmonary veins and left atrial appendage draining and being continuous with the main body of the coronary sinus. When proximal coronary sinus stenosis occurs this vein can be fur-

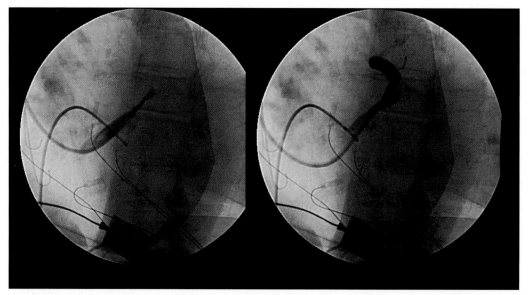

Figure 11.18 Coronary sinus stenosis in a patient with no previous intracardiac procedure. The vein was dilated and allowed passage of a pacing lead. Reproduced from [52] with permission. © Mayo Foundation for Medical Education and Research.

ther enlarged. When large, lead manipulation in this coronary sinus can be difficult, with the lead continuously engaging the atrial branches, particularly the persistent left superior vena cava. Conversely, the left superior vena cava can be used to gain rather easy access to the coronary sinus and the leads subsequently will have to be manipulated into a ventricular vein to maintain stability.

Dual coronary sinus

Rare duplication of the coronary sinus has been described [25]. This is often a result of either a malformed or occluded portion of the coronary sinus, wherein large atrial or ventricular tributaries further enlarge to reconstitute the primary venous circulation of the heart. When the primary abnormality is corrected, such as reformation of the lumen after thrombus resolution, the appearance of parallel coronary sinuses arises. True duplication also occurs; however, this is very rare.

Complete occlusion of a coronary sinus vein because of a circumferential valve

When this occurs the venous drainage for that site of the ventricle from the time of development occurs either via a thebesian vein or collateral veins. The lumen of the coronary vein itself is atretic. However, when a lead is placed through an anastomotic vein, the lead may come through this atretic vein up to the valve at the ostium of the coronary sinus. This can be mistaken for coronary venous system perforation or dissection.

Atrial opening of the coronary sinus

When a semilunar thebesian valve covers the inferior portion of the coronary sinus ostium or proximal coronary sinus stenosis occurs and the ostium is reconstituted via an atrial vein, the opening into the coronary sinus vasculature is through a site in the atrium that is superior and posterior to the usual ostium of the coronary sinus. Cannulation of such veins can be difficult and coronary arterial angiography with venous phase imaging may be required to identify the remaining ostium of the coronary sinus system. Deflectable catheters placed on the atrial septum and gradually advanced towards the posterior tricuspid annulus will often engage these unusual ostia.

Coronary sinus opening into the right ventricle

This occurs as a very rare anomaly but is more commonly seen after congenital heart surgery, particularly certain procedures for Ebstein's anomaly. Here the reconstructed tricuspid valve is placed more atrially thereby having drainage of the coronary sinus into the basal right ventricular septum. In such patients atrial angiography performed with adenosine will fail to visualize the coronary sinus. Manipulation of a catheter from the ventricle towards the atrium or coronary arterial angiography will reveal the true course of the coronary veins.

Iatrogenic causes of coronary sinus variation

Both cardiovascular surgery and radiofrequency ablation may produce unusual variation in the coronary venous vasculature. Radiofrequency ablation for AV node reentry or epicardial accessory pathways may heal with the formation of coronary sinus stenosis. Mitral valve surgery both because of the annular changes and placement of sutures may produce highly abnormal coursing of the coronary veins with intermittent partial stenosis. Coronary sinus perforation as well dissection can occur with either ablation or lead manipulation in the coronary veins. Dissections tend to occur in the main body of the coronary sinus and may propagate more distally, particularly with added catheter manipulation. Spontaneous propagation to occlusion of the coronary veins is very infrequent because of the low flow state in the coronary veins. In cases that we have observed, the dissection does not propagate into the secondary tributaries of the coronary veins. This is likely because of the even lower flow state of these secondary tributaries.

Variceal coronary venous tree

Very large coronary veins can be seen in certain patients (Fig. 11.19). These may be an isolated and anatomical anomaly or seen in the setting of severe congestive heart failure. The most common associations that should be excluded are persistent left superior vena cava, coronary artery to vein fistulous formation and isolated multiple diverticula [14–17].

Understanding the typical coronary venous anatomy and encountered variation (Table 11.1) should

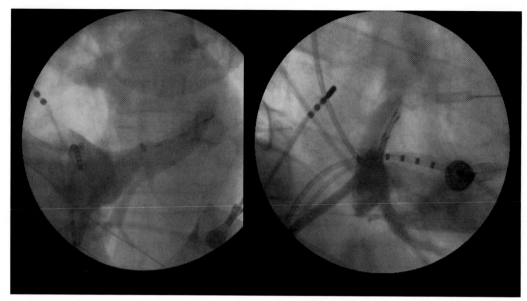

Figure 11.19 A large aneurysmal coronary sinus with relatively normal tributaries. Sometimes the coronary sinus itself is small with variceal or diverticular branches. Reproduced from [52] with permission. © Mayo Foundation for Medical Education and Research.

Table 11.1 Salient anatomical features for implantation of a coronary sinus lead

---

1 Multiple veins drain the lateral wall and usually robust anastomoses occur

2 The true posterior ventricular vein arises close to the middle cardiac vein and is the most consistently oblique or horizontal vein in the heart allowing access to the left ventricular free wall

3 Intramyocardial tributaries of the lateral veins frequently exist and can be utilized to avoid phrenic nerve stimulation

4 Atrial myocardial sleeves occur in the coronary veins sometimes causing atrial pacing when the ventricular lead is placed too basally in the coronary venous vasculature

5 A large thebesian vein usually signifies a sub-eustachian pouch whereas the absent thebesian vein may be associated with muscle bundles (pectinates) coursing into the coronary sinus

6 The phrenic nerve typically courses lateral to the left atrial appendage crossing superficial to the great cardiac vein forming variable relations with the lateral, posterior branches of the anterolateral and anterior branches of the posterolateral cardiac veins

7 Relationships of coronary venous anatomy to coronary arterial anatomy include:
   • The course of the anterior intraventricular vein is similar to the left anterior descending coronary artery and the primary anterolateral tributary to the anterior ventricular vein is analogous to the first diagonal branch of the left anterior descending coronary artery
   • The great cardiac vein is the accompanying vein of the circumflex coronary artery and is usually superficial to the artery
   • The posterior ventricular vein regardless of the nature of its origin courses directly to the lateral wall and accompanies the posterolateral branches of the right coronary artery

---

allow enhanced facility with sheath and lead manipulation in the coronary sinus and placement of left ventricular sinus pacing leads.

References

1 Abraham WT. Cardiac resynchronization therapy for heart failure: biventricular pacing and beyond. *Curr Opin Cardiol* 2002; **17**: 346–352.

2 Gerber TC, Kantor B, Keelan PC, Hayes DL, Schwartz RS, Holmes DR. The coronary venous system: An alternate portal to the myocardium for diagnostic and therapeutic procedures in invasive cardiology. *Curr Interv Cardiol Rep* 2000; **2**: 27–37.

3 Grzybiak M. Morphology of the coronary sinus and contemporary cardiac electrophysiology. *Folia Morphol* 1996; **55**: 272–273.

4 Linde C, Leclercq C, Rex S *et al.* Long-term benefits of biventricular pacing in congestive heart failure: results from the MUltisite STimulation in cardiomyopathy (MUSTIC) study. *J Am Coll Cardiol* 2002; 40: 111–118.

5 Alonso C, Leclercq C, d'Allonnes FR *et al.* Six year experience of transvenous left ventricular lead implantation for permanent biventricular pacing in patients with advanced heart failure: technical aspects. *Heart* 2001; **86**: 405–410.

6 D'Cruz IA, Shala MB, Johns C. Echocardiography of the coronary sinus in adults. *Clin Cardiol* 2000; **23**: 149–154.

7 Gerber TC, Sheedy PF, Bell MR *et al.* Evaluation of the coronary venous system using electron beam computed tomography. *Int J Cardiovasc Imag* 2001; **17**: 65–75.

8 Ortale JR, Gabriel EA, Iost C, Marquez CQ. The anatomy of the coronary sinus and its tributaries. *Surg Radiol Anat* 2001; **23**: 15–21.

9 Cendrowska-Pinkosz M, Urbanowicz Z. Analysis of the course and the ostium of the oblique vein of the left atrium. *Folia Morphol* 2000; **59**: 163–166.

10 Ludinghausen M. Clinical anatomy of cardiac veins. *Surg Radiol Anat* 1987; **9**: 159–168.

11 Antz M, Otomo K, Arruda M *et al.* Electrical conduction between the right atrium and the left atrium via the musculature of the coronary sinus. *Circulation* 1998; **98**: 1790–1795.

12 Asirvatham S, Packer DL. Evidence of electrical conduction within the coronary sinus musculature by non-contact mapping. *Circulation* 1999; **100** (suppl 1): I-850.

13 Chauvin M, Shah DC, Haissaguerre M, Marcellin L, Brechenmacher C. The anatomic basis of connections between the coronary sinus musculature and the left atrium in humans. *Circulation* 2000; **101**: 647–652.

14 Guiraudon GM, Guiraudon CM, Klein GJ, Sharma AD, Yee R. The coronary sinus diverticulum: a pathologic entity associated with the Wolff-Parkinson-White syndrome. *Am J Cardiol* 1988; **62**: 733–735.

15 Ludinghausen M, Ohmachi N, Boot C. Myocardial coverage of the coronary sinus and related veins. *Clin Anat* 1992; **5**: 1–15.

16 Meisel E, Pfeiffer D, Engelmann L *et al.*, Investigation of coronary venous anatomy by retrograde venography in patients with malignant ventricular tachycardia. *Circulation* 2001; **104**: 442–447.

17 Sun Y, Arruda M, Otomo K *et al.* Coronary sinus-ventricular accessory connections producing posteroseptal and left posterior accessory pathways: incidence and electrophysiological identification. *Circulation* 2002; **106**: 1362–1367.

18 Dobosz PM, Kolesnik A, Aleksandrowicz R, Ciszek B.

Anatomy of the valve of the coronary (thebesian valve). *Clin Anat* 1995; **8**: 438–439.

19 Duda B, Grzybiak M. Variability of valve configuration in the lumen of the coronary sinus in the adult human hearts. *Folia Morphol* 2000; **59**: 207–209.

20 Hellerstein HK, Orbison JL. Anatomic variations of the orifice of the human coronary sinus. *Circulation* 1951; **3**: 514–523.

21 Kuta W, Grzybiak M, Nowicka E. The valve of the coronary sinus (thebesian) in adult human hearts. *Folia Morphol* 2000; **58**: 263–274.

22 Santoscoy R, Walters HL 3rd, Ross RD, Lyons JM, Hakimi M. Coronary sinus ostial atresia with persistent left superior vena cava. *Ann Thorac Surg* 1996; **61**: 879–882.

23 Ansari A. Anatomy and clinical significance of ventricular thebesian veins. *Clin Anat* 2001; **14**: 102–110.

24 Maros TN, Racz L, Plugor S, Maros TG. Contributions to the morphology of the human coronary sinus. *Anat Anz* 1983; **154**: 133–144.

25 Duda B, Grzybiak M. Main tributaries of the coronary sinus in the adult human heart. *Folia Morphol* 1998; **57**: 363–369.

26 Hwang C, Wu TJ, Doshi RN, Peter CT, Chen PS. Vein of marshall cannulation for the analysis of electrical activity in patients with focal atrial fibrillation. *Circulation* 2000; **101**: 1503–1505.

27 Kim DT, Lai AC, Hwang C, Fan LT, Karagueuzian HS, Chen PS, Fishbein MC. The ligament of Marshall: a structural analysis in human hearts with implications for atrial arrhythmias. *J Am Coll Cardiol* 2000; **36**: 1324–1327.

28 Gensini GG, Digiorgi S, Coskun O, Palacio A, Kelly AE. Anatomy of the coronary circulation in living man; coronary venography. *Circulation* 1965; **31**: 778–784.

29 Gilard M, Mansourati J, Etienne Y, Larlet JM, Truong B, Boschat J, Blanc JJ. Angiographic anatomy of the coronary sinus and its tributaries. *Pacing Clin Electrophysiol* 1998; **21**: 2280–2284.

30 Micklos TJ, Proto AV. CT demonstration of the coronary sinus. *J Comput Assist Tomogr* 1985; **9**: 60–64.

31 Maurer G, Punzengruber C, Haendchen RV, Torres MA, Heublein B, Meerbaum S, Corday E. Retrograde coronary venous contrast echocardiography: assessment of shunting and delineation of regional myocardium in the normal and ischemic canine heart. *J Am Coll Cardiol* 1984; **4**: 577–586.

32 von Ludinghausen M. Clinical anatomy of cardiac veins, Vv. cardiacae. *Surg Radiol Anat* 1987; **9**: 159–168.

33 Schaffler GJ, Groell R, Peichel KH, Rienmuller R. Imaging the coronary venous drainage system using electron-beam CT. *Surg Radiol Anat* 2000; **22**: 35–39.

34 Ruengsakulrach P, Buxton BF. Anatomic and hemodynamic considerations influencing the efficiency of retrograde cardioplegia. *Ann Thorac Surg* 2001; **71**: 1389–1395.

35 Sethna DH, Moffitt EA. An appreciation of the coronary circulation. *Anesth Analg* 1986; **65**: 294–305.

36 Meinertz T. [A study of coronary sinus (v. cava cran. sin.), the middle cardiac vein and the aortic arch as well as ductus (lig.) Botalli in a number of mammal hearts]. *Gegenbaurs Morphol Jahrb* 1966; **109**: 473–500.

37 Scherf D, Harris R. Coronary sinus rhythm. *Am Heart J* 1946; **32**: 443.

38 Silver MA, Rowley NE. The functional anatomy of the human coronary sinus. *Am Heart J* 1988; **115**: 1080–1084.

39 Wit AL, Cranefield PF. Triggered and automatic activity in the canine coronary sinus. *Circ Res* 1977; **41**: 434–445.

40 Aronson RS, Cranefield PF, Wit AL. The effects of caffeine and ryanodine on the electrical activity of the canine coronary sinus. *J Physiol* 1985; **368**: 593–610.

41 Borman MC, Meek WJ. Coronary sinus rhythm. Rhythm subsequent to destruction by radon of the sino-auricular nodes in dogs. *Arch Intern Med* 1931; **47**: 957.

42 Giudici M, Winston S, Kappler J *et al.* Mapping the coronary sinus and great cardiac vein. Pacing Clin Electrophysiol 2002; **25**: 414–419.

43 Olgin JE, Jayachandran JV, Engesstein E, Groh W, Zipes DP. Atrial macroreentry involving the myocardium of the coronary sinus: a unique mechanism for atypical flutter. *J Cardiovasc Electrophysiol* 1998; **9**: 1094–1099.

44 Takatsuki S, Mitamura H, Ieda M, Ogawa S. Accessory pathway associated with an anomalous coronary vein in a patient with Wolff-Parkinson-White syndrome. *J Car-*

diovasc Electrophysiol 2001; **12**: 1080–1082.

45 Volkmer M, Antz M, Hebe J, Kuck KH. Focal atrial tachycardia originating from the musculature of the coronary sinus. *J Cardiovasc Electrophysiol* 2002; **13**: 68–71.

46 Boyden PA, Cranefield PF, Gadsby DC, Wit AL. The basis for the membrane potential of quiescent cells of the canine coronary sinus. *J Physiol* 1983; **339**: 161–183.

47 Katritsis D, Ioannidis JP, Giazitzoglou E, Korovesis S, Anagnostopoulos CE, Camm AJ. Conduction delay within the coronary sinus in humans: implications for atrial arrhythmias. *J Cardiovasc Electrophysiol* 2002; **13**: 859–862.

48 Scherlag BJ, Yeh BK, Robinson MJ. Inferior interatrial pathway in the dog. *Circ Res* 1972; **31**: 18–35.

49 Adatia I, Gittenberger-de Groot AC. Unroofed coronary sinus and coronary sinus orifice atresia. Implications for management of complex congenital heart disease. *J Am Coll Cardiol* 1995; **25**: 948–953.

50 Peterson LR, Peterson LF, Rattray TA, Quillen JE. Images in cardiovascular medicine. Sinus node artery fistula. *Circulation* 1998; **97**: 499–500.

51 Zanoschi C. [Malformations of the coronary sinus]. *Rev Med Chir Soc Med Nat Iasi* 1986; **90**: 749–752.

52 Wang PJ, Hayes DL. Implantable defibrillators and combined ICD-resynchronization therapy in patients with heart failure. In: Hayes DL, Wang PJ, Sackner-Bernstein J, Asirvatham S, eds. *Resynchronization and Defibrillation for Heart Failure: A Practical Approach*. Blackwell Publishing, Oxford, 2004: 177–208.

Chapter 12

Surgical approaches to epicardial left ventricular lead implantation for biventricular pacing

Joseph J. DeRose, Jr, MD *& Jonathan S. Steinberg,* MD

Introduction

Prospective randomized trials have demonstrated improvements in ventricular function, exercise capacity, quality of life, and mortality among patients undergoing cardiac resynchronization therapy (CRT) via biventricular pacing [1–5]. Transvenous biventricular pacing is performed by placing standard endocardial right atrial and right ventricular leads. The left ventricular (LV) lead can be inserted percutaneously by taking advantage of the fact that the coronary sinus is the major venous drainage for the left-sided coronary arteries. By cannulating the orifice of the coronary sinus in the right atrium, an epicardial pacing lead can be fed into the coronary sinus venous tributaries and onto the surface of the left ventricle. However, technical limitations owing to individual coronary sinus and coronary venous anatomy result in a 10–15% failure rate of LV lead placement [3, 6] when performed in this manner. Lead dislodgement contributes to an additional 5–10% late failure rate of LV lead capture and sensing [6, 7].

Although the response from percutaneous biventricular pacing can be dramatic, the overall response rate in previous large, prospective randomized trials ranges from 69% to 72%. The reason for this incomplete response is likely multifactorial and remains incompletely defined. Nonetheless, it does appear that appropriate LV site stimulation remains critical for complete LV resynchronization [8, 9]. Optimal

resynchronization is most likely to be achieved by pacing posterolateral sites on the left ventricle and more anterior sites may actually worsen resynchronization [9, 10]. LV leads placed by percutaneous coronary sinus cannulation are inserted in anterior sites, lateral sites, and posterolateral sites in fairly equal distribution and are primarily determined by the presence or absence of acceptable coronary sinus venous tributaries.

When percutaneous lead placement is unsuccessful, rescue therapy for these frail patients has typically involved direct surgical approaches to the LV epicardial surface. The range of procedures has included approaches as invasive as median sternotomy or thoracotomy [7, 11, 12] to a totally endoscopic procedure with the use of robotics [13–17]. Although used predominantly in the setting of coronary sinus (CS) lead failure, these approaches do offer direct access to the LV surface, and reliable LV lead insertion can be performed with a near 100% success rate. Access to the entire LV surface also provides a unique opportunity for detailed LV mapping and precise site-directed resynchronization [18].

Techniques of surgical epicardial lead placement

Open surgical approaches to epicardial lead placement

Traditional surgical access to the epicardial surface of the LV is performed via full sternotomy. This has historically been the preferred approach for right ventricular and right atrial epicardial pacemaker lead placement in pediatric patients. Sternotomy has been a particularly helpful approach in patients with congenital or surgically corrected anatomy (i.e. Fontan) who do not have endovascular access to the right atrium or right ventricle [19]. Access to the left ventricle through a sternotomy, however, does require significant cardiac manipulation. The techniques for accessing the posterolateral surface of the heart through a sternotomy are well known to cardiac surgeons versed in off pump coronary bypass grafting. Nonetheless, the morbidity of this approach, especially in the setting of prior cardiac surgery, may be restrictive in these sometimes frail heart failure patients who warrant CRT. A limited lower hemisternotomy with unilateral division of the sternum into the 3rd or 4th interspace, can be used to access the left ventricle in a more minimally invasive fashion [20]. However, the surgical approach to the posterolateral surface of the left ventricle is very difficult through this exposure, especially in reoperative situations.

Thoracotomy incisions have been used most commonly for LV epicardial lead implantation. These incisions provide more direct access to the left ventricle without significant cardiac manipulation. A formal rib spreading thoracotomy can be used in all situations for the fullest exposure to the posterolateral wall. However, this approach does carry a significant morbidity with a real recuperative phase.

In order to minimize the trauma of a formal thoracotomy, minimally invasive cardiac surgeons have developed limited thoracotomy approaches to access particular parts of the LV surface. Limited anterior or lateral thoracotomy with or without rib spreading is an excellent minimally invasive approach for exposure of the anterior wall and is used commonly for minimally invasive revascularization of the left anterior descending artery [7, 12, 21]. The incision is made below and just lateral to the nipple and a soft tissue retractor can be used in some patients for adequate exposure without the use of a rib spreader (Fig. 12.1). Access to the lateral wall and posterolateral wall is possible with some cardiac displacement. The use of special screw-in tools has helped in accessing the posterolateral surface through these small thoracotomy incisions [11] (Fig. 12.2).

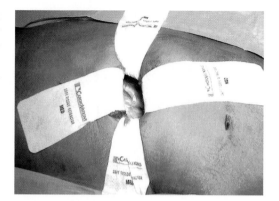

Figure 12.1 Non-rib spreading anterior thoracotomy with the aid of a minimally invasive soft tissue retractor.

Endoscopic approaches to left ventricular lead placement

Totally endoscopic approaches to the LV surface have the advantage of eliminating chest wall retraction and rib spreading and, therefore, shortening post-operative recovery and significantly decreasing post-operative pain. More importantly, however, these video-assisted approaches also allow access to the entire LV surface with excellent visualization.

Thoracoscopy

Thoracoscopic approaches to the pericardium have been used in the past for both diagnostic and therapeutic interventions. Thoracoscopy involves the use of a camera which is placed through a chest wall port ranging in size from 5 mm to 10 mm. All structures found within the chest cavity can be well visualized, including the lung, pleura, esophagus, mediastinum, pericardium, and heart. Surgery is performed with long, specially designed instruments that are placed through additional small ports in the chest.

Thoracoscopy for LV lead placement has been championed by many groups [7, 12, 21, 22]. A number of different approaches exist, including placement of the ports in anterolateral and posterolateral positions. The dexterity with which surgery can be performed is variable and suturing fine leads on the LV surface can be challenging. As such, the placement of screw-in leads with the use of introducing tools is the preferred implantation technique when thoracoscopy is performed. Similarly, fine dissection necessary to free the heart and lung from surrounding structures in the re-operative setting can also be difficult. Nonetheless, global LV access

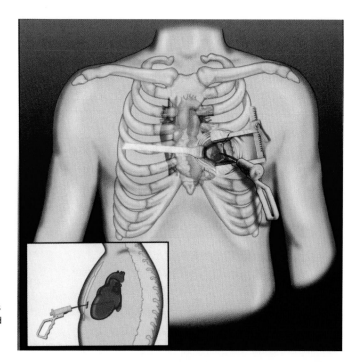

Figure 12.2 The screw-in tool manufactured by Medtronic helps access the posterolateral wall through a limited rib spreading lateral thoracotomy. Pic provided by Medtronic Inc.

and LV mapping are facilitated with the endoscopic approach and site-directed lead placement can be easily accomplished.

Robotics

Robotically assisted approaches to biventricular pacing aim to combine the dexterity advantages of open surgery with the minimally invasive and exposure advantages of thoracoscopic surgery. The daVinci robotic system (Intuitive Surgical Incorporated, Sunnyvale, California, USA) is composed of a surgeon control console and a surgical arm unit that positions and directs the micro-instruments (Fig. 12.3A). Unlike standard thoracoscopic instruments, these specialized "EndoWrist" instruments have a full 7 degrees of freedom, simulating the motion of a human wrist at the operative site (Fig. 12.3B). Insertion of the instruments into the chest cavity is performed through two 8 mm ports. A third 10 mm port is used to insert the endoscope. The instruments are controlled by a surgeon who sits at the operating console away from the operative field. Computer interfacing allows for scaled motion, eliminating tremor, and providing for incredibly accurate surgical precision through these small ports. The surgeon views the surgery through the eyepiece in the surgical console which provides high-definition, magnified, real three-dimensional vision.

For LV lead insertion, the patient is positioned in a full, left posterolateral thoracotomy position and the robot is introduced in the posterior axillary line [15]. A separate working port is used for introduction of the leads. The fine, scaled motion of the robotic arms allows for facile dissection of the pericardium from the epicardium as well as easy identification of bypass grafts when prior cardiac surgery has been performed. The robotic facilitation similarly allows for implantation of all types of leads as suturing is easily done. The three-dimensional endoscopic view gives the surgeon complete access to all surfaces of the LV for mapping and implantation (Fig. 12.4).

Lead types

A number of different epicardial leads have been used for right ventricular (RV) pacing over the past 25 years. Historically, steroid eluting leads have had greater durability that non-steroid eluting "fishhook" type leads or screw-in leads. Presently, the only steroid eluting epicardial leads for use in the

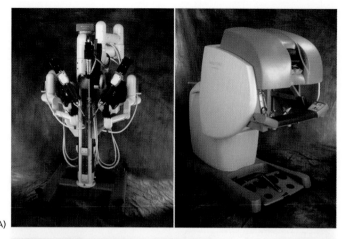

(A)

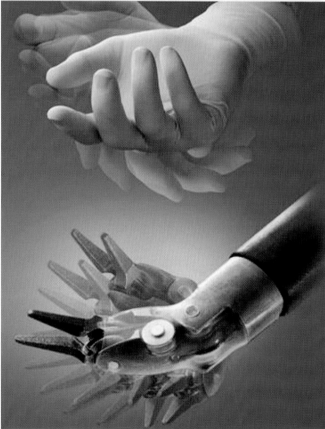

(B)

Figure 12.3 (A) Photograph of the daVinci surgical system showing the surgical arm unit on the left and the surgeon control console on the right. (B) Figure demonstrating the EndoWrist instrument capabilities. Each instrument has seven ranges of motion approximating the movement of a human wrist.

United States are secured by sewing them onto the heart with fine sutures (Fig. 12.5). These leads require exposure of bare myocardium in the target zone in order to achieve adequate pacing thresholds and do require finer dexterity when placed via an endoscopic approach.

The leads that can be placed without sutures are composed of a conducting screw that is secured into

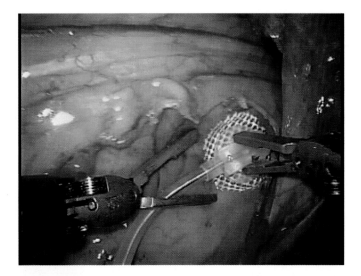

Figure 12.4 Operative photograph of robotic left ventricular lead placement. The pericardium is divided posterior to the phrenic nerve exposing the obtuse marginal vessels on the posterolateral wall of the left ventricle. A two-turn, helical screw-in lead is being placed by the console surgeon.

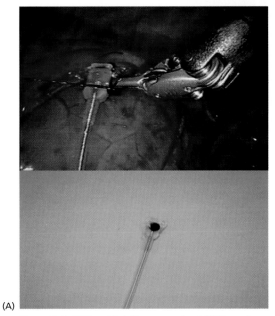

(A)

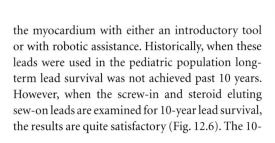

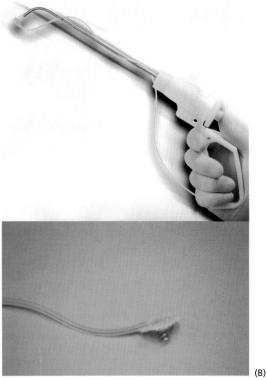

(B)

Figure 12.5 (A) Steroid eluting sew-on lead. (B) Screw-in lead.

the myocardium with either an introductory tool or with robotic assistance. Historically, when these leads were used in the pediatric population long-term lead survival was not achieved past 10 years. However, when the screw-in and steroid eluting sew-on leads are examined for 10-year lead survival, the results are quite satisfactory (Fig. 12.6). The 10-year lead survival of the screw-in lead is 92% and the steroid eluting lead nears 96%. These lead survivals far outlast the life expectancy of most elderly class III or IV heart failure patients and are very reason-

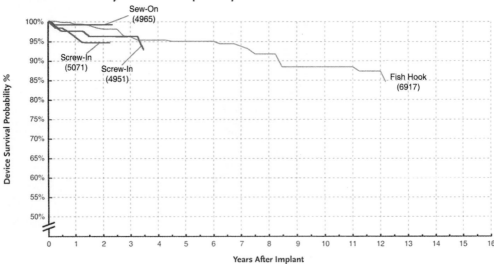

Figure 12.6 Ten-year lead survival for steroid eluting and screw-in leads. Image provided by Medtronic Inc.

able alternatives to epicardial coronary sinus leads. Nonetheless, the active development of steroid eluting screw-in leads promises to produce more durable epicardial leads for simple surgical epicardial lead placement.

Left ventricular mapping

Surgical access to the LV surface should allow for optimal lead placement in all patients. The target zone for optimal LV lead placement should correspond to the latest point of both electrical and mechanical activation. Historically, this has been labeled as the posterolateral wall midway between the base and the apex of the left ventricle. With pre-operative imaging, the area of latest mechanical activation can now be more accurately localized. As discussed in great detail elsewhere in the book (Chapter 6), the technique of tissue Doppler imaging (TDI) can be used to characterize the contraction of myocardial segments in time [9, 23–25]. By color-coding the segments, the target area of the left ventricle can be easily identified and more specifically defined. Three-dimensional echocardiography can also be used to evaluate 16–32 "voxels" of LV myocardium and to track their contraction in time [26, 27]. Multiple contraction waveforms can

be imaged on line and the latest point of mechanical activation can be localized. These pre-operative imaging techniques allow for documentation of dyssynchrony in those patients evaluated for CRT with a widened QRS on baseline ECG. However, these techniques may also serve in the future to identify dyssynchrony in heart failure patients with no evidence of intraventricular conduction delay on baseline ECG.

Pre-operative LV mapping is presently used by several groups for site localization. However, intra-operative LV mapping may provide an even more accurate tool for optimal LV lead placement. On-line TDI via transesophageal echocardiography (TEE) can be performed with temporary LV pacing during robotic approaches to the left ventricle (Fig. 12.7). More elegant intra-operative mapping has been performed with a conductance catheter placed into the left ventricle via a femoral artery puncture with resultant construction of pressure–volume loops [21, 28]. These procedures provide very detailed mapping of even small portions of the posterolateral wall with sometimes significant differences in stroke work and dP/dt. Although still experimental, it is hoped that the data collected from such detailed intra-operative mapping will improve our ability to maximize CRT response rate.

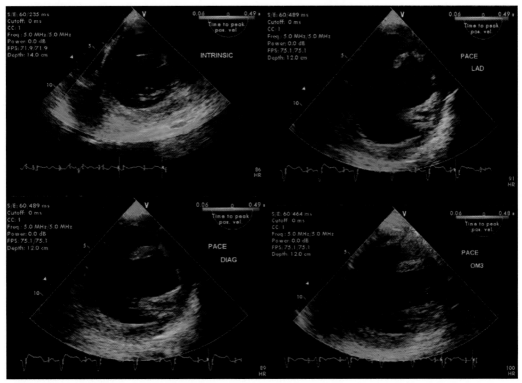

Figure 12.7 Transesophogeal echocardiogram with tissue Doppler imaging of intra-operative mapping during robotic LV lead insertion. Late mechanical activation is coded red and earlier activation in green. Notice that pacing at more posterolateral sites results in more complete resynchronization.

Outcomes of surgical left ventricular lead placement for cardiac resynchronization therapy

Most series of surgical epicardial lead placement have been reported in the setting of prior failure of CS lead insertion. As such, the majority of these patients are highly selected and represent a different population than the patients undergoing primary implantation. Nonetheless, a body of literature has been established over the past four years that accurately describes both peri-operative morbidity and short-term response rate with surgical epicardial lead placement through a variety of approaches.

Navia and colleagues reported on 41 patients undergoing minimally invasive lead placement following failed CS lead insertion [12]. Twenty-three of these patients underwent mini-thoracotomy, and 18 underwent an endoscopic approach (14 thoracoscopic and four robotic-posterior approach). The patient population described was quite ill, with 46%

of the patients in hospital with a heart failure exacerbation. Of note, a pre-operative LV mapping protocol of TDI was used in order to target the optimal site of LV pacing. Similarly, post-operative echocardiography-guided optimization of LV pacing was performed on post-operative day 2. All patients had two LV leads successfully placed and there were no endoscopic conversions. Seventy-eight per cent of patients were extubated in the operating room. Two patients had prolonged respiratory failure. Mean ICU stay was 1.5 days and hospital stay was 4 days. There was no difference between mini-thoracotomy patients and endoscopic patients in terms of length of stay or extubation time. Over a six-month follow-up there were six deaths and 34 clinical responders for an overall response rate of 73%. Interestingly, both responders and non-responders had documentation of resynchronization via TDI. Despite resynchronization, it is postulated that other factors, including severe ventricular systolic and diastolic dysfunction, can impact heavily on clinical outcome.

Our group at St. Luke's-Roosevelt Hospital Center in New York has reported extensively on the short- and medium-term follow-up of robotic LV lead placement for biventricular pacing [13, 15–17]. Between 2002 and 2005, 60 patients have undergone robotic LV lead placement [16]. The majority of these patients have had robotic LV lead implantation for a failure of CS lead placement (83%). The operative results have been similar to those described by other groups with a 100% success rate for LV lead placement and a very low conversion rate to mini-thoracotomy (3%). All patients in this robotic series have been extubated in the operating room and median ICU and hospital lengths of stay have been 0.5 days and 1.5 days respectively. The last 20 patients in this series have undergone pre-operative TDI site localization and post-operative TDI pacing optimization. Post-operative morbidity has included one episode of pneumonia and two patients with intercostal neuropathy. No patients required re-intubation and there were no episodes of respiratory failure. Significant ventricular remodeling has been observed over the mean follow-up of 16.7 ± 9.5 months (range, 3–36 months) with statistically significant improvements in systolic LV internal dimension index and diastolic LV internal dimension index. Improvements in LV ejection fraction and New York Heart Association (NYHA) class have also been observed. The three-month clinical response rate has been 81%. Over the 36-month follow-up there have been four deaths (all of whom were initial non-responders). There have been three non-responders who remain alive with heart failure, one non-responder who underwent heart transplantation and four patients who worsened after an initial response for an overall response rate of 75% over the mean 17-month follow-up.

Although no prospective, randomized comparison has yet been performed between surgical epicardial LV lead placement and CS lead placement, Mair *et al.* have reported results on a retrospective comparison [7]. The study group included 79 patients undergoing CS lead insertion and 16 patients undergoing LV epicardial lead placement through a limited left lateral thoracotomy. The patients undergoing surgically placed LV leads included nine patients with failed CS leads and seven patients undergoing primary implant. All patients undergoing surgical placement of the epicardial LV lead achieved posterolateral lead placement as opposed to only 70% in the transvenous CS group. Length of stay was not statistically different between the two groups. Over a mean follow-up of 16 months, CS lead thresholds were significantly higher than surgically placed epicardial leads with seven CS leads having a pacing threshold of >4 V/0.5 ms versus no epicardial leads with a pacing threshold greater than 1.8 V/0.5 ms. In follow-up, 25 CS lead-related complications occurred, compared with one in the surgical group.

Specific considerations and troubleshooting

All minimally invasive surgical options for LV lead placement require general endotracheal anesthesia. Selective single lung ventilation allows for complete cardiac access and is a requirement for thoracoscopic or robotic lead insertion. As such, all patients requiring surgical LV lead placement with underlying pulmonary disease require pulmonary function tests in order to determine their suitability for single lung ventilation. A history of prior cardiac surgery including the arrangement of coronary bypass grafts should be obtained in order to allow for safe cardiac dissection. A posterior approach with the robot is especially helpful in this re-operative situation. Anticoagulation should be held prior to either endoscopic or open approaches as hematoma is prone to develop along the path of lead tunneling when the patient is anticoagulated.

Lead surveillance is performed in a similar manner as for CS leads. However, the presence of a back-up LV lead in the device pocket should allow for rapid lead exchange should LV lead failure be a concern. Pocket and device infections should be dealt with aggressively. All intravascular hardware should be removed and epicardial leads can easily be extracted endoscopically.

Conclusions

In summary, the outcome data of surgically placed LV epicardial leads appear to compare favorably to those for CS lead insertion. Nonetheless, post-operative morbidity varies based on surgical approach. Minimally invasive options including robotics and thoracoscopy appear to carry a post-operative morbidity similar to CS lead placement and are excellent minimally invasive rescue procedures. An ongoing prospective randomized trial comparing TDI-directed robotic LV lead insertion with CS lead insertion hopes to clarify the role of surgical LV lead implantation in primary biventricular implantation.

References

1 Cazeau S, LeClerq C, Lavergne T *et al.* Effects of multisite biventricular pacing in patients with heart failure and intraventricular conduction delay. *N Engl J Med* 2001; **344**: 873–880.

2 Auricchio A, Stellbrink C, Butter C *et al.* Pacing Therapies in Congestive Heart Failure II Study Group; Guidant Heart Failure Research Group. Clinical efficacy of cardiac resynchronization therapy using left ventricular pacing in heart failure patients stratified by severity of ventricular conduction delay. *J Am Coll Cardiol* 2003; **87**: 119–120.

3 Abraham WT, Fischer WG, Smith AL *et al.* Cardiac resynchronization in chronic heart failure. *N Engl J Med* 2002; **346**: 1845–1853.

4 Cleland JG, Daubert JC, Erdmann E, Freemantle N *et al.* Cardiac Resynchronization-Heart Failure (CARE-HF) Study Investigators. The effect of cardiac resynchronization on morbidity and mortality in heart failure. *N Engl J Med* 2005; **352**: 1539–1549.

5 Linde C, Braunschweig F, Gadler F, Bailleul C, Daubert JC. Long-term improvements in quality of life by biventricular pacing in patients with chronic heart failure: results from the Multisite Stimulation in Cardiomyopathy study (MUSTIC). *Am J Cardiol* 2003; **91**: 1090–1095.

6 Alonso C, Leclercq C, d'Allones FR *et al.* Six year experience of transvenous left ventricular lead implantation for permanent biventricular pacing in patients with advanced heart failure: technical aspects. *Heart* 2001; **86**: 405–410.

7 Mair H, Sachweh J, Meuris B *et al.* Surgical epicardial left ventricular lead versus coronary sinus lead placement in biventricular pacing. *Eur J Cardiothorac Surg* 2005; **27**: 235–242.

8 Butter C, Auricchio A, Stellbrink C *et al.* Effect of resynchronization therapy stimulation site on the systolic function of heart failure patients. *Circulation* 2001; **104**: 3026–3029.

9 Ansalone G, Giannantoni P. Ricci R, Trambaiolo P, Fedele F, Santini M. Doppler myocardial imaging to evaluate the effectiveness of pacing sites in patients receiving biventricular pacing. *J Am Coll Cardiol* 2002; **39**: 489–499.

10 Rossillo A, Verma A, Saad EB *et al.* Impact of coronary sinus lead position on biventricular pacing: mortality and echocardiographic evaluation during long-term follow-up. *J Cardiovasc Electrophysiol* 2004; **15**: 1120–1125.

11 Doll N, Opfermann UT, Rastan AJ *et al.* Facilitated minimally invasive left ventricular epicardial lead placement. *Ann Thorac Surg* 2005; **79**: 1023–1025.

12 Navia JI, Atik FA, Grimm RA. Minimally invasive left ventricular epicardial lead placement: Surgical techniques for heart failure resynchronization therapy. *Ann Thorac Surg* 2005; **79**: 1536–1544.

13 DeRose JJ, Jr., Ashton RC, Jr., Belsley S *et al.* Robotically-assisted left ventricular epicardial lead implantation for biventricular pacing. *J Am Coll Cardiol* 2003; **41**: 1414–1419.

14 Jansens JL, Jottrand M, Preumont N, Stoupel E, de Canniere D. Robotic-enhanced biventricular resynchronization: an alternative to endovenous cardiac resynchronization therapy in chronic heart failure. *Ann Thorac Surg* 2003; **76**: 413–417.

15 DeRose JJ, Jr., Belsley S, Swistel DG, Shaw R, Ashton RC, Jr. Robotically-assisted left ventricular epicardial lead implantation for biventricular pacing: The posterior approach. *Ann Thorac Surg* 2004; **77**: 1472–1474.

16 DeRose JJ, Jr., Kypson AP. Robotic arrhythmia surgery and resynchronization. *Am J Surg* 2004; **188** (4A suppl 1): 104S–111S.

17 DeRose JJ, Jr., Balaram S, Ro C *et al.* Two-year follow-up of robotic biventricular pacing demonstrates excellent lead stability and improved response rates. *Innovations* 2005 (in press).

18 Steinberg JS, DeRose JJ. The rationale for nontransvenous leads and cardiac resynchronization devices. *Pacing Clin Electrophysiol* 2003; **26**: 2211–2212.

19 Cohen MI, Vetter VL, Wernovsky G *et al.* Epicardial pacemaker implantation and follow-up in patients with a single ventricle after the Fontan operation. *J Thorac Cardiovasc Surg* 2001; **121**: 804–811.

20 Sako H, Hadama T, Shigemitsu O *et al.* An implantation of DDD epicardial pacemaker through ministernotomy in a patient with a superior vena cava occlusion. *Pacing Clin Electrophysiol* 2003; **26**: 778–780.

21 Maessen JG, Phelps B, Dekker ALAJ, Dijkman B. Minimal invasive epicardial lead implantation: Optimizing cardiac resynchronization with a new mapping device for epicardial lead placement. *Eur J Cardiothorac Surg* 2004; **25**: 894–896.

22 Mair H, Jansens JL, Lattouf OM, Reichart B, Dabritz S. Epicardial lead implantation techniques for biventricular pacing via left lateral thoracotomy, video-assisted thoracoscopy, and robotic approach. *Heart Surg Forum* 2003; **6**: 412–417.

23 Penicka M, Bartunek J, De Bruyne B *et al.* Improvement of left ventricular function after cardiac resynchronization therapy is predicted by tissue Doppler imaging

echocardiography. *Circulation* 2004; **109**: 978–983.

24 Lafitte S, Garrigue S, Perron JM *et al.* Improvement in left ventricular wall synchronization with multisite ventricular pacing in heart failure: a prospective study using Doppler tissue imaging. *Eur J Heart Failure* 2004; **6**: 203–212.

25 Yu CM, Fung WH, Lin H, Zhang Q, Sanderson JE, Lau CP. Predictors of left ventricular reverse remodeling after cardiac resynchronization therapy for heart failure secondary to idiopathic dilated or ischemic cardiomyopathy. *Am J Cardiol* 2003; **91**: 684–688.

26 Burri H, Lerch R. Visualization of cardiac resynchronization using real-time three-dimensional echocardiogra-

phy. *Heart Rhythm* 2005; **2**: 447–448.

27 Krenning BJ, Szili-Torok T, Voormolen MM *et al.* Guiding and optimization of resynchronization therapy with dynamic three-dimensional echocardiography and segmental volume – time curves: a feasibility study. *Eur J Heart Failure* 2004; **6**: 619–625.

28 Dekker ALAJ, Phelps B, Dijkman B *et al.* Epicardial left ventricular lead placement for cardiac resynchronization therapy: Optimal pace site selection with pressure-volume loops. *J Thorac Cardiovasc Surg* 2004; **127**: 1641–1647.

SECTION 5

Clinical trials – an overview

CHAPTER 13

Clinical trials – an overview*

David L. Hayes, MD *& William T. Abraham,* MD, FACP, FACC, FAHA

Introduction

In the early days of cardiac resynchronization therapy (CRT), some physicians argued that CRT was being embraced clinically without the necessary randomized clinical trial data to support such a novel therapy. However, most would agree that any deficit of clinical trial data has now been overcome.

To date, more than 4000 patients have been included in completed randomized clinical trials of CRT. This chapter will address several aspects of cardiac resynchronization clinical trial data, such as:
• Trends and generalizations of available trial data
• Summaries of individual clinical trials
• Ongoing or planned clinical trials.

Trends in completed cardiac resynchronization therapy trials

Trials can be discussed in terms of design, endpoints, and therapies included. Table 13.1 shows the completed trials that will be discussed in this chapter and notes the patient inclusion criteria regarding QRS width, underlying rhythm, New York Heart Association (NYHA) functional class, and whether an implantable cardioverter defibrillator (ICD) was indicated.

The inclusion criteria for clinical trials of CRT have been relatively narrow; this has resulted in convincing data for those criteria included, such as NYHA functional class III or IV, wide QRS, normal sinus rhythm, and biventricular pacing configuration. Present guidelines restrict the use of CRT or CRT-D defibrillators to this highly selected patient population (Fig. 13.1). However, the narrow criteria result in very limited trial data to support broader parameters or more relaxed criteria, such as NYHA class I or II, narrow (normal) QRS, underlying rhythm of atrial fibrillation, and left ventricular (LV) pacing-only configuration.

Predominantly, patients with NYHA functional classes III and IV congestive heart failure have been included. A minority of patients have been in functional class II. The notable exception among trials was the InSync ICD II study, which enrolled only patients in class II [1]. Given the importance of determining the effectiveness of CRT in functional classes I and II, several ongoing trials include patients in these functional classes (see Cardiac Resynchronization Therapy Trials Under Way or Planned).

Normal sinus rhythm has been a criterion for inclusion in all but one of the studies included in Table 13.1. Exceptions include the atrial fibrillation arm of the MUSTIC trial [2], which enrolled 43 patients in chronic atrial fibrillation, and the RD-CHF trial [3]. Although more data are emerging regarding the application of CRT in patients with chronic atrial fibrillation, they are not yet available. All trials included in Table 13.1 have required a QRS width of 120 ms or greater. The earliest trials assessed the safety and efficacy of CRT pacemakers (CRT-P).

*Portions of this chapter were previously published in Abraham WT. *Curr Opin Cardiol* 2002; **17**: 346–52 and Abraham WT, Hayes DL. *Circulation* 2003; **108**: 2596–2603. Used with permission.
© Mayo Foundation for Medical Education and Research.

Table 13.1 Patient enrollment criteria for completed trials of cardiac resynchronization therapy

Study (no. of patients)	Patient characteristics			
	NYHA class	QRS width (ms)	Underlying rhythm	ICD indication
MUSTIC-SR (N = 58) [15]	III	>150	NSR	No
MUSTIC-AF (N = 43) [2]	III	>200	AF	No
PATH-CHF (N = 41) [13]	III, IV	≥120	NSR	No
MIRACLE (N = 453) [16]	III, IV	≥130	NSR	No
CONTAK-CD (N = 490) [17]	II-IV	≥120	NSR	Yes
MIRACLE-ICD (N = 369) [18]	III, IV	≥130	NSR	Yes
COMPANION (N = 1520) [19]	III, IV	≥120	NSR	No
PATH-CHF II (N = 86) [14]	III, IV	≥120	NSR	Both
MIRACLE-ICD II (N = 186) [1]	II	≥130	NSR	Yes
CARE-HF (N = 813) [20]	III, IV	≥120	NSR	No
RD-CHF (N = 44) [3]	III, IV	NK	AF and NSR	No

AF, atrial fibrillation; CRT, cardiac resynchronization therapy; ICD, implantable cardioverter defibrillator; NK, not known; NSR, normal sinus rhythm; NYHA, New York Heart Association.

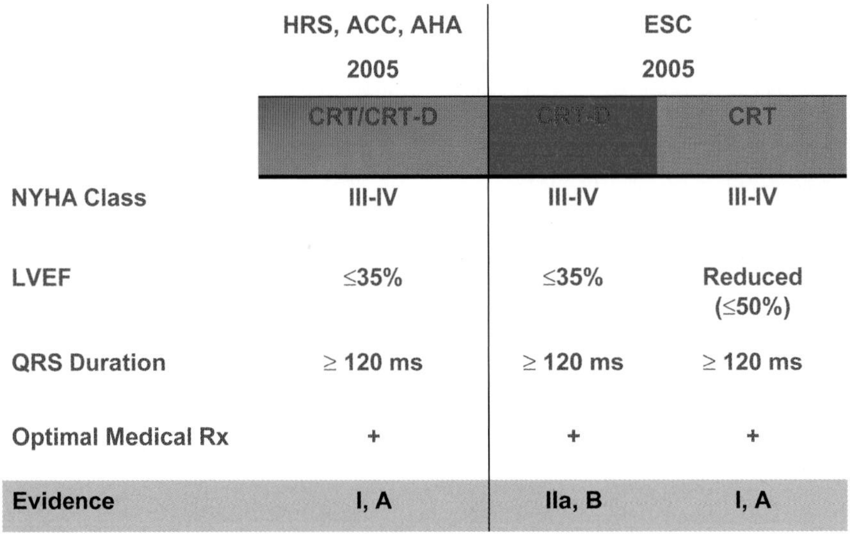

	HRS, ACC, AHA 2005	ESC 2005	
	CRT/CRT-D	CRT-D	CRT
NYHA Class	III-IV	III-IV	III-IV
LVEF	≤35%	≤35%	Reduced (≤50%)
QRS Duration	≥ 120 ms	≥ 120 ms	≥ 120 ms
Optimal Medical Rx	+	+	+
Evidence	I, A	IIa, B	I, A

Figure 13.1 Current implant criteria for cardiac resynchronization therapy (CRT) and CRT-D (defibrillation). HRS, Heart Rhythm Society; ACC, American College of Cardiology; AHA, American Heart Association; ESC, European Society of Cardiology.

As CRT-D devices became available, patients with an indication for ICD were included, and trials assessed the safety and efficacy of CRT-D and the effect of CRT on the occurrence of potentially malignant ventricular arrhythmias.

Most trials have relied on primary endpoints reflecting functional status, specifically the 6-Minute Walk Test, NYHA functional class, and quality of life. More recent trials have used "composite" endpoints including outcomes such as cardiac mortality, all-cause mortality, and hospitalization for congestive heart failure. Some of the more common secondary endpoints include peak oxygen consumption (Vo_2), LV ejection fraction

(LVEF), LV volumes, degree of mitral regurgitation, number of hospitalizations, neurohormonal levels, and volume indices.

Randomized clinical trials of CRT have been relatively consistent in showing improvement in the 6-Minute Walk Test, NYHA functional class, and quality of life assessed with the Minnesota Living With Heart Failure Questionnaire (MLHFQ). Some exceptions exist and will be detailed by individual trial.

Relative consistency in some secondary endpoints also has been found. In the studies assessing peak Vo_2, with the exception of InSync ICD II in which only patients in class II were enrolled, consistent improvement has been seen in this endpoint. Echocardiographic variables, specifically LV end-diastolic dimension (LVEDD), have consistently shown a decrease in LV dimensions, which suggests reverse LV remodeling. When mitral regurgitation has been assessed, it has decreased after CRT.

When hospital admission for congestive heart failure has been used as an endpoint all but one major study, CONTAK-CD, have demonstrated a lower rate of hospitalizations.

Many acute (temporary) and chronic (device implantation) observational and cohort studies of cardiac resynchronization were crucial in setting the stage for subsequent randomized clinical trials. A considerable number of trials have now been completed and each one has contributed to the evolution of CRT. Table 13.2 describes a selection of the observational and cohort trials believed to have been critical to the evolution of CRT [4–12]. Table 13.3 describes three major randomized clinical trials.

All together, the gain in life expectancy and, in particular, the reduction in hospitalization after CRT (Fig. 13.2) are as large as those observed in pharmacologic and other non-pharmacologic approaches evaluated for the treatment of patients with advanced heart failure (Fig. 13.3). As in the other therapies, these improvements may correspond to a favorable cost-effectiveness ratio for CRT (Figs 13.4 and 13.5). A preliminary economic analysis from the COMPANION study has concluded that CRT is a cost-effective intervention. The modestly higher up-front cost of implanting a CRT device was offset by the substantial decrease in hospitalization within the first year of treatment (Fig. 13.5). Long-term data are missing, and true comparative data between CRT and CRT-D are not yet available. At present, it is debatable whether COMPANION results can be translated to other, somewhat less sick patients or to patients with different CRT indications. Thus data from other ongoing or new designed prospective randomized trials may help further define patient cohorts that may benefit from CRT. Moreover, formal cost-effectiveness analyses, yet to be done, of existing CRT trials may provide additional information regarding the cost implications of these therapies.

PATH-CHF trials

The PATH-CHF (Pacing Therapies in Congestive Heart Failure) trial was a single-blind, randomized, crossover, controlled trial designed to evaluate the acute hemodynamic effects and assess the long-term clinical benefit of right ventricular (RV), LV, and biventricular pacing in patients with moderate-to-severe chronic heart failure and interventricular conduction block [13]. During the crossover periods, patients were assigned to two different pacing modes (best univentricular vs. biventricular pacing), each lasting four weeks with a four-week control phase in between. This was followed by a chronic pacing phase. The effects of pacing both on Vo_2 at peak exercise and at anaerobic threshold during cardiopulmonary exercise testing and on 6-Minute Walk distance were selected as primary endpoints of this study. Secondary endpoints were changes in NYHA class, quality of life (assessed by the MLHFQ), and hospitalization frequency. Changes in LVEF, cardiac output, and filling pattern were also assessed by echocardiography.

Forty-one patients were enrolled. Aortic pulse pressure and dP/dt were measured at baseline and during acute pacing. Acutely, biventricular and LV pacing increased dP/dt and pulse pressure more than did RV pacing ($P < 0.01$). Chronic results were encouraging, with slight improvement in all primary and secondary endpoints during pacing [13]. Statistically significant decreases in end-systolic and end-diastolic volumes were also shown. However, the results are weakened by the small number of patients studied, the single-blind design, and the observation that functional endpoints did not re-

Table 13.2 Observational trials of cardiac resynchronization therapy in heart failure

Author	Patients	Improvement
Cazeau et al. [4] (1994)	Six-week technical feasibility study of four-chamber pacing in a 54-year-old with NYHA class IV heart failure, LBBB, 200 ms PR interval, and interatrial conduction delay	Yes (clinical status)
Foster et al. [5] (1995)	Acute study of biventricular pacing in 18 post-operative coronary revascularization patients	Yes (hemodynamics)
Cazeau et al. [6] (1996)	Eight patients with wide QRS and end-stage heart failure; comparing the effect of various ventricular pacing sites (RV apex, RVOT, RV apex-LV pacing, RVOT-LV pacing); follow-up period 3–17 months	Yes (hemodynamics and functional status, in patients with LV or biventricular pacing only)
Blanc et al. [7] (1997)	Acute hemodynamic study comparing the effect of various ventricular pacing sites (RV apex, RVOT, LV, or biventricular pacing) in 27 patients with severe heart failure with first-degree AV block and/or an IVCD	Yes (hemodynamics, in patients with LV or biventricular pacing only)
Kass et al. [8] (1999)	Acute hemodynamic study comparing the effect of various ventricular pacing modes (RV apex, RV septal, LV free wall, or biventricular pacing) in 18 patients with advanced heart failure	Yes (hemodynamics, in patients with LV or biventricular pacing only)
Saxon et al. [9] (1998)	Study of biventricular pacing in 11 postoperative cardiac surgery patients with depressed LV function	Yes (hemodynamics)
Gras et al. [10] (1998)	(InSync Study, interim results, three-month follow-up) European and Canadian multicenter trial of biventricular pacing in 68 patients with dilated cardiomyopathy, IVCD, and NYHA class III or IV heart failure	Yes (quality of life, NYHA class, 6-Minute Walk distance)
Leclercq et al. [11] (1998)	Acute hemodynamic study comparing single-site RV DDD pacing with biventricular pacing in 18 patients with NYHA class III or IV heart failure	Yes (hemodynamics, for biventricular pacing only)
Gras et al. [12] (2002)	(InSync Study, final analysis, long-term follow-up) 117 patients (103 were successfully implanted with a CRT device) with idiopathic or ischemic dilated cardiomyopathy, NYHA class III or IV heart failure, LV dysfunction, and an IVCD	Yes (quality of life, NYHA class, 6-Minute Walk distance)

AV, atrioventricular; CRT, cardiac resynchronization therapy; IVCD, intraventricular conduction delay; LBBB, left bundle branch block; LV, left ventricular; NYHA, New York Heart Association; RV, right ventricular; RVOT, RV outflow tract. Modified from Abraham and Hayes [23]. Used with permission.

turn to baseline during the "pacing off" control or washout period (most likely due to the rather short four weeks of washout).

PATH-CHF II was a prospective, randomized, crossover study assessing univentricular versus biventricular pacing with both acute and chronic measurements [14]. The study included 86 patients with congestive heart failure, NYHA functional class II to IV, LV systolic dysfunction, peak ≤ 18 mL/kg per min, normal sinus rhythm, and a QRS interval greater than 120 ms. The study used equal numbers of patients in two groups with long (>150 ms) or short (120–150 ms) baseline QRS interval. The groups

were compared during a three-month period of active (univentricular) pacing and a three-month period of inactive (ventricular inhibited) pacing. The primary endpoints included peak Vo_2 followed by anaerobic threshold, distance walked in 6 min, and MLHFQ quality-of-life score.

Twelve patients were withdrawn before assignment and 17 could not complete both study periods. The short QRS group did not improve in any endpoint with active pacing. For the patients with long QRS, several measurements improved over baseline; peak Vo_2 increased by 2.46 mL/kg per min ($P < 0.001$), the anaerobic threshold increased

Table 13.3 Design and results of randomized clinical trials of cardiac resynchronization therapy

Trial	Design	No. of patients	Endpoints		Results
			Primary	Secondary	
PATH-CHF [13]	Crossover	41	Peak V_{O_2}, 6MW	Hospitalizations, NYHA class, QOL	Chronic improvement in 6MW, QOL, and NYHA class
MUSTIC-SR [15]	Crossover	58	6MW	NYHA class, QOL, peak V_{O_2}, worsening CHF, patient preference, total mortality	Sustained improvement in 6MW, NYHA class, QOL, and peak V_{O_2} Hospitalizations reduced with CRT, $P < 0.05$
MUSTIC-AF [2]	Crossover	43	6MW	NYHA class, QOL, peak V_{O_2}, worsening CHF, patient preference, total mortality	Sustained improvement in 6MW, NYHA class, QOL, and peak V_{O_2} Fewer hospitalizations with CRT
MIRACLE [16]	Parallel arms	453	6MW, NYHA class, QOL	Peak V_{O_2}, exercise time, LVEF, LVEDD, MR, QRS duration, clinical composite response	Sustained improvement in all three primary endpoints
MIRACLE-ICD [18]	Parallel arms	369	6MW, NYHA class, QOL	Peak V_{O_2}, exercise time, clinical composite response	Improvement in QOL and functional class; no improvement in 6MW
COMPANION [19]	Parallel arms	1520	Composite endpoint was time to death from or hospitalization for any cause	All-cause mortality, cardiac morbidity, maximal exercise	CRT and CRT-D reduced the risk of the primary endpoint

(Continued.)

Table 13.3 (Continued.)

Trial	Design	No. of patients	Endpoints Primary	Secondary	Results
CARE-HF [20]	Open-label randomization to control vs. CRT device	813	Composite of death from any cause and hospitalization for a major cardiovascular event that is unplanned	All-cause mortality; all-cause mortality and unplanned hospitalizations for or with heart failure; days alive and not in hospital for unplanned cardiovascular cause during the minimum period of follow-up; days alive and not in hospital for any reason during the minimum period of follow-up; NYHA class at 90 days; QOL at 90 days; patient status at end of study	CRT improved symptoms and QOL and reduced complications and risk of death
PATH-CHF II [14]	Crossover (no pacing vs. LV pacing)	86	Peak V_{O_2} anaerobic V_{O_2}, 6MW	QOL, NYHA class	Exercise tolerance, 6MW, and QOL improved
MIRACLE-ICD II [1]	Parallel arms	186	V_{O_2}	V_E/V_{O_2}, NYHA class, QOL, 6MW, LV volumes, LVEF, composite clinical response	Improvement in QOL, functional status, and exercise capacity
CONTAK-CD [17]	Crossover and parallel controlled	490	6MW, NYHA class, QOL	Composite of mortality, CHF, hospitalizations, VT, and VF	Slightly decreased morbidity and mortality end point; improvement in exercise capacity, QOL, and NYHA class
RD-CHF [3]	Crossover of patients already paced with class III or IV CHF (RV vs. biventricular pacing)	44	6MW, NYHA class, QOL	QRS width, hospitalizations	In previously paced patients, upgrading from RV to biventricular pacing improves symptoms and exercise tolerance

CHF, congestive heart failure; CRT, cardiac resynchronization therapy; CRT-D, CRT-defibrillator; ICD, implantable cardioverter defibrillator; LV, left ventricular; LVEDD, LV end-diastolic dimension; LVEF, LV ejection fraction; 6MW, 6-Minute Walk Test; MR, mitral regurgitation; NYHA, New York Heart Association; QOL, quality of life; RV, right ventricular; V_E, minute ventilation; VF, ventricular fibrillation; V_{O_2}, oxygen consumption; VT, ventricular tachycardia.

Hazard Ratio

MIRACLE N=461 0.58 [EF≤0.35, NYHA ≥III, no PM Indication]

MIRACLE ICD N=362 0.69 [EF≤0.35, NYHA ≥III, ICD Indication]

COMPANION (CRT-P) N=1520 0.65 [EF≤0.30, NYHA ≥III, recent Hospitalization, no ICD, no PM Indication]

COMPANION (CRT-D) 0.60

CARE-HF N=813 0.63 [EF≤0.30, NYHA ≥III, recent Hospitalization, no ICD, no PM Indication]

0.4 0.6 0.8 1.0 1.2 1.4 1.6 1.8

CRT Better ⟵

Figure 13.2 Hazard plot of five trials demonstrating effect of cardiac resynchronization therapy (CRT) on death, heart failure hospitalizations, and need for intravenous (i.v.) medications versus controls. CRT-D, CRT defibrillator; CRT-P, CRT pacemaker; EF, ejection fraction; ICD, implantable cardioverter defibrillator; NYHA, New York Heart Association; PM, pacemaker.

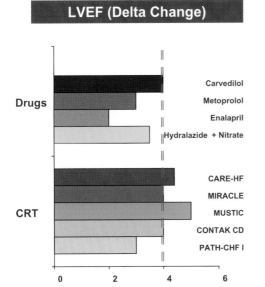

LVEF (Delta Change)

Drugs: Carvedilol, Metoprolol, Enalapril, Hydralazide + Nitrate

CRT: CARE-HF, MIRACLE, MUSTIC, CONTAK CD, PATH-CHF I

0 2 4 6

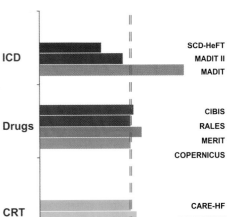

Mortality (Risk Reduction)

ICD: SCD-HeFT, MADIT II, MADIT

Drugs: CIBIS, RALES, MERIT, COPERNICUS

CRT: CARE-HF, COMPANION

0 20 40 60

Figure 13.3 The effect of cardiac resynchronization therapy (CRT) on change in left ventricular ejection fraction (LVEF) and mortality (i.e. risk reduction) is shown compared with pharmacologic therapies and implantable cardioverter defibrillator (ICD) therapy only.

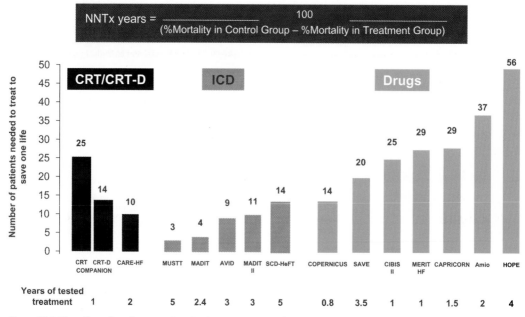

$$\text{NNTx years} = \frac{100}{(\%\text{Mortality in Control Group} - \%\text{Mortality in Treatment Group})}$$

Figure 13.4 The effect of cardiac resynchronization therapy (CRT) or CRT-D (defibrillation) compared with pharmacologic therapies and implantable cardioverter defibrillator (ICD) therapy alone in terms of number of patients needed to treat to save one life.

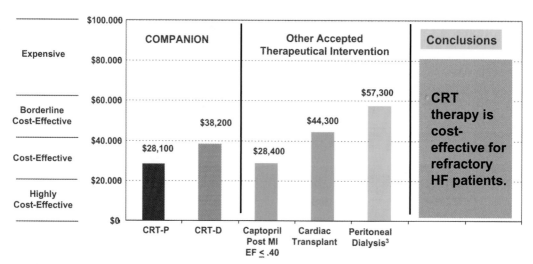

Figure 13.5 Cost-effectiveness of cardiac resynchronization therapy with a pacemaker or defibrillator (CRT-P and CRT-D) as demonstrated in the COMPANION trial vs. cost-effectiveness of the use of Captopril post-myocardial infarction (MI) with a left ventricular ejection fraction (EF) less than 40%, cardiac transplant, and peritoneal dialysis. HF, heart failure.

by 1.55 mL/kg per min ($P < 0.001$), the distance walked in 6 min increased by 47 m ($P = 0.03$), and the quality-of-life score improved by 8.1 points ($P = 0.004$). The investigators concluded that in patients with a long QRS (>150 ms), chronic congestive heart failure, and LV systolic dysfunction, LV pacing significantly improves exercise tolerance and quality of life.

MUSTIC-SR (Multisite Stimulation in Cardiomyopathies – Sinus Rhythm)

The MUSTIC trial was also a single-blind, randomized, crossover evaluation of CRT [15]. Sixty-seven patients were enrolled, 58 were randomly assigned, and 47 completed both phases of the study. Inclusion criteria were normal sinus rhythm, no indication for pacing, NYHA class III congestive heart failure, optimized drug therapy, LVEF less than 35%, LVEDD greater than 60 mm, intraventricular conduction delay (IVCD) (QRS >150 ms), and 6-Minute Walk of less than 450 m. Each phase of the study then lasted three months. Patients were randomly assigned to active cardiac resynchronization or to no pacing and then crossed over to the alternative study assignment. The primary endpoint was the change in distance walked in 6 min, and secondary endpoints included change in quality of life, NYHA class, peak Vo_2, hospital admissions, worsening heart failure, total mortality, and patient preference for pacing mode. Significant improvement was shown in all primary and secondary endpoints with pacing. For example, during the active pacing phase the mean distance walked in 6 min was 23% greater than during the inactive pacing phase ($P < 0.001$).

MUSTIC-AF

A second MUSTIC trial (MUSTIC-AF) evaluated similar endpoints in heart failure patients with atrial fibrillation and ventricular dyssynchrony due to a paced QRS duration of more than 200 ms [2]. Although the number of patients completing the MUSTIC-AF trial was smaller, significant improvements were seen in the following primary and secondary endpoints: 6-Minute Walk ($P = 0.05$); peak Vo_2 ($P = 0.04$); and hospitalizations ($P \leq 0.001$). Although quality of life improved with biventricular pacing, statistical significance was not met ($P = 0.11$).

MIRACLE (Multicenter InSync Randomized Clinical Evaluation)

MIRACLE was the first prospective, randomized, double-blind, parallel-controlled clinical trial designed to validate the results from previous cardiac resynchronization studies and to further evaluate the therapeutic efficacy and mechanisms of benefit of CRT [16]. Primary endpoints were NYHA class, quality-of-life score (using the MLHFQ), and 6-Minute Walk distance. Secondary endpoints included assessments of a composite clinical response, cardiopulmonary exercise performance, neurohormone and cytokine levels, QRS duration, cardiac structure and function, and various measures of worsening heart failure and combined morbidity and mortality.

The MIRACLE trial began in October 1998 and was completed late in 2000. Four hundred and fifty-three patients with moderate to severe symptoms of heart failure associated with LVEF less than 35% and a QRS duration longer than 130 ms were randomly assigned (double-blind) to cardiac resynchronization ($n = 228$) or to a control group ($n = 225$) for six months while conventional therapy for heart failure was maintained [16]. Compared with the control group, patients receiving CRT had a significant improvement in quality-of-life score (−18.0 vs. −9.0 points, $P = 0.001$), 6-Minute Walk distance (+39 vs. +10 m, $P = 0.005$), change in NYHA functional class (−1 vs. 0, $P < 0.001$), treadmill exercise time (+81 vs. +19 s, $P = 0.001$), peak Vo_2 (+1.1 vs. +0.1 mL/kg per min, $P < 0.01$), and LVEF (+4.6% vs. −0.2%, $P < 0.001$).

Patients randomly assigned to CRT had significant improvement in a composite clinical heart failure response endpoint compared with control subjects, which suggests an overall improvement in heart failure clinical status. In addition, when compared with the control group, fewer patients in the cardiac resynchronization group required hospitalization (8% vs. 15%) or intravenous medications (7% vs. 15%) for the treatment of worsening heart failure (both $P < 0.05$). In the CRT group, the 50% decrease in hospitalization was accompanied by a significant decrease in length of stay, resulting in a 77% decrease in total days hospitalized over six months compared with the control group. Implantation of the device was unsuccessful in 8% of patients.

VENTAK-CHF/CONTAK-CD

The VENTAK-CHF/CONTAK-CD study was also a randomized, controlled, double-blind study comparing active CRT versus no pacing [17]. The initial design was that of a three-month crossover trial; this was later changed to a six-month parallel-controlled study design. The device used in the study combines ICD capabilities with biventricular pacing. Patients included had NYHA functional class II–IV heart failure, LVEF of 35% or less, QRS duration longer than 120 ms, and an accepted indication for an ICD. The primary endpoint was a composite of mortality, hospitalizations for heart failure, and episodes of ventricular tachycardia or ventricular fibrillation.

A total of 581 patients were enrolled, 248 into the three-month crossover study and 333 into the six-month parallel-controlled trial; 490 patients were eventually randomly assigned. For the primary composite endpoint, the resynchronization group had a slight but non-significant improvement. However, peak Vo_2, 6-Minute Walk distance, quality of life, and NYHA class were significantly improved in the active pacing group compared with control subjects, particularly in the NYHA class III and IV subgroup of patients. Decreases in LV end-systolic and end-diastolic dimensions were also seen in this trial.

MIRACLE-ICD

The design of the MIRACLE-ICD study was nearly identical to that of the MIRACLE trial [18]. MIRACLE-ICD was a prospective, multicenter, randomized, double-blind, parallel-controlled clinical trial intended to assess the safety and clinical efficacy of another combined ICD and cardiac resynchronization system in patients with dilated cardiomyopathy (LVEF ≤35%, LVEDD >55 mm), NYHA class III or IV heart failure (a cohort of class II patients was also enrolled), IVCD (QRS >130 ms), and an indication for an ICD. Primary and secondary efficacy measures were essentially the same as those evaluated in the MIRACLE trial but also included measures of ICD function (including the efficacy of anti-tachycardia therapy with biventricular pacing).

In a cohort of 369 patients randomly assigned to ICD on and CRT off ($n = 182$) or ICD on and CRT activated ($n = 187$), those with the CRT activated showed significant improvements in quality of life, NYHA class, exercise capacity (by cardiopulmo-nary exercise testing only), and composite clinical response compared with control subjects. The magnitude of improvement was comparable to that seen in the MIRACLE trial, suggesting that heart failure patients with an ICD indication benefit as much from CRT as those patients without an indication for an ICD. Of interest, the efficacy of biventricular anti-tachycardia pacing was significantly greater than that seen in the univentricular (RV) configuration. This observation suggests another potential benefit of a combined ICD plus resynchronization device in such patients.

COMPANION

The Comparison of Medical Therapy, Pacing, and Defibrillation in Heart Failure (COMPANION) trial was a multicenter, prospective, randomized, controlled clinical trial that assessed optimal pharmacologic therapy alone or with CRT using a pacemaker or a combination pacemaker–defibrillator in patients with dilated cardiomyopathy, IVCD, NYHA class III or IV heart failure, and no indication for a device [19]. Optimal pharmacologic therapy in all patients included diuretics (if needed), angiotensin-converting enzyme inhibitors (or angiotensin II receptor blockers if not tolerated), beta blockers (unless not tolerated or contraindicated), and spironolactone (unless not tolerated).

The trial design called for random assignment of 2200 patients into one of three treatment groups: group I (440 patients) receiving optimal medical care only, group II (880 patients) receiving optimal medical care and biventricular pacing alone, and group III (880 patients) receiving optimal medical care and a combined heart failure/bradycardia/tachycardia ICD device. The primary endpoint of the COMPANION trial was a combination of all-cause mortality and all-cause hospitalization. Secondary endpoints included several measures of cardiovascular morbidity. The trial was terminated prematurely after assignment of 1520 patients at the recommendation of an independent data and safety monitoring board.

Over 12–16 months, the primary composite endpoint of all-cause death or any hospitalization was decreased by approximately 20% with use of either device therapy compared with pharmacologic therapy alone. Further, a "pacing only" resynchronization device reduced the risk of death from any cause (secondary endpoint) by 24% ($P = 0.06$) and a resynchronization device with defibrillation reduced the risk by 36% ($P = 0.003$).

RD-CHF (upgrading from RV pacing in previously paced patients with severe heart failure and LV systolic dysfunction)

This randomized trial included patients with a standard pacemaker with RV pacing and NYHA class III or IV heart failure, an aortic pre-ejection delay greater than 180 ms or an interventricular delay greater than 40 ms [3]. Although this study has made important contributions to CRT research, it has not yet been published in manuscript form. Patients were randomly assigned in three-month crossover periods to RV pacing or biventricular pacing. Forty-four patients were enrolled, of whom 21 were in normal sinus rhythm and 23 in atrial fibrillation. With biventricular pacing, QRS width decreased significantly ($P < 0.001$), NYHA functional class improved from a baseline of 3.2 ± 0.4 to 2.1 ± 0.5 (2.6 ± 0.7 with RV pacing), 6-Minute Walk Test improved (baseline, 278 ± 127 m; RV pacing, 325 ± 149 m; biventricular pacing, 386 ± 99 m; $P = 0.001$), and quality of life improved (baseline, 49 ± 20; RV pacing, 40 ± 26; biventricular pacing, 29 ± 33; $P < 0.001$) [3].

The investigators concluded that in previously paced heart failure patients with poor LV function, upgrading from RV to biventricular pacing significantly improves symptoms and exercise tolerance. They also showed fewer heart failure hospitalizations in the biventricular pacing group.

CARE-HF

The Cardiac Resynchronization–Heart Failure Trial (CARE-HF) was designed to examine the long-term mortality and morbidity of patients with serious LV systolic dysfunction and clinical congestive heart failure (NYHA class III and IV heart failure) [20]. Total enrollment was 813 patients followed up for a mean of 29.4 months. A total of 159 patients in the CRT group reached the primary endpoint of "time to death from any cause or an unplanned hospitalization for a major cardiovascular event," whereas 224 patients in the medical therapy-only group reached the primary endpoint ($P < 0.001$). The secondary endpoint was death from any cause:

82 deaths in the CRT group vs. 120 in the medically treated group ($P < 0.002$).

Other parameters that improved in the CRT group included a decrease in interventricular mechanical delay, area of the mitral regurgitant jet, and end-systolic volume index, and an increase in the LVEF in the CRT group. The CRT group also showed improvement in quality of life, both MLHFQ and European Quality of Life-5 Dimensions score. All of these comparisons reached $P < 0.01$. Thus, the CARE-HF study showed, for the first time, a decrease in mortality with CRT alone (i.e. without defibrillation).

MIRACLE-ICD II

The hypothesis in the MIRACLE-ICD II trial was that CRT would limit disease progression and improve exercise capacity in patients with less severe heart failure (NYHA functional class II) [1]. A total of 186 patients were enrolled, with inclusion criteria of NYHA class II, QRS of 130 ms or greater, LVEF of 35% or less, LVEDD of 55 mm or greater, no bradycardia, ICD indicated, and optimal medical therapy.

Quality of life improved in the CRT group ($P = 0.01$). Peak Vo_2 increased by 1.1 mL/kg per min in the CRT group and 0.1 mL/kg per min in the control group ($P = 0.04$). Although 6-Minute Walk distance did not improve with CRT ($P = 0.36$), the treadmill exercise duration increased by 56 s in the CRT group and decreased by 11 s in the control group ($P < 0.001$). LV size, LV function, overall clinical status, survival, and hospitalization for heart failure were not significantly different in the two groups.

Synthesis of completed cardiac resynchronization therapy trial data

Several reviews and meta-analyses of CRT trial data have been published [21–26]. A review of nine trials was published by McAlister and colleagues [21] that sought to determine the safety and efficacy of CRT in patients with congestive heart failure and advanced systolic dysfunction. The review included a detailed analysis and comparison of the following outcomes of CRT versus control in the nine trials with available data: cardiac mortality, non-cardiac mortality, all-cause mortality, heart failure hospitalizations, 6-Minute Walk Test, NYHA functional class, and quality of life.

All-cause mortality data were available from all nine trials (considering the two arms of the MUSTIC trial together); the meta-analysis showed mortality to be significantly decreased by CRT (Fig. 13.6). Seven trials reported mortality from progressive heart failure and the data favored CRT. However, overall cardiac deaths were not significantly decreased by CRT when data from six trials were analyzed. CRT did not influence non-cardiac deaths.

The pooled data from six trials favored fewer heart failure hospitalizations in patients receiving CRT. This result is consistent with an earlier meta-analysis including four randomized controlled trials [22].

The 6-Minute Walk Test was measured as an endpoint in eight trials, and CRT resulted in improvement with a weighted mean difference of 28 m (range 16–40 m) when all symptomatic patients were included. When limited to patients with class III or IV heart failure, the 6-Minute Walk increased by a mean of 30 m (range 18–42 m).

Only four of the trials assessed included NYHA functional class as an endpoint. In this group, 58% of patients with CRT improved by at least one functional class as compared with 37% of controls. Neither MIRACLE-ICD nor RD-CHF reported this endpoint in such a way that it could be pooled with the other four trials, but both of these trials also reported an improvement in NYHA functional class.

Seven of the trials (considering MUSTIC as one trial) used the MLHFQ to assess quality of life (Fig. 13.7). Overall, significant improvement was seen with CRT, with a 7.6-point improvement in this scale. When only class III and IV patients were included, there was an 8-point improvement.

This review underscores the major lessons learned from the entire CRT trial experience:

1 Survival benefits appear to be largely due to a decrease in progressive heart failure. CARE-HF, designed to assess mortality benefit in patients with CRT-P only, did demonstrate a mortality reduction even without defibrillation capability.

2 That 58% of patients had improved NYHA functional class by at least one grade is very appealing to most patients with clinical heart failure symptoms. However, the placebo effect of placing a device is powerful – 37% of control patients had a one-class

improvement in NYHA functional status. This once again underscores the importance of performing randomized clinical trials.

Cardiac resynchronization therapy trials under way or planned

Additional trials are needed to refine CRT patient selection and optimization. Broad categories of controversy include biventricular versus LV (univentricular) pacing, which functional classes should receive CRT (NYHA class I and II vs. III and IV), and whether LV dyssynchrony should be a criterion for cardiac resynchronization versus traditional QRS width requirements. Controversies also exist regarding atrial pacing versus atrial sensing during cardiac resynchronization and the effect of CRT on atrial arrhythmias.

The trials described below are not intended to be exhaustive. Many other trials are under way and multiple registries also will certainly yield valuable clinical information.

Left ventricular versus biventricular pacing

Multiple studies are under way that will compare the effectiveness of biventricular pacing versus LV pacing only.

- B-LEFT (*Biventricular vs. Left Univentricular Pacing With ICD in Heart Failure Patients*): B-LEFT is a prospective, randomized, double-blind, parallel-controlled study that compares optimized biventricular pacing with LV pacing alone.
- DECREASE-HF (*Device Evaluation of CONTAK RENEWAL 2 and EASYTRAK 2 – Assessment of Safety and Effectiveness in Heart Failure*): Enrolling patients with standard indication for CRT and with a primary endpoint of Vo_2, this study attempts to show the implications of interventricular timing in patients with ICD. Patients are randomly assigned to CRT, CRT with LV offset, or LV pacing only. Inclusion criteria include NYHA class III or IV, LVEF of 35% or less, QRS of 150 ms or more, PR interval of 320 ms or less, P wave duration less than 150 ms, and creatinine level of 2.5 mg/dL or less in patients with or at high risk for spontaneous or inducible life-threatening ventricular arrhythmias [27].

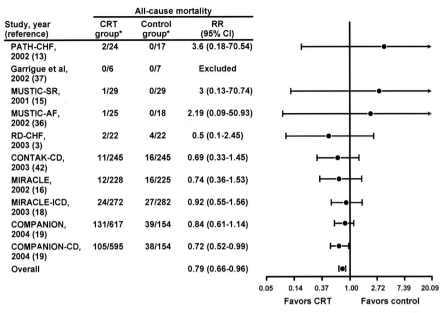

	All-cause mortality		
Study, year (reference)	CRT group*	Control group*	RR (95% CI)
PATH-CHF, 2002 (13)	2/24	0/17	3.6 (0.18-70.54)
Garrigue et al, 2002 (37)	0/6	0/7	Excluded
MUSTIC-SR, 2001 (15)	1/29	0/29	3 (0.13-70.74)
MUSTIC-AF, 2002 (36)	1/25	0/18	2.19 (0.09-50.93)
RD-CHF, 2003 (3)	2/22	4/22	0.5 (0.1-2.45)
CONTAK-CD, 2003 (42)	11/245	16/245	0.69 (0.33-1.45)
MIRACLE, 2002 (16)	12/228	16/225	0.74 (0.36-1.53)
MIRACLE-ICD, 2003 (18)	24/272	27/282	0.92 (0.55-1.56)
COMPANION, 2004 (19)	131/617	39/154	0.84 (0.61-1.14)
COMPANION-CD, 2004 (19)	105/595	38/154	0.72 (0.52-0.99)
Overall			0.79 (0.66-0.96)

Figure 13.6 All-cause mortality with CRT versus controls. CI, confidence interval; CRT, cardiac resynchronization therapy; RR, relative risk. *No. of deaths/no. of patients in the study. (Modified from McAlister et al [21]. Used with permission.)

	Quality of life				
	CRT group		Control group		Wt mean diff in MLHFQ score (95% CI)
Study, year (reference)	N	Mean±SD MLHFQ score	N	Mean±SD MLHFQ score	
PATH-CHF, 2002 (13)	41	25.2±10.6	41	28.1±11.2	−2.9 (−6.4 to 0.6)
MUSTIC-AF, 2002 (36)	39	−9.9±21.3	39	−5.5±21.7	−4.4 (−11.2 to 2.4)
MUSTIC-SR, 2001 (15)	45	−17.4±21.6	45	−3.8±22.4	−13.6 (−20.0 to −7.2)
CONTAK-CD, 2003 (42)	234	−5.2±19.8	225	−4.5±20.2	−0.7 (−4.4 to 3.0)
MIRACLE, 2002 (16)	213	−18.0±28.6	193	−9.0±22.9	−9.0 (−14.0 to −4.0)
MIRACLE-ICD, 2003 (18)	162	−18.3±23.2	153	−13.1±22.7	−5.2 (−10.3 to −0.1)
COMPANION, 2004 (19)	459	−25.0±−26.0	104	−12.0±23.0	−13.0 (−18.0 to −8.0)
COMPANION-CD, 2004 (19)	479	−26.0±28.0	103	−12.0±23.0	−14.0 (−19.1 to −8.9)
Overall					−7.6 (−11.5 to −3.8)

Figure 13.7 Quality of life with CRT versus controls. CI, confidence interval; CRT, cardiac resynchronization therapy; MLHFQ, Minnesota Living With Heart Failure Questionnaire; Wt, weighted. Modified from McAlister *et al.* [21] with permission.

- *BELIEVE (Biventricular Versus LV Pacing)*: This randomized pilot study of biventricular versus LV pacing alone included patients with LVEF of 35% or less, LVEDD of 55 mm or more, and QRS of 130 ms or more. The primary endpoints were echocardiographic indices (LVEF, left atrial and LV dimensions, interventricular mechanical delay, and Doppler measurements) and freedom from device complications [28]. Publication of this study is pending, but the results showed no difference between biventricular and LV pacing (Maurizio Gaspirini, personal communication).

Utility of left ventricular dyssynchrony measurements

- *DESIRE (DESynchronization as Indication for Resynchronization)*: This trial attempts to identify responders to CRT as defined by electromechanical echocardiographic measurements and to determine if dyssynchrony measurements can be used for patient selection. The study will include patients with severe heart failure, with dilated cardiomyopathy of idiopathic or ischemic etiology, and without any conventional pacing indication, but the patients must have an indication for CRT. The protocol assesses CRT by echocardiography and evaluates its effectiveness through a composite criterion combining mortality, morbidity, and functional status. It evaluates safety by reporting adverse events [29].
- *PROSPECT (Predictors of Response to CRT)*: PROSPECT is a prospective, multicenter, non-randomized study with an aim of identifying echocardiographic measures of dyssynchrony and evaluating their ability to predict response to CRT [30]. Enrollment of over 400 patients has been completed. The primary response criteria are improvement in the heart failure Clinical Composite Score and LV reverse remodeling.
- *RETHINQ (Resynchronization Therapy in Normal QRS)*: This multicenter trial evaluates the safety and efficacy of CRT in patients with an approved ICD indication, NYHA class III congestive heart failure, and a QRS duration of less than 130 ms, and with evidence of mechanical dyssynchrony by echocardiography. The primary efficacy endpoint is peak Vo_2, and secondary endpoints include assessment of quality of life and NYHA functional class (McGuire J, personal communication, July 2005).

Timing of cardiac resynchronization therapy and functional class

- *BLOCK-HF (Biventricular Versus RV Pacing in Heart Failure Patients With Atrioventricular Block)*: BLOCK-HF began enrollment in 2003 [31]. This trial includes patients with NYHA class I–III and advanced atrioventricular (AV) block who are not currently indicated for CRT with an LVEF of 45% or less. The objective is to assess whether biventricular pacing limits the clinical progression of heart failure when compared with atrial synchronous RV pacing. The primary endpoint is a composite of mortality, morbidity, and cardiac function. An enrollment of up to 1200 patients is planned.
- *REVERSE (Resynchronization ReVErses Remodeling in Systolic LV Dysfunction)*: REVERSE began enrolling patients in 2004 [32]. Included will be patients who are NYHA class I and previously symptomatic and class II patients with QRS of 120 ms or more, LVEF of 40% or less, LVEDD of 55 mm or more, without bradycardia, with or without ICD indication, and receiving optimal medical therapy. The trial will assess whether CRT limits the clinical progression of heart failure. The primary endpoint is a clinical composite response [33]. LV end-systolic volume index is a key secondary endpoint.
- *MADIT-CRT (Multicenter Automatic Defibrillator Implantation Trial – Cardiac Resynchronization Therapy)*: The objective of this trial is to determine whether CRT-D decreases the combined endpoint of all-cause mortality or heart failure events when compared with ICD alone. Patients will be class I or II with ischemic heart disease, with one or more documented myocardial infarction or one or more coronary artery bypass graft surgery or percutaneous coronary intervention [34]. Events must have occurred more than 90 days before enrollment. Also eligible are patients with non-ischemic heart disease including dilated cardiomyopathy with a low LVEF and increased ventricular volume, with ventricular compliance that is normal or increased. All patients must have a stable medical regimen, LVEF of 30% or less, QRS duration of 130 ms or longer, and nor-

mal sinus rhythm, and be older than 21 years. Exclusion criteria include existing indication for CRT, pacemaker, or ICD therapy, NYHA class I with non-ischemic heart failure, NYHA class III or IV, and myocardial infarction within 90 days. Enrollment began in 2005.

- *BIOPACE (Biventricular Pacing for AV Block to Prevent Cardiac Desynchronization)*: This study aims to evaluate whether patients with a standard pacing indication benefit from biventricular pacing for the prevention of LV remodeling. Patients must have an indication for pacing but no specific LVEF or QRS duration. Endpoints include patient survival time, 6-Minute Walk, and quality of life [35].

Atrial rhythm status and cardiac resynchronization therapy

In addition to MUSTIC-AF, other investigations have assessed some aspects of CRT in patients with atrial fibrillation. In an early single-center study [36], right univentricular versus biventricular pacing was compared in patients with atrial fibrillation. Thirty-seven patients completed both crossover phases. In the intention-to-treat analysis, no significant difference was observed. However, in the patients with effective therapy, the mean distance walked increased by 9.3% with biventricular pacing (374 ± 108 vs. 342 ± 103 m with right univentricular pacing; $P = 0.05$). Peak Vo_2 increased by 13% ($P = 0.04$), hospitalizations decreased by 70%, and 85% of the patients had a preference for biventricular pacing ($P < 0.001$).

The investigators concluded that compared with standard VVIR pacing, biventricular pacing seems to improve exercise tolerance in patients with NYHA class III heart failure with chronic atrial fibrillation and wide-paced QRS complexes.

Clinical and hemodynamic differences between LV and biventricular pacing were compared in another small study of patients with chronic atrial fibrillation and severe heart failure (mean LVEF, 24%; QRS width, >140 ms) in patients who had undergone His bundle ablation. The design was a prospective, single-blind, randomized study with crossover and included 13 patients. It was concluded that during symptom-limited exercise tests and activities of daily living, resynchronization pro-

vided better hemodynamic performance than left univentricular pacing [37].

Other studies include the following:

- *The PAVE (Post AV Nodal Evaluation) Study* compared biventricular versus RV standard pacing in patients with chronic atrial fibrillation who had undergone AV nodal ablation [38]. Patients were NYHA class I, II, and III. The study showed that, in this population of patients with chronic atrial fibrillation after AV nodal ablation, CRT resulted in a statistically significant improvement in functional capacity determined by exercise duration, 6-Minute Walk, and peak Vo_2 compared with standard RV pacing. The final manuscript for the PAVE study is still pending publication.

- *PEGASUS-CRT (Pacing Evaluation – Atrial Support Study in Cardiac Resynchronization Therapy)*: The objective of this interesting study is to investigate the effect of a CRT-D device programmed to DDD-70 or DDDR-40 to DDD-40. The primary goal is to assess the effect of atrial support pacing on the endpoint of a clinical composite score consisting of all-cause mortality, heart failure events, NYHA class, and a "global assessment" tool. Secondary endpoints include quality of life, arrhythmia rates, and the effect of lead positions [39].

- *CHAMP (CHF Atrial Monitoring and Pacing)*: This study seeks to determine the effect of CRT on atrial arrhythmias. Enrolling patients with NYHA class III and IV symptoms, the primary endpoint is the burden of atrial fibrillation. Atrial fibrillation burden will be determined by diagnostic data provided by the pacemaker. Secondary atrial fibrillation-related endpoints include onset mechanisms, number and duration of atrial fibrillation episodes, and the average sinus rhythm duration.

- *Canadian AF/CHF Study*: The Canadian AF/CHF study includes patients with a history of atrial fibrillation and an LVEF of 35% or less. The primary endpoint is cardiovascular mortality, and secondary endpoints are all-cause mortality, stroke, quality of life, and hospitalization.

- *APAF (Assessment of CRT in Patients With Permanent Atrial Fibrillation)*: APAF will include patients with permanent atrial fibrillation and refractory heart failure. The study compares a strategy of delayed CRT based on clinical indications versus early CRT based on echocardiographic stratification. Eligible patients are those who have successfully received AV nodal ablation and CRT. Patients are randomly assigned to RV apical pacing and delayed CRT versus optimal CRT, defined as the shortest intra-LV delay obtained with tissue Doppler echocardiography among RV-, LV-, and biventricular-optimized interventricular interval. Endpoints are acute echocardiographic comparison, quality of life, and exercise tolerance, with a composite endpoint of CRT clinical failure [40].

• *The OPSITE (Optimal Pacing SITE) trial* assessed RV pacing versus CRT with both LV and biventricular pacing [41]. Patients enrolled were undergoing AV nodal ablation and pacing for chronic atrial fibrillation. Although quality of life and exercise capacity improved as a result of the ablation and regularization of ventricular rate, biventricular or LV pacing did not provide significant benefit over RV pacing.

Incorporating sensors in cardiac resynchronization therapy

Other techniques are beginning to emerge to assess newer techniques to optimize CRT programming. These techniques will be the basis of additional trials. An example of such a trial is the CLEAR (Clinical Evaluation of Advanced Resynchronization) trial. This trial uses a sensor, the PEA or peak endocardial acceleration sensor, to determine optimal AV and interventricular intervals versus more traditional echocardiographic techniques to optimize the AV interval.

Summary

The discipline of cardiac resynchronization has advanced rapidly as a result of excellent clinical trial data. The trials have resulted in wide acceptance of CRT in patients with standard criteria. We have clearly not yet perfected our patient selection criteria or patient management after CRT. Additional trials that are under way or planned should help with both selection and management.

References

1 Abraham WT, Young JB, Leon AR *et al.* Multicenter In-Sync ICD II Study Group. Effects of cardiac resynchro-nization on disease progression in patients with left ventricular systolic dysfunction, an indication for an implantable cardioverter-defibrillator, and mildly symptomatic chronic heart failure. *Circulation* 2004; **110**: 2864–2868.

2 Linde C, Leclercq C, Rex S *et al.* Long-term benefits of biventricular pacing in congestive heart failure: results from the MUltisite STimulation in cardiomyopathy (MUSTIC) study. *J Am Coll Cardiol* 2002; **40**: 111–118.

3 Leclercq C, Cazeau S, Lellouche D *et al.* Upgrading from right-ventricular pacing to biventricular pacing in previously paced patients with advanced heart failure: a randomized controlled study [abstract]. *Eur Heart J* 2003; **24**(abstract suppl): 364.

4 Cazeau S, Ritter P, Bakdach S *et al.* Four chamber pacing in dilated cardiomyopathy. *Pacing Clin Electrophysiol* 1994; **17**: 1974–1979.

5 Foster AH, Gold MR, McLaughlin JS. Acute hemodynamic effects of atrio-biventricular pacing in humans. *Ann Thorac Surg* 1995; **59**: 294–300.

6 Cazeau S, Ritter P, Lazarus A *et al.* Multisite pacing for end-stage heart failure: early experience. *Pacing Clin Electrophysiol* 1996; **19**: 1748–1757.

7 Blanc JJ, Etienne Y, Gilard M *et al.* Evaluation of different ventricular pacing sites in patients with severe heart failure: results of an acute hemodynamic study. *Circulation* 1997; **96**: 3273–3277.

8 Kass DA, Chen CH, Curry C *et al.* Improved left ventricular mechanics from acute VDD pacing in patients with dilated cardiomyopathy and ventricular conduction delay. *Circulation* 1999; **99**: 1567–1573.

9 Saxon LA, Kerwin WF, Cahalan MK *et al.* Acute effects of intraoperative multisite ventricular pacing on left ventricular function and activation/contraction sequence in patients with depressed ventricular function. *J Cardiovasc Electrophysiol* 1998; **9**: 13–21.

10 Gras D, Mabo P, Tang T *et al.* Multisite pacing as a supplemental treatment of congestive heart failure: preliminary results of the Medtronic Inc. InSync Study. *Pacing Clin Electrophysiol* 1998; **21**: 2249–2255.

11 Leclercq C, Cazeau S, Le Breton H *et al.* Acute hemodynamic effects of biventricular DDD pacing in patients with end-stage heart failure. *J Am Coll Cardiol* 1998; **32**: 1825–1831.

12 Gras D, Leclercq C, Tang AS, Bucknall C, Luttikhuis HO, Kirstein-Pedersen A. Cardiac resynchronization therapy in advanced heart failure: the multicenter InSync clinical study. *Eur J Heart Failure* 2002; **4**: 311–320.

13 Auricchio A, Stellbrink C, Sack S *et al.* Pacing Therapies in Congestive Heart Failure (PATH-CHF) Study Group. Long-term clinical effect of hemodynamically optimized cardiac resynchronization therapy in patients with heart failure and ventricular conduction delay. *J Am Coll Car-*

diol 2002; **39**: 2026–2033.

14 Auricchio A, Stellbrink C, Butter C *et al.* Pacing Therapies in Congestive Heart Failure II Study Group; Guidant Heart Failure Research Group. Clinical efficacy of cardiac resynchronization therapy using left ventricular pacing in heart failure patients stratified by severity of ventricular conduction delay. *J Am Coll Cardiol* 2003; **42**: 2109–2116.

15 Cazeau S, Leclercq C, Lavergne T *et al.* Multisite Stimulation in Cardiomyopathies (MUSTIC) Study Investigators. Effects of multisite biventricular pacing in patients with heart failure and intraventricular conduction delay. *N Engl J Med* 2001; 344: 873–880.

16 Abraham WT, Fisher WG, Smith AL *et al.* MIRACLE Study Group. Multicenter InSync Randomized Clinical Evaluation. Cardiac resynchronization in chronic heart failure. *N Engl J Med* 2002; **346**: 1845–1853.

17 Lozano I, Bocchiardo M, Achtelik M *et al.* VENTAK CHF/CONTAK CD Investigators Study Group. Impact of biventricular pacing on mortality in a randomized crossover study of patients with heart failure and ventricular arrhythmias. *Pacing Clin Electrophysiol* 2000; **23**: 1711–1712.

18 Young JB, Abraham WT, Smith AL *et al.* Multicenter InSync ICD Randomized Clinical Evaluation (MIRACLE ICD) Trial Investigators. Combined cardiac resynchronization and implantable cardioversion defibrillation in advanced chronic heart failure: the MIRACLE ICD Trial. *JAMA* 2003; **289**: 2685–2694.

19 Bristow MR, Saxon LA, Boehmer J *et al.* Comparison of Medical Therapy, Pacing, and Defibrillation in Heart Failure (COMPANION) Investigators. Cardiac-resynchronization therapy with or without an implantable defibrillator in advanced chronic heart failure. *N Engl J Med* 2004; **350**: 2140–2150.

20 Cleland JG, Daubert JC, Erdmann E *et al.* Cardiac Resynchronization-Heart Failure (CARE-HF) Study Investigators. The effect of cardiac resynchronization on morbidity and mortality in heart failure. *N Engl J Med* 2005; **352**: 1539–1549.

21 McAlister FA, Ezekowitz JA, Wiebe N *et al.* Systematic review: cardiac resynchronization in patients with symptomatic heart failure. *Ann Intern Med* 2004; **141**: 381–390. Erratum in: *Ann Intern Med* 2005; **142**: 311.

22 Bradley DJ, Bradley EA, Baughman KL *et al.* Cardiac resynchronization and death from progressive heart failure: a meta-analysis of randomized controlled trials. *JAMA* 2003; **289**: 730–740.

23 Abraham WT, Hayes DL. Cardiac resynchronization therapy for heart failure. *Circulation* 2003; **108**: 2596–2603.

24 Desai AS, Fang JC, Maisel WH, Baughman KL. Implantable defibrillators for the prevention of mortality in patients with nonischemic cardiomyopathy: a meta-analysis of randomized controlled trials. *JAMA* 2004; **292**: 2874–2879.

25 Cazeau S, Alonso C, Jauvert G, Lazarus A, Ritter P. Cardiac resynchronization therapy. *Europace* 2004; **5** (suppl 1): S42–S48.

26 Al-Khatib SM, Sanders GD, Mark DB *et al.* Expert panel participating in a Duke Clinical Research Institute-sponsored conference. Implantable cardioverter defibrillators and cardiac resynchronization therapy in patients with left ventricular dysfunction: randomized trial evidence through 2004. *Am Heart J* 2005; **149**: 1020–1034.

27 De Lurgio DB, Foster E, Higginbotham MB, Larntz K, Saxon LA. A comparison of cardiac resynchronization by sequential biventricular pacing and left ventricular pacing to simultaneous biventricular pacing: rationale and design of the DECREASE-HF clinical trial. *J Card Failure* 2005; **11**: 233–239.

28 Gasparini M, Bocchiardo M, Lunati M *et al.* Left ventricular stimulation alone (LEFT) significantly increased ejection fraction (EF) at 1 year follow-up: preliminary results from the BELIEVE multi-center randomized study [abstract]. *Heart Rhythm* 2004; **1** (suppl): S69.

29 Cardiac Resynchronization Therapy (CRT). DESIRE. ELA Medical c2003 [cited 17 August 2005]. Available from: http: //www.elamedical.com/cadres/clinical_txt.htm.

30 Yu CM, Abraham WT, Bax J *et al.* PROSPECT Investigators. Predictors of response to cardiac resynchronization therapy (PROSPECT): study design. *Am Heart J* 2005; **149**: 600–605.

31 Medtronic begins study evaluating potential for biventricular pacing to inhibit heart failure progression: BLOCK HF clinical trial compares biventricular pacing with right ventricular pacing in people with early to mid-stage heart failure. Minneapolis, Minnesota: Medtronic, Inc; 2005 [cited 2005 August 24]. Available from: http: //wwwp.medtronic.com/Newsroom/NewsReleaseDetails.do?itemId=1096991155516&lang=en_US.

32 Linde C, Gold M, Abraham WT, Daubert JC, the REVERSE study group. Rationale and design of a randomised controlled clinical study to assess if cardiac resynchronisation therapy can slow disease progression in mild to moderate heart failure: the Resynchronisation reVerses Remodelling in aSymptomatic left vEntricular dysfunction (REVERSE) study. *Am Heart J* 2005 (in press).

33 Packer M. Proposal for a new clinical end point to evaluate the efficacy of drugs and devices in the treatment of chronic heart failure. *J Card Failure* 2001; **7**: 176–182.

34 Moss, AJ, Brown MW, Cannom DS *et al.* Multicenter automatic defibrillator implantation trial-cardiac resynchronization therapy (MADIT-CRT): design and clinical protocol. *Ann Noninvasive Electrocardiol* 2005; **10** (4

Suppl): 34–43.

35 Seloken ZOK [homepage on the Internet]. AstraZeneca Group of Companies; c2005 [cited 31 August 2005]. Congress reports: implantable devices for heart failure I. Available from: http://www.seloken.com/3430_49642. aspx.

36 Leclercq C, Walker S, Linde C *et al.* Comparative effects of permanent biventricular and right-univentricular pacing in heart failure patients with chronic atrial fibrillation. *Eur Heart J* 2002; **23**: 1780–1787.

37 Garrigue S, Bordachar P, Reuter S *et al.* Comparison of permanent left ventricular and biventricular pacing in patients with heart failure and chronic atrial fibrillation: prospective haemodynamic study. *Heart* 2002; **87**: 529–534.

38 Doshi R, Daoud E, Fellows C, Turk K, Duran A, Hamdan M. PAVE: the first prospective, randomized study evaluating BV pacing after ablate and pace therapy. Read at the American College of Cardiology Annual Scientific Session 2004, New Orleans, Louisiana, 7 to 10 March 2004.

39 Clinical trials/research: Hoag Heart and Vascular Institute. Hoag Heart & Vascular Institute, Newport Beach, California [cited 31 August 2005]. Available from: http://www.hoaghospital.org/HeartandVascular/ClinicalTrialsResearch.html.

40 APAF: Assessment of cardiac resynchronization therapy in patients with permanent atrial fibrillation. U.S. ClinicalTrials.gov [updated 1 August 2005; cited 31 August 2005]. Available from: http://clinicaltrials.gov/ct/show/NCT00111527?order=1.

41 Brignole M, Gammage M, Puggioni E *et al.* Comparative assessment of right, left, and biventricular pacing in patients with permanent atrial fibrillation. *Eur Heart J* 2005; **26**: 637–638.

42 Higgins SL, Hummel JD, Niazi IK *et al.* Cardiac resynchronization therapy for the treatment of heart failure in patients with intraventricular conduction delay and malignant ventricular tachyarrhythmias. *J Am Coll Cardiol* 2003; **42**: 1454–1459.

6 SECTION 6

Follow-up

CHAPTER 14

Troubleshooting

Christophe Leclercq, MD, PhD, FESC, *Philippe Mabo,* MD & *J. Claude Daubert,* MD, FESC

Introduction

Cardiac resynchronization therapy (CRT) is now a well-recognized treatment in patients with advanced and drug refractory heart failure with left ventricular (LV) systolic dysfunction and evidence of ventricular dyssynchrony defined by a QRS duration equal to or greater than 120 ms [1, 2]. CRT improves symptoms, exercise tolerance, and quality of life [3–7]. More importantly, recent trials specifically designed to evaluate the effects of CRT on morbidity and mortality showed a significant reduction in hospitalization rate and especially hospitalization for decompensated heart failure and a significant reduction in overall mortality and sudden cardiac death even when CRT is not associated with ventricular defibrillation features [6, 8]. Finally, the different cost-effectiveness analyses demonstrate that CRT is attractive for health care despite the price of the devices [8, 9]. The recent European and US guidelines for the treatment of chronic heart failure recommend CRT in advanced heart failure patients (New York Heart Association (NYHA) class III and IV) despite optimal drug treatment, poor LV function and dilated left ventricle and wide QRS above 120 ms on surface ECG with a high level of recommendation for improving symptoms, and hospitalization (IA) as well as for mortality (IB) [1, 2]. So, we can reasonably assume that the number of implantations of CRT devices will dramatically increase in the next few years.

The first step in the process of implantation of a CRT device (CRT pacemaker (CRT-P) or CRT defibrillator (CRT-D)) is the selection of the patients. So far, the US and European guidelines have based the selection of CRT patients on the inclusion criteria of the major clinical trials. The second step is the implantation of the CRT device, mostly using the transvenous approach with the LV lead inserted into a tributary coronary sinus vein. The third step is the optimization of the atrioventricular (AV) delay to provide the optimal LV filling and in some cases the optimal interventricular delay before hospital discharge. This very important step based on echocardiographic techniques will be discussed in Chapter 17. The last step is the long-term follow-up. Indeed, a patient with a CRT-P or a CRT-D has to be followed up very carefully. The follow-up of these patients does not consist only in an "electric" follow-up. The patients are primarily patients with severe heart failure with evidence of atrioventricular, inter- and intraventricular dyssynchronies. The complexity of CRT devices and the need for careful management of these severe patients emphasize the need for a multidisciplinary approach. A triple "association" is usually recommended: a heart failure physician to assess clinically and biologically the patient's hemodynamic condition, an echocardiographer with expertise in the field of cardiac dyssynchrony, and finally an electrophysiologist to evaluate the proper functioning of the device and the delivery of CRT. Careful medical management and monitoring of the CRT patients before, during but also after implantation would increase the efficacy of CRT and decrease the complications rates. In this chapter we will focus on the functioning of the device and the delivery of CRT during the follow-up and the different troubleshooting which may occur.

Initial device programming

After the implantation of the CRT device, the initial programming includes the choice of the pacing mode (VDD, DDD, DDDR, or VVIR in case of permanent atrial fibrillation), lower and upper rates limits, the AV delay during atrial sensing and atrial pacing and heart rate limits to activate anti-tachycardia therapy in case of implantation of a CRT-D. Most available data in the literature consider patients with normal sinus rhythm with atrial-synchronous biventricular pacing (VDD mode). However, some patients with associated sinus node dysfunction or atrial chronotropic incompetence require sensor-driven pacing modes (DDDR mode). A recent study demonstrated that systematic atrial pacing might worsen ventricular function (DDD mode) as compared to VDD mode with atrial sensing [10]. These results suggest that atrial pacing or sensor-driven pacing should not be activated systematically and that an evaluation of the increase in heart rate during exercise should be performed. Usually the AV delay is programmed in the operating room empirically with a range of 80–120 ms during atrial sensing with an additional offset of 30–50 ms during atrial pacing.

In-hospital monitoring

After the implantation of the device, procedure-related complications have to be carefully checked. Potential complications of implantation of CRT devices include those associated with conventional pacing and implantable cardioverter defibrillators (ICDs): pneumothorax, hemothorax, pocket hematoma, cardiac perforation or tamponade, and arrhythmias [11–14]. However some complications occur specifically with CRT devices and are related to the implantation of the LV lead into a tributary vein of the coronary sinus, such as coronary sinus dissection and coronary sinus perforation, phrenic nerve stimulation and finally LV lead dislodgement requiring a careful analysis of the chest X-ray and the surface ECG to ensure biventricular capture (see below) [11–14]. Moreover, these severe heart failure patients are hemodynamically unstable and the occurrence of a hemodynamic deterioration after a long procedure, sometimes with general anesthesia, has to be monitored very carefully. In the case of hemodynamic instability in relation to cardiac perforation, coronary sinus perforation and pericardial effusion which may require percutaneous drainage

or surgical procedure should be systematically discussed [11–14]. After implantation careful monitoring with continuous telemetry to detect pacing or sensing problems, hemodynamic instability, or arrhythmias may be recommended for 1–2 days. In case of worsening of fluid overload, additional diuretics might be necessary for a few days, especially when contrast agent was injected for coronary sinus venogram.

During hospitalization, confirmation of biventricular capture has to be assessed daily by analyzing the surface ECG and comparing it with the ECG templates recorded at the time of implant. Atrial and ventricular threshold data for both pacing and sensing have to be recorded before hospital discharge, providing a reference for further follow-up. Finally a chest X-ray is usually performed as a reference for the next follow-up.

Long-term monitoring

Cardiac resynchronization therapy is an additive treatment beside the pharmacological therapy, which may include angiotensin-converting enzyme (ACE) inhibitors, beta blockers, diuretics, aldosterone antagonists and angiotensin receptor blockers. As previously mentioned, a close collaboration between general practitioner, heart failure physician, echocardiographer, and electrophysiologist is needed to optimize the global care of the CRT patients. Beside the functional evaluation of the patients and the continuous optimization of the pharmacological treatment (especially the increase in ACE inhibitors and beta blocker dosage) and the conventional follow-up of a pacemaker or an ICD, the follow-up of the CRT device has three goals: to ensure proper device functioning, especially the permanent biventricular capture, to diagnose significant events, especially atrial and ventricular arrhythmias, and finally the survey of device- or therapy-related complications [11–14]. Moreover, an echocardiography has to be performed regularly to assess the quality of AV, interventricular, and left intraventricular synchronicity and if necessary to re-optimize the AV delay and eventually the interventricular delay.

In the case of deterioration of the hemodynamic condition, especially after a period of initial improvement, loss of resynchronization has to be suspected. Many causes can induce the loss of resynchronization, such as lead dislodgement, increase in pacing threshold, non-optimal device programming and/or occurrence of atrial or ventricular arrhythmias which may interfere with resynchronization [15, 16].

Loss of biventricular capture

CRT is based on a simultaneous or sequential biventricular pacing. In CRT patients, the left ventricle has to be continuously paced as well as the right ventricle to improve outcome; this means that biventricular pacing has to be delivered in all situations including exercise. As shown in Table 14.1, many other reasons than an increase in LV pacing threshold can cause the loss of biventricular capture.

The right ventricle is paced endocardially whereas the left ventricle is paced epicardially, usually through an LV lead inserted into a tributary vein of the coronary sinus. This means that the LV lead may be separated from the myocardium by structures such as the venous wall, epicardial fat, or myocardial fibrosis, resulting in a decrease in the conduction velocity [17]. As a consequence of the differences between the endocardial and epicardial pacing, the LV pacing thresholds are generally higher than endocardial right ventricular (RV) pacing thresholds with an increase in chronaxie [17].

Ten years ago, biventricular pacing was delivered with a Y-adaptor inserted in the ventricular port of a conventional DDD pacemaker with a high risk of

Table 14.1 Causes of loss of permanent or temporary biventricular pacing

Increase in LV or RV pacing thresholds
Left ventricular lead dislodgement
Right ventricular lead dislodgement
Non-optimal AV delay
Atrial tachyarrhythmias with rapid ventricular rate
Low maximal tracking rate
Frequent ventricular premature beats
Atrial undersensing
T Wave oversensing
Far-field atrial sensing
Ventricular double counting
Post-premature ventricular contraction extension of PVARP

LV, left ventricular; RV, right ventricular; AV, atrioventricular; PVARP, post-ventricular atrial refractory period.

increase in pacing thresholds. The first generation of biventricular pacemakers included the Y-adaptor in the connecting system, which improved technical issues. Now, almost all the devices available have two separate ventricular ports allowing independent programming of the left and right ventricular pacing and making it easier to evaluate both ventricular pacing thresholds.

When to suspect the loss of biventricular capture?

The loss of biventricular capture may be suspected in various clinical situations:
- The most frequent situation is a hemodynamic deterioration occurring after a period of significant clinical improvement. The patient complains of an increase in dyspnea during exercise or at rest, and an increase in body weight associated with limb edema.
- The loss of biventricular capture may be responsible in some cases of acute or sub-acute pulmonary edema. However, other causes of clinical deterioration in these heart failure patients have to be suspected such as drug treatment or low-salt diet non-compliance, infection, myocardial ischemia, or the natural evolution of the cardiomyopathy.
- Finally, the loss of biventricular capture may be asymptomatic and diagnosed during a scheduled follow-up with the analysis of QRS complexes on surface ECG, or it may be suspected from data from the device indicating a low biventricular pacing rate.

How to detect a loss of biventricular capture?

The diagnosis of loss of biventricular capture is quite easy if it is permanent and is usually performed with the analysis of the QRS complexes on surface ECG. If the loss of biventricular capture is transient, the diagnosis is much more difficult and may require different techniques such as exercise testing or evaluation of the percentage of biventricular pacing obtained from Holter monitoring capabilities of the biventricular devices, or a 24-h Holter monitoring.

Electrocardiographic follow-up of biventricular pacemakers

In patients selected on the basis of the current guidelines, biventricular pacing is usually associated with

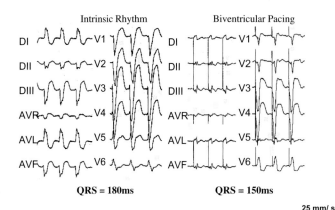

Figure 14.1 Twelve-lead surface ECG illustrating the reduction in QRS width from 180 ms with intrinsic rhythm to 150 ms with biventricular pacing. Please also note the change in the QRS axis shifting from a left axis deviation to a normal axis.

a significant decrease in QRS duration of on average 20–40 ms in the main clinical trials, but also changes in the QRS axis (Fig. 14.1) [3–7]. The MUSTIC trial has shown that the reduction of QRS width remains stable over time [18]. As illustrated in Fig. 14.2, the loss of LV or RV pacing mode is generally easy to diagnose on surface ECG. Generally, the lost of biventricular capture is due to the lost of LV pacing with a higher pacing threshold, with an aspect of uni-right ventricular pacing on surface ECG.

Biventricular pacing has given a new dimension to the electrocardiographic assessment of pacemaker function [19–23]. With uni-right ventricular pacing, the role of 12-lead ECG was minor. Biventricular pacing has provided a new interest in the 12-lead paced ECG, which is an indispensable tool in the assessment of cardiac resynchronization [19].

During the implantation procedure a 12-lead ECG should be recorded to identify the ECG pattern of intrinsic rhythm, RV pacing, LV pacing, and

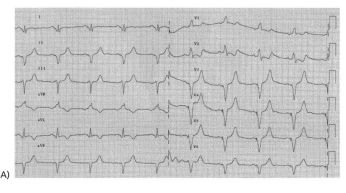

(A)

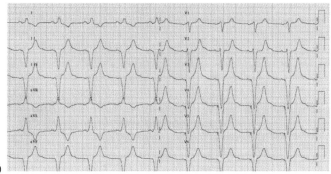

(B)

Figure 14.2 (A) Twelve-lead ECG with biventricular pacing. (B) Twelve-lead ECG in the same patient one month later showing the loss of LV capture associated with hemodynamic deterioration after an initial hemodynamic improvement. The loss of LV capture was due to a LV lead dislodgement requiring a re-positioning. (25 mm/s.)

Spontaneous Rhythm   **RVP**   **LVP**   **BVP**

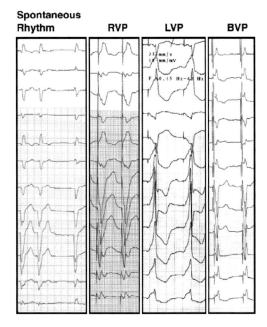

Figure 14.3 Twelve-lead surface ECG illustrating QRS pattern with spontaneous sinus rhythm, right (RVP), left (LVP), and biventricular pacing (BVP) in a heart failure patient with permanent atrial fibrillation and left bundle branch block. Reproduced from Garrigue *et al.* [21] with permission from Blackwell Publishing Ltd.

biventricular pacing (Fig. 14.3). This is of major importance to demonstrate the differences between the different pacing configurations and to be used for further evaluation during the follow-up. Loss of capture of one ventricular lead will change the morphology of 12-lead paced ECG to the other functional pacing lead pattern. The analysis of the axis in the frontal plane may also be helpful to diagnose the loss of the capture of one ventricle [19, 20].

With the first generation of devices with a common ventricular output, the diagnosis of the loss of one ventricular capture (usually the LV capture first during threshold testing) required continuous recording of 12-lead surface ECG and telemetered markers and intracardiac electrocardiogram (Fig. 14.4). With both ventricular captures, the evoked response of the ventricular electrocardiogram shows a monomorphic complex different from the two complexes observed with the native left bundle branch block (LBBB) or left intraventricular conduction delay (IVCD) [22, 23]. When the loss of a ventricular capture occurs, the pattern of the ECG is

that observed with the persistent contralateral pacing lead.

In the new generation of CRT devices with independent ventricular ports, the evaluation of pacing threshold of the right and left ventricular pacing leads is easier, and it is possible to measure the right and left ventricular pacing thresholds independently as illustrated in Fig. 14.5.

ECG patterns with LV pacing with a lead inserted into the coronary sinus

A right bundle branch block pattern (RBBB) is usually observed in lead V1 (Fig. 14.6). The recommended LV pacing site for CRT is the lateral or posterior site. LV lateral or posterior pacing produces in most cases a RBBB pattern with a right axis deviation. With apical LV lead positioning V4–V6 are typically negative whereas V4–V6 leads are generally positive with more basal sites [19, 21–23]. When the LV lead is implanted into the middle cardiac vein, a RBBB pattern is frequently observed but in some cases a LBBB pattern may be displayed due to an entry into the right ventricle from the septum. The great cardiac vein is not recommended for CRT but in some cases is the only available site for anatomic considerations. In this case LV pacing generates a RBBB pattern with axis deviation to the right inferior quadrant [19, 21].

ECG patterns with biventricular pacing

The comparison of the morphology and duration of the QRS complexes on 12-lead surface ECG with those obtained at the time of implant or during previous follow-up is useful to diagnose the loss of biventricular capture. The analysis of the frontal plane axis of the paced QRS may be useful to determine the loss of one of the two ventricular captures during threshold testing. When the loss of LV capture is the first we may observe a greater positivity of the QRS in lead I and a greater negativity of the QRS in lead III with a clockwise axis shift. In case of loss of the RV capture a greater negativity of the QRS occurs in lead I as well as a greater positivity of the QRS in lead III with a counterclockwise axis shift [19–21].

In the early days of CRT, the RV lead was positioned at the RV apex. Now, in some centers, the RV lead is often positioned either at the RV outflow tract or in the mid interventricular septum. With these

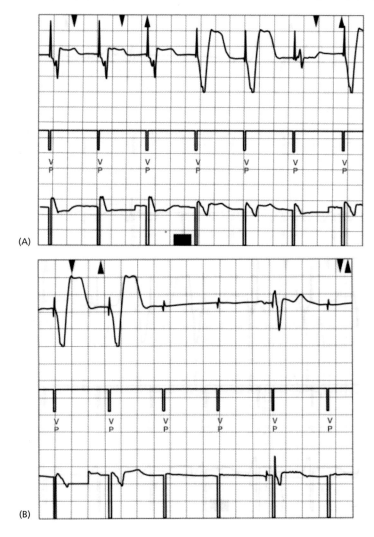

Figure 14.4 (A): Ventricular pacing threshold with progressive decrease in ventricular pacing output. The first three complexes show a biventricular capture. The two following QRS complexes show loss of LV capture with only RV pacing. The next complex is a fusion beat between RV pacing and intrinsic conduction. (B) Further decrease in ventricular output results in loss of RV capture with the occurrence of intrinsic rhythm. Reproduced from Asirvatham [20] with permission from Blackwell Ltd

two locations, the frontal plane paced QRS axis is more often directed to the right inferior quadrant with a more negative QRS in lead I.

Recently, Ammann *et al.* proposed an algorithm based on the analysis of the R-S ratio on leads V1 and I on the surface ECG with a sensitivity of 94% and a specificity of 93% in CRT patients with a RV lead placed at the RV apex [24]. Diotallevi *et al.* proposed an algorithm for verifying biventricular capture based on evoked-response morphology with high specificity and sensitivity [25].

Anodal pacing

Today, bipolar LV leads are available allowing a real bipolar configuration between the tip electrode (cathode) and the ring electrode (anode). However, many patients have a unipolar LV lead. In this case, the tip electrode of the LV lead is the cathode and the proximal electrode of the bipolar RV lead is used as the anode for LV pacing, creating a common anode for LV and RV pacing. In the case of delivery of high current density at the common cathode, an anodal capture may be observed, generating a biventricular ECG pattern slightly different from real biventricular capture [26–30]. This anodal capture disappears during threshold testing or with real unipolar biventricular pacing (Fig. 14.7). This phenomenon was usually observed with the first generations of biventricular pacemakers without separate ventricular ports but may also be observed with a separate

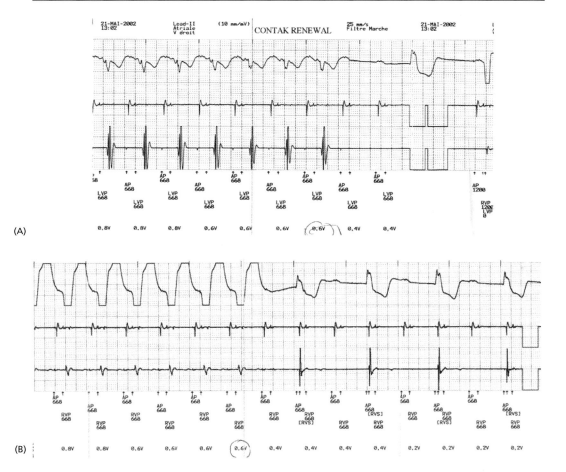

Figure 14.5 (A) Measurement of LV pacing threshold with a CRT pacemaker with independent ventricular ports. The pacing threshold is at 0.6 V with a pulse width at 0.5 ms. (B)

Measurement of RV pacing threshold in the same patient. The RV pacing threshold is measured at 0.6 V with a pulse width at 0.5 ms.

Figure 14.6 Different QRS patterns according to LV pacing site. (A) Twelve-lead surface ECG during spontaneous sinus rhythm (SR). (B) Twelve-lead ECG during LV pacing (LVP) from the lateral wall (lat). (C) Twelve-lead ECG during LV pacing from the anterior (ant) wall. (D) LV pacing lead location for (B) and (C) in veins of the coronary sinus. Reproduced from Garrigue *et al.* [21] with permission from Blackwell Publishing Ltd.

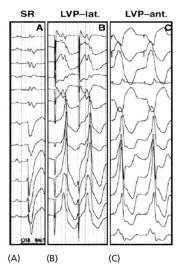

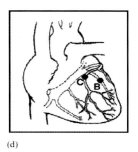

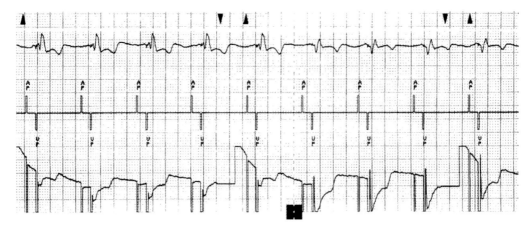

Figure 14.7 Example of an anodal capture during biventricular pacing. The anodal capture present on the left disappears on the right with the decrease in common ventricular output. Reproduced from Garrigue et al. [21] with permission from Blackwell Publishing Ltd.

ventricular ports device. It may interfere with an optimized interventricular interval evaluated during an echo study providing simultaneous and not sequential biventricular pacing.

Ventricular fusion beats

In patients with sinus rhythm and a relatively short PR interval, a ventricular fusion phenomenon between the intrinsic QRS complex and the biventricular complex may lead to misinterpretation of the ECG (Fig. 14.8) [26]. This emphasizes the importance of the programming of an adequate AV delay not only at rest but also during exercise.

Long-term ECG biventricular changes

Several studies have shown that the QRS width with biventricular pacing does not change over time if the lead's position remains stable. For instance, in the MUSTIC trial at one-year follow-up the biventricularly paced QRS width was similar to those measured at the time of implant [18]. By contrast, when switching off the device, some authors found that the spontaneous QRS duration significantly decreased over time after several months of biventricular pacing [31].

Evaluation of the ECG during an exercise test

In a patient implanted with a CRT device, the assessment of permanent biventricular capture should always require an exercise test. There are many rea-

sons why a permanent biventricular capture may disappear during exercise, such as loss of atrial sensing, frequent premature ventricular contractions (PVCs), atrial tachyarrhythmia, and spontaneous AV conduction more rapid than the programmed AV delay. Generally, right and left ventricular pacing are programmed in bipolar mode to avoid potential pectoral stimulation generating spikes with low amplitude on surface ECG. To better identify atrial and ventricular spikes, reprogramming ventricular and atrial pacing into unipolar mode may be useful, as illustrated in Fig. 14.9. The shape of atrial and ventricular complexes is similar with the two pacing modes (unipolar and bipolar). The analysis of ventricular complexes is of major importance to assess the permanent biventricular capture during exercise. Changes of the QRS complexes during exercise may suggest, as illustrated in Fig. 14.10, the loss of one ventricular capture.

Both the programmed AV delay at rest and the adaptation of the AV delay during exercise have to be assessed carefully. Figure 14.11 shows adequate programming of AV delay at rest and during exercise. By contrast, in Fig. 14.12, the rate adaptive AV delay is not optimized during exercise, resulting in the loss of LV capture. The loss of biventricular capture during exercise due to a too long programmed AV delay may also be assessed using the telemarkers of the device (Fig. 14.13). In patients with permanent atrial fibrillation and without AV node ablation, exercise testing has to be performed to verify

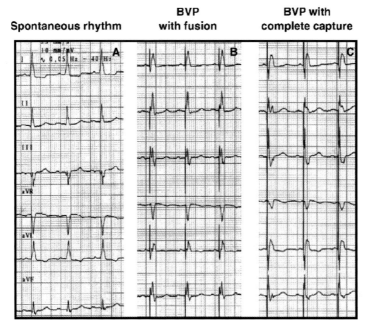

Figure 14.8 Ventricular fusion during biventricular pacing (BVP). (A) Spontaneous ventricular depolarization. Surface ECG from a patient with severe congestive heart failure showing sinus rhythm, partial left bundle branch block and QRS duration of 125 ms. (B) Ventricular fusion. ECG from the same patient after receiving a BVP device. The atrioventricular (AV) delay was fixed at 120 ms and the paced QRS shortened to 115 ms. The slight change in QRS morphology strongly suggests a fusion phenomenon with spontaneous ventricular depolarization. (C) Pure biventricular depolarization. The AV delay was programmed to 80 ms, resulting in a longer QRS duration of 130 ms. The QRS morphology is quite different from that in (B) and similar to that obtained with biventricular VVI pacing, confirming complete biventricular capture. The shorter AV delay therefore eliminated ventricular fusion with spontaneous ventricular depolarization. Reproduced from Garrigue et al. [21] with permission from Blackwell Publishing Ltd.

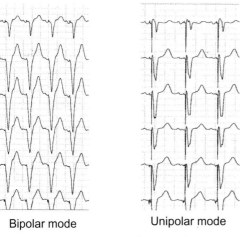

Figure 14.9 Temporary switching from a bipolar configuration (left) to a unipolar configuration (right) during exercise testing to improve the identification of the ventricular spikes.

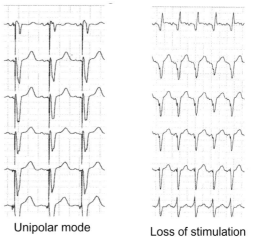

Figure 14.10 Biventricularly paced QRS complexes with unipolar configuration at rest (left). During exercise test the loss of biventricular capture was diagnosed by the modifications of the QRS complexes and the loss of ventricular spikes (right). (25 mm/s)

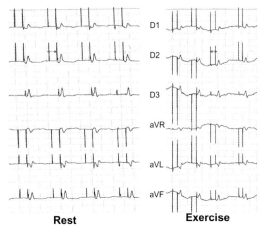

Rest | Exercise

Figure 14.11 Surface ECG recording at rest with unipolar atrial and ventricular spikes and an AV delay of 150 ms (left). During exercise heart rate increases and the AV delay shortens, providing a permanent biventricular capture (right).

permanent biventricular capture. In these patients, a biventricular capture at rest may not be a sufficient marker of permanent biventricular capture because intrinsic AV conduction may inhibit biventricular capture due to a higher spontaneous ventricular rate than the pacemaker rate driven by the rate-adaptative sensor (Fig. 14.14).

Deterioration of hemodynamic conditions during exercise is sometimes secondary not to a loss of ventricular capture but to a loss of atrial sensing, requiring a reprogramming of the atrial sensitivity (Fig. 14.15).

Finally, the evaluation of a patient with a rate-adaptative pacemaker has to consider the type of rate-adaptative sensor. For example, patients implanted with an activity sensor may exhibit a lack of increase of heart rate during an exercise performed on a cyclo-ergometer. An exercise test performed on a treadmill in the same patient without changing the sensor programming demonstrates a better adaptation of the heart rate (Fig. 14.16).

(A)
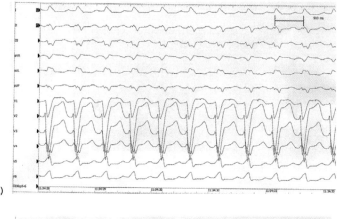

(B)
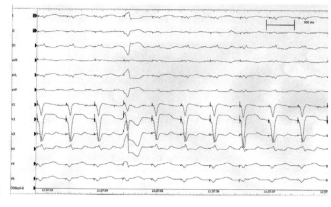

Figure 14.12 (A) Twelve-lead surface ECG recorded during an exercise test in a patient implanted with a CRT pacemaker. The patient did not improve after CRT implantation and the pacemaker interrogation showed a low percentage of paced ventricles of about 60%. An exercise test performed on a treadmill showed that the programmed AV delay was longer than that of the spontaneous PR interval, resulting in loss of cardiac resynchronization therapy. (B) In the same patient programming a shorter AV delay during exercise resulted in permanent biventricular capture during exercise, associated with a significant improvement in symptoms.

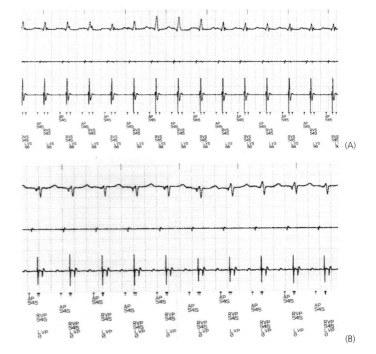

Figure 14.13 (A) Six-Minute Hall Walk Test performed in a patient implanted with a biventricular pacemaker. Inadequate programming of the AV delay resulted in the absence of biventricular pacing as illustrated by the ECG channel and the marker channels. AP, atrial pace; RVS, right ventricular sense; LVS, left ventricular sense. (B) Optimization of the AV delay provided a permanent biventricular capture with right ventricular (RVP) and left ventricular (LVP) pacing.

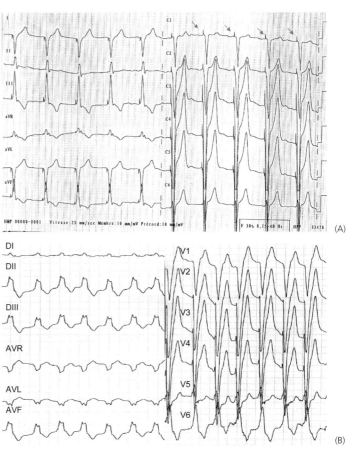

Figure 14.14 (A) Twelve-lead surface ECG in a patient with permanent atrial fibrillation implanted with a biventricular pacemaker. At rest, biventricular pacing is provided with QRS duration of 130 ms. The patient complained of fatigue as soon as he started exercising. (B) Twelve-lead ECG in the same patient during treadmill exercise test. Intrinsic ventricular rate with a left bundle branch block pattern was observed resulting in the loss of cardiac resynchronization therapy. After AV node ablation the patient was permanently paced in both ventricles, resulting in a functional improvement.

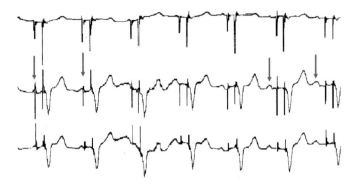

Figure 14.15 Example of a loss in atrial sensing during exercise (arrows) in a heart failure patient during an exercise test. Surface ECG at rest showed an appropriate detection of the atria. Increase in atrial sensing resulted in an appropriate detection of the atrial signal during further exercise test.

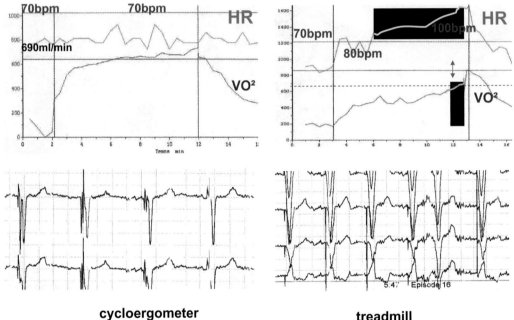

cycloergometer   treadmill

Figure 14.16 This figure displays the importance of the choice of the exercise test in patients with sensor-driven pacemakers. On the left panel with an exercise test performed on a cyclo-ergometer the sensor was not activated and the heart rate (HR) remained below 70 bpm. By contrast, when the exercise test was performed on a treadmill, the sensor was activated with a significant increase in heart rate (right).

24-Hour Holter monitoring

The 24-h Holter monitor may be useful for assessing permanent and complete biventricular capture during daily activities. A very careful analysis of the QRS complexes is required.

Device memories

Device memories give the percentage of sensed and paced events in the atria and ventricles. A high percentage of right and left ventricular sensed events suggests that biventricular capture is not permanent. However, a high percentage of biventricular paced events does not mean that cardiac resynchronization therapy is well delivered, for example in the case of fusion with the intrinsic ventricular activation or in the case of an increase in biventricular pacing thresholds.

Causes of loss of biventricular capture and solutions

Left ventricular lead dislodgement

The first cause of permanent loss of LV pacing is

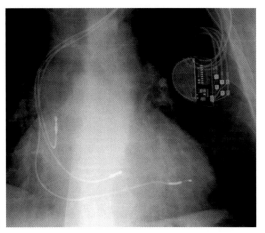

(A)

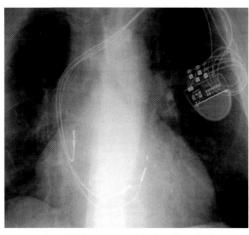

(B)

Figure 14.17 (A) Chest X-ray of a patient implanted with a biventricular defibrillator. The atrial lead is placed in the right appendage, the RV lead in the mid interventricular septum and the LV lead into the lateral vein of the

coronary sinus. (B) Anteroposterior chest X-ray in the same patient 2 days later showing a dislodgement of the LV lead now located into the body of the coronary sinus.

the dislodgement of the LV lead. A LV lead dislodgement is reported in 2–10% of cases in the different studies [3–7, 11–14]. As illustrated in Fig. 14.17, LV lead dislodgement may require a re-operation, especially if the pacing threshold becomes too high. If the increase of LV pacing threshold is moderate an increase in the LV output may be a solution to avoid a re-operation with the risk of complications such as infection. The repositioning of the LV lead should be discussed when the pacemaker is replaced in case of battery depletion for example. In some cases, the chest X-ray does not show any significant dislodgement, suggesting a so-called micro-dislodgement or an exit block or an inhibition of ventricular capture due to a tuning problem.

Upper rate behavior in biventricular devices

A common reason for loss of biventricular capture is related to sensing close to the maximal tracking rate [26, 32, 33]. Upper rate behavior of biventricular pacemakers may be Wenckebach or 2:1, as defined by the programmed upper tracking rate and the total atrial refractory period (TARP). In the case of an atrial rate exceeding the upper tracking rate but below the 2:1 rate, a pacemaker Wenckebach occurs. Two-to-one block occurs in situations where every other atrial event falls in the post-ventricular atrial refractory period (PVARP). The upper tracking limit is defined by the TARP,

equal to the summation of the AV delay and the PVARP.

In CRT devices with ventricular sensing using a composite ECG from both the left and right ventricles, the TARP during biventricular pacing and the TARP during intrinsic rhythm are quite different. In spontaneous ventricular beats, the CRT device often double counts the ventricular ECG, resetting the ventricular refractory period and the PVARP by the latest ventricular activation. In this case the TARP during biventricular pacing is longer than that during ventricular sensing with a difference equal to the interventricular delay. For example, during biventricular pacing with a single counting of the ventricular ECG and with an AV delay of 120 ms and a PVARP of 300 ms, the atrial tracking will occur at rates up to 142 bpm. In the case of occurrence of an intrinsic ventricular beat with double ventricular counting and an interventricular delay of 150 ms the TARP will be equal to 570 ms, generating a 2:1 block at rates greater than 105 bpm. The same phenomenon may occur in the case of loss of LV capture generating a ventricular double counting. This extends the PVARP by an interval equal to the IVCD, resulting in the occurrence of 2:1 block at relatively low ventricular rates [17, 32, 33].

The practical consequence of the increase of the TARP during intrinsic rhythm is that a lack of ventricular pacing may occur at heart rates slower than the heart rates theoretically predicted by addition of the AV delay to the PVARP. This phenomenon may occur especially in cases of PVC with an automatic extension of the PVARP to 400 ms. Following a PVC, the next atrial event falls within the PVARP and so the next ventricular stimulus will be inhibited, resulting in a non-paced QRS. This non-paced QRS is double counted and the next PVARP is extended by an interval equal to the IVCD. This continuous resetting of the PVARP by an interval equal to the IVCD perpetuates intrinsic rhythm. Specific

algorithms of new CRT devices by shortening the PVARP at high rates allow maintaining tracking even in the TARP with intrinsic rhythm (Figs 14.18 and 14.19). The potential disadvantage of this feature is the possibility of promoting pacemaker-mediated tachycardia [26, 32].

Pre-empted Wenckebach upper rate response

In a conventional Wenckebach upper rate response,

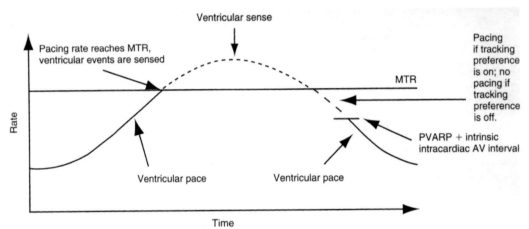

Figure 14.18 Atrial tracking preference in the Guidant Renewal CRT ICD allows tracking to occur even during the intrinsic total atrial refractory period by retracting the post-ventricular atrial refractory period (PVARP) when a second atrial event occurs in PVARP, thus allowing the maximal tracking rate (MTR) to be achieved. Courtesy of Guidant Corporation.

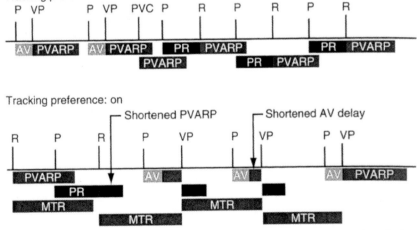

Figure 14.19 Atrial tracking preference function of the Guidant Renewal ICD. If two successive cycles occur in which a sensed RV event is preceded by an atrial event that occurs in post-ventricular atrial refractory period (PVARP), the PVARP shortens until normal atrial tracking is restored. The atrial electrogram is tracked at rates up to the maximum tracking rate (MTR). At rates above MTR, atrial tracking preference is disabled. Courtesy of Guidant Corporation.

a dual-chamber pacemaker delivers a ventricular stimulus only at the completion of the upper rate interval driven by the atria. The AV delay initiated by a sensed P wave increases progressively because the ventricular channel waits to deliver its output at the end of the upper rate interval. In the case of a P wave sensed in the post-ventricular atrial period, a pause occurs and the ventricular paced sequence repeats itself. In patients with a CRT indication, the Wenckebach upper rate response induces sequences with no evident paced complexes. In patients with normal or near-normal sinus nodes function and AV conduction the Wenckebach upper rate response takes the form of a repetitive pre-empted process which consists of an attempted Wenckebach upper response with each cycle, associated with continual partial or incomplete extension of the programmed AV interval (Fig. 14.20) [26, 32]. The process starts with a traditional Wenckebach upper rate response characterized by a gradual prolongation of the atrial sensed, ventricular paced interval and fusion of the ventricular paced beat and the intrinsic QRS with a progressive decrease in the contribution of the ventricular paced beat.

In the so-called pre-empted Wenckebach upper rate response, the spontaneous QRS complex continually occurs before completion of the upper rate interval. It is therefore sensed by the device, and ventricular pacing is pre-empted. This form of upper rate response is more likely observed in patients with relative normal AV conduction, a short programmed AV delay, a relatively slow programmed upper rate (driven by the atria) and a sinus rate greater than the programmed upper rate. Moreover, this phenomenon occurs more often on exercise or in circumstances with high adrenergic tone. The occurrence of a pre-empted Wenckebach response in CRT patients defeats the aim of this therapy based on a permanent capture of both ventricles [26, 32].

Atrial arrhythmias

In patients with severe heart failure, atrial arrhythmias and especially atrial fibrillation (AF) occur in up to 40% of cases, with a significant correlation with the severity of the heart failure [34–38]. The occurrence of AF in CRT patients may have major hemodynamic consequences due to the loss of the atrial contribution to cardiac output. AF may also

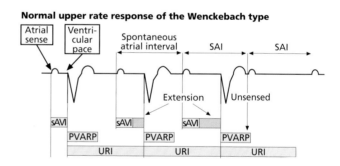

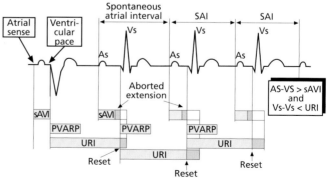

Figure 14.20 (A) Normal pacemaker Wenckebach response. (B) Repetitive pre-empted Wenckebach upper rate response. See text for details. As, atrial sense; Vs, ventricular sense; sAVI, AV delay after sensing; PVARP, post-ventricular refractory period; URI, upper rate interval; SAI, spontaneous atrial interval. Reproduced from Barold et al. [26] with permission from Blackwell Publishing Ltd.

interfere with the programming capabilities of the device. Atrial arrhythmias may result in loss of biventricular pacing in the case of a rapid ventricular rate or induce an excessively rapid ventricular pacing during arrhythmias tracking. They may also be the cause of poor resynchronization in up to 20% of CRT patients [15].

In the case of paroxysmal AF, mode-switching activation may avoid a rapid ventricular rate. If the mode switch is programmed on, a mode switch episode begins at the onset of an atrial tachyarrhythmia. In a mode switch episode, the device switches from the programmed mode (DDD or DDR) to a non-tracking mode (DDIR). This ensures that an inappropriate atrial rate does not influence the ventricular rate. For example in the Medtronic InSync Sentry device, mode switch detects an atrial tachyarrhythmia (AT) if the A–A median (the median of the last 12 A–A intervals) exceeds the programmable atrial detect rate and satisfies the AF/AT evidence criterion. When an atrial tachyarrhythmia is detected, the device smoothly reduces the ventricular pacing rate from the atrial synchronous rate to the sensor-indicated rate. The smooth rate reduction prevents an abrupt drop in the ventricular rate (Fig. 14.21). The termination of atrial tachyarrhythmia is detected when the atrial rate is less than or equal to the upper tracking rate. After the atrial tachyarrhythmia ends, the device returns to either DDD or DDDR mode.

To optimize AV synchrony some algorithms were recently developed to prevent triggering of atrial tachyarrhythmias. For example, non-competitive atrial pacing (NCAP) delays an atrial pace scheduled to fall within the relative atrial refractory period to prevent the occurrence of atrial tachycardia. Using the NCAP interval parameter, it is possible to program how long to delay an atrial pace if a refractory atrial event is sensed within the PVARP: if an atrial pace is scheduled to occur during the NCAP interval, the atrial pace is delayed until the NCAP interval expires. If no atrial pace is scheduled to be delivered during the NCAP interval, timing is not affected (Fig. 14.22).

However, preventing competitive atrial pacing may be obtained by reprogramming pacing parameters as illustrated in Fig. 14.23. For example, by programming an upper sensor rate at 120 bpm with an AV delay of 180 ms and a PVARP of 310 ms, the minimal interval between the end of the PVARP and the next atrial pace is 10 ms. In this case, an atrial pace is delivered immediately after an atrial refractory period, which may trigger an atrial tachycardia. In the same patient, with programming the upper sensor rate at 100 bpm with an AV delay of 100 ms and a shorter PVARP at 200 ms, the minimum interval between the end of the PVARP and the next atrial pace is 300 ms, so that an intrinsic atrial event occurs after the shorter PVARP interval is sensed (Fig. 14.23).

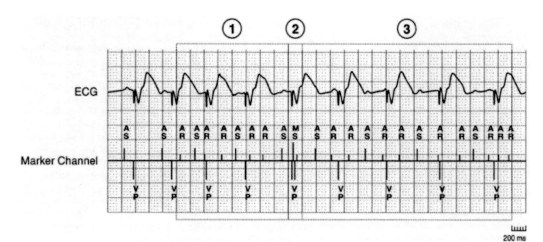

Figure 14.21 Mode switch of the Medtronic InSync Sentry. (1) An atrial tachyarrhythmia starts, causing rapid ventricular pacing in response. (2) The onset of atrial tachyarrhythmia occurs, and mode switch changes the pacing mode to DDIR. (3) The device gradually changes from the faster ventricular pacing rate to the slower sensor-indicated rate. Reprinted with the permission of Medtronic, Inc. © 2005 Medtronic, Inc.

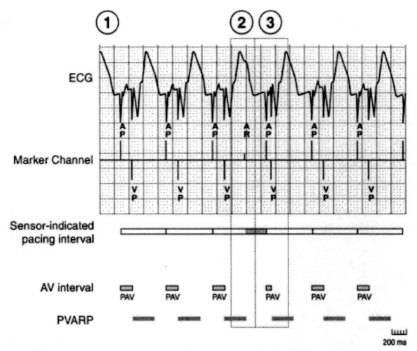

Figure 14.22 Non-competitive atrial pacing operation of the Medtronic InSync Sentry. (1) The device is pacing at the upper sensor rate of 120 per min. (2) An atrial refractory event occurs, starting a non-competitive atrial pacing (NCAP) interval (300 ms in this case). (3) After the NCAP interval expires, the device paces the atrium and then paces the ventricle after a shortened paced AV interval. Reprinted with the permission of Medtronic, Inc. © 2005 Medtronic, Inc.

New features are available in the most recent devices to increase the percentage of ventricular pacing with little or no increase in the daily mean heart rate and so to promote delivery of CRT during AF/AT episodes. Conducted atrial fibrillation response regularizes the ventricular rate by adjusting the pacing escape interval after each ventricular event. The escape interval increases or decreases, depending on whether the preceding events were paced or sensed. The result is a higher percentage of ventricular pacing at an average rate that closely matches the patient's own ventricular response (Figs 14.24 and 14.25). These types of algorithm are operating only in non-tracking modes. Therefore, when a DDD or DDDR mode is programmed, the conducted AF response operates only during a mode switch.

Permanent atrial fibrillation

Because almost all the clinical trials designed to examine the efficacy of CRT included patients with stable sinus rhythm, the presence of a permanent atrial fibrillation being an exclusion criterion, only few data on the CRT efficacy in patients with per-

manent atrial fibrillation are available. Moreover, these data were obtained from non-controlled and non-randomized studies except the MUSTIC AF study and the OPSITE trial [39, 40].

The MUSTIC AF study included 49 patients in a prospective, randomized trial with two three-month crossover periods. The patients were in permanent atrial fibrillation requiring ventricular pacemaker implantation due to a slow ventricular rate, either spontaneous or induced by AV node radiofrequency ablation. Biventricular pacing mode was compared with uni-right ventricular pacing mode. The results of the MUSTIC AF trial underlined the major importance of permanent biventricular capture as a prerequisite of CRT efficacy. Because of a higher than expected drop-out rate, only 37 patients completed the two crossover periods. The intention-to-treat analysis did not show any significant difference between the two pacing modes for the 6-Minute Walk distance, the quality of life or the peak oxygen uptake [39]. Analyzing the 24-h Holter recordings and pacemaker files showed that some patients without AV ablation had a low per-

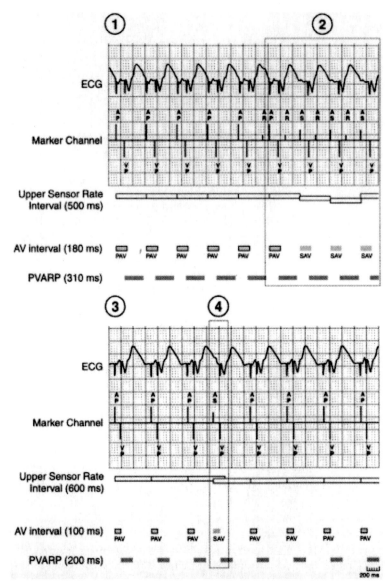

Figure 14.23 Preventing competitive atrial pacing by reprogramming pacing parameters. (1) With pacing occurring at the upper sensor rate of 120 per min, A–V intervals = 180 ms, and PVARP = 310 ms, the minimum interval between the end of PVARP and the next atrial pace is 10 ms. (2) An atrial pace is delivered immediately after an atrial refractory event, causing competitive atrial pacing, which triggers an atrial tachyarrhythmia. (3) With pacing occurring at the upper sensor rate of 100 per min, A–V intervals = 100 ms, and PVARP = 200 ms, the minimum interval between the end of PVARP and the next atrial pace is 300 ms. (4) An intrinsic atrial event occurs after the shorter PVARP interval and is sensed. Reprinted with the permission of Medtronic, Inc. © 2005 Medtronic, Inc.

centage of paced ventricular cycles (less than 50%). By contrast, all the other patients had a permanent or almost permanent biventricular capture between 97% and 100%. In the sub-group of permanent biventricularly paced patients, biventricular pacing significantly improved the 6-Minute Walk distance and the peak oxygen uptake but also significantly reduced the number of all-causes and heart failure hospitalizations [39].

In permanent atrial fibrillation, the permanent biventricular capture has to be assessed both at rest and during exercise as previously discussed. Usually in patients with permanent atrial fibrillation without spontaneous or radiofrequency-induced

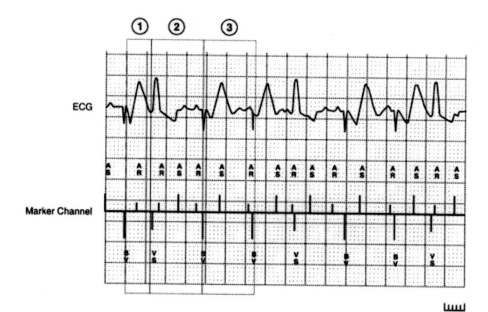

Figure 14.24 Conducted atrial fibrillation response operation of the Medtronic InSync Sentry. (1) BV–AR–VS sequence causes pacing rate to increase by 1 per min if response level is programmed to low or medium. (2) VS–BV sequence causes pacing rate to be unchanged. (3) BV–BV sequence causes pacing rate to decrease by 1 per min. Reprinted with the permission of Medtronic, Inc. © 2005 Medtronic, Inc.

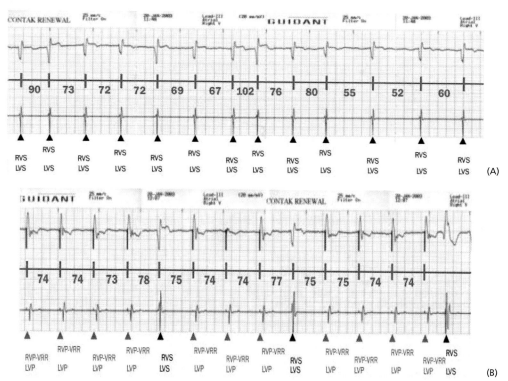

Figure 14.25 (A) Patient with a CRT device and permanent atrial fibrillation with spontaneous ventricular rate from 55 to 102 bpm. The ventricular rate regularization algorithm is not activated and the patient is not paced in right and left ventricles so the cardiac resynchronization is not achieved. (B) The same patient after switching on the ventricular rate regularization (VRR). The patient is biventricularly paced in 84% of the cardiac cycles with a more regular heart rate. Courtesy of Guidant Corporation.

AV block, the rate control is obtained using beta blockers, calcium blockers, or digoxin, alone or in combination. At rest, the rate control with these drugs is effective but may not be sufficient as soon as the patient starts exercise. The use of calcium blockers is discouraged in general due to its negative inotrophic effect which might impact negatively on survival. In these patients with a low percentage of paced ventricular cycles a radiofrequency AV node ablation may be recommended to optimize the CRT delivery. Some authors proposed the AV ablation systematically at the time of implant or one month later after verification of the proper functioning of the device.

Classically, to provide CRT in patients with permanent atrial fibrillation, a conventional dual-chamber pacemaker was implanted with the LV lead connected to the atrial port and the RV lead to the ventricular port. The pacemaker is programmed in DDDR mode with the shortest available AV delay to achieve biventricular pacing. Figures 14.26 and 14.27 illustrate the loss of biventricular capture due to inadequate programming. The pacemaker was programmed in DDDR mode with an AV delay of 30 ms. However the AV hysteresis was programmed, resulting in a prolongation of the AV delay of 52 ms, the right ventricle was sensed and the patient was paced only in the left ventricle. This case illustrates

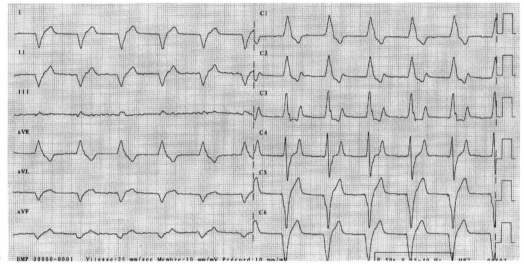

(A)

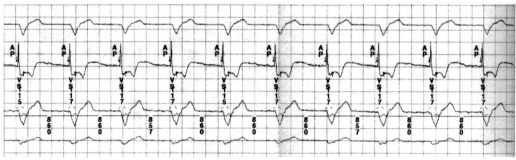

(B)

Figure 14.26 (A) Twelve-lead ECG in a patient with permanent atrial fibrillation implanted with a standard dual-chamber pacemaker. An AV node ablation was performed at the time of implant to ensure permanent biventricular capture. The surface ECG shows a right bundle branch block due to uni-left ventricular pacing. (B) Markers from the pacemaker show that the patient is paced in the left ventricle (AP), the LV lead being connected to the atrial port and the RV lead to the ventricular port. The AV delay was set at 30 ms. The right ventricle is sensed (VS). The AV delay hysteresis was not disabled resulting in a prolongation of the AV delay with the loss of biventricular capture with no pacing in the right ventricle.

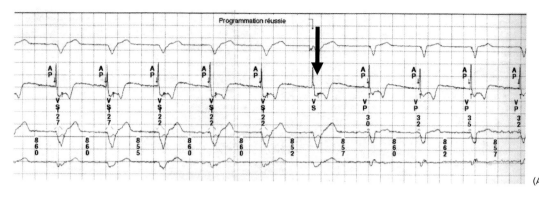

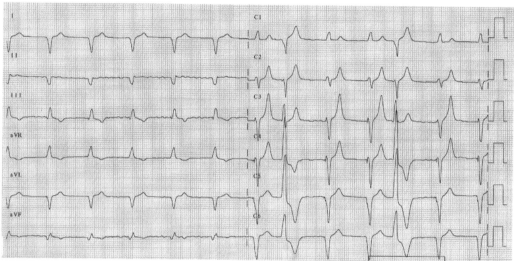

Figure 14.27 (A) The same patient as in Fig. 14.26. By switching off the AV delay hysteresis (arrow) both left and right ventricles were paced (AP and VP). (B) The 12-lead ECG displays biventricular pacing complexes.

the limitations of conventional dual-chamber pacemakers and therefore suggests the implantation of a real triple-chamber pacemaker and plugging the atrial port in permanent atrial fibrillation patients. Moreover, the triple-chamber devices allow capabilities of a better V-V interval optimization when necessary than a conventional dual-chamber pacemaker.

Premature ventricular contractions

Another potential cause of loss of cardiac resynchronization is the presence of frequent premature ventricular contractions (PVCs).

The occurrence of a PVC is defined by the device as a sensed ventricular event following a ventricular event without an intervening atrial event. Usually the detection of the PVC generates an extension of the PVARP of 400 ms, for example to avoid pace-

maker-mediated tachycardia. With the extension of the PVARP, the retrograde P wave occurs during the atrial refractory period and so inhibits tracking to the ventricle, resulting in the occurrence of a spontaneous QRS complex [26]. This spontaneous QRS may be double-counted and the subsequent PVARP is delayed by an interval equal to the IVCD. Intrinsic conduction leads to intrinsic conduction, resulting in a permanent loss of biventricular capture. In order to resume atrial tracking and CRT delivery, atrial events have to fall outside the intrinsic TARP (equal to intrinsic PR interval plus PVARP). Some algorithms temporally shorten the PVARP and so reduce the TARP, which may resume atrial tracking and CRT delivery (Fig. 14.28). In some devices, a ventricular event detected during the AV interval may trigger an immediate ventricular pacing with a 2.5 ms V–V pace delay.

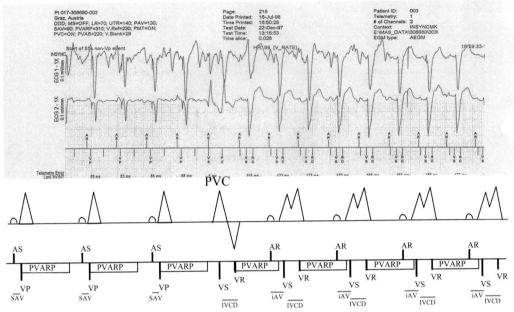

Figure 14.28 Loss of biventricular capture after premature ventricular complex (PVC). After the PVC, the device lengthens the post-ventricular atrial refractory period to 400 ms and the following atrial event falls within the refractory period, resulting in inhibition of biventricular capture and the occurrence of intrinsic rhythm. Reprinted with the permission of Medtronic, Inc. © 2001 Medtronic, Inc.

A PVC is generally followed by a long pause. These short–long interval sequences may generate in some cases spontaneous ventricular arrhythmias. To eliminate these short–long sequences some algorithms have been developed to stabilize the ventricular rate. Figure 14.29 shows a constant rate-smoothing algorithm.

Slow ventricular tachycardia

In CRT patients with dilated cardiomyopathy, slow

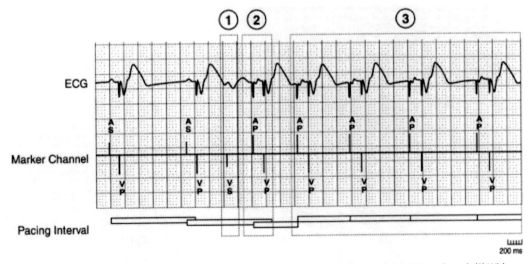

Figure 14.29 Ventricular rate stabilization of the Medtronic Insync Sentry. (1) A PVC occurs, causing a short V–V interval. (2) VRS paces the ventricle at the previous V–V interval plus the programmed interval increment (and schedules the atrial pace early to maintain AV synchrony). (3) With each successive VRS pace, the pacing interval increases by the programmed interval increment. Reprinted with the permission of Medtronic, Inc. © 2005 Medtronic, Inc.

ventricular tachycardia may occur and be responsible for loss of biventricular capture. Moreover, there is an interaction between CRT and ICD tachycardia detection zones without the possibility of antitachycardia pacing to resume the slow ventricular tachycardia (VT). For CRT ICD, the lowest programmable VT detection zone is 5 bpm above the maximal tracking rate. This may result in trade-offs between the rates of CRT delivery and the slowest detected VT. For example, a patient with a monomorphic VT at 130 bpm will require programming of the VT detection rate to 120 bpm. With this VT detection rate, CRT will be limited to tracking of atrial rates <115 bpm. With an increase in the maximal tracking rate, for example up to 140 bpm, the slow VT at 130 bpm will not be detected. Thus, in patients with slow VT, alternative VT therapies such as antiarrhythmic drugs or radiofrequency ablation can be proposed to provide effective CRT at physiologic rates.

Double counting of ventricular electrocardiogram

In the first generation of biventricular pacing, with parallel dual cathodal biventricular systems, pacing and sensing occur simultaneously in the two ventricles. Double counting may be observed during spontaneous complex (with generally LBBB and normal or almost normal AV conduction) [41, 42]. Double counting is less commonly observed in the case of the loss of LV capture with persistence of RV capture. The magnitude of temporal separation of RV and LV ECGs depends on the interventricular delay as well as the location of the ventricular leads. In the CONTAK CD trial, double counting was observed in about 7% of cases [43]. The consequences of double counting may be ventricular inhibition and so resynchronization, but also inappropriate shocks in the case of biventricular ICDs.

Conventional dual-chamber ICDs modified with a Y-adaptor have been used in an "off-label" fashion for biventricular pacing [26]. In such a system sinus tachycardia, supraventricular tachycardia, and ventricular tachycardia below the cutoff point might generate double counting (Figs 14.30 and 14.31). One of the solutions was to prolong the ventricular blanking period but the side effect was a reduction in the ability to detect a ventricular tachyarrhythmia.

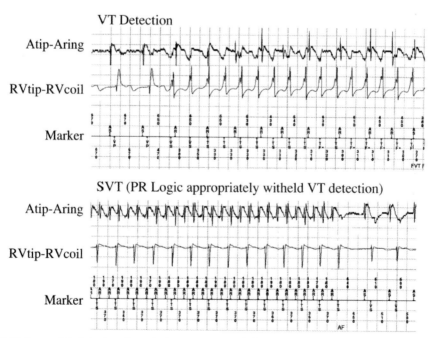

Figure 14.30 Appropriate detection of ventricular tachycardia (VT) in the top panel and supraventricular tachycardia (SVT) in the bottom panel by a biventricular cardioverter defibrillator that senses ventricular activity only from the right ventricle. The atrial and ventricular ECGs are displayed on top and the markers at the bottom of each panel. Reproduced from Barold *et al.* [26] with permission from Blackwell Publishing Ltd.

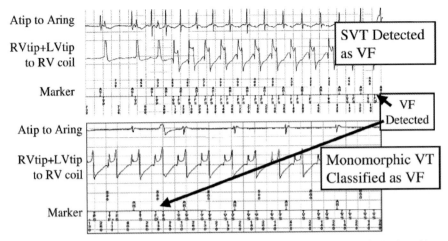

Figure 14.31 Double counting of supraventricular tachycardia (SVT) by an "off-label" biventricular implantable cardioverter defibrillator (ICD) using a conventional ICD with a Y-adaptor to produce a dual cathodal system. The atrial and ventricular ECGs are displayed on top and the markers at the bottom. Top panel. The device interprets the SVT as ventricular fibrillation (VF). Bottom panel. The device interprets slow VT as ventricular fibrillation. Reproduced from Barold et al. [26] with permission from Blackwell Publishing Ltd.

Some algorithms to prevent double counting are available in the most recent devices, such as the ventricular sense response or the interventricular refractory period.

The ventricular sense response provides cardiac resynchronization in the presence of ventricular sensing by allowing a ventricular sensed event to trigger a biventricular paced event. The detected signal triggers an immediate output delivered to both ventricles. The triggered output is ineffective if the ventricle sensing is initiated during the physiologically refractory period. The triggered mode results in an output delivered to the other ventricle as long as the maximum rate response is not exceeded. When this function is enabled, the risk of double counting is prevented (Fig. 14.32).

The interventricular refractory period prevents the restart of the ventricular refractory period, post-ventricular atrial blanking and refractory periods, and upper rate timers when a second sensed depolarization is seen following a paced or sensed event (Fig. 14.33). This function is not required during monochamber sensing but may be useful with biventricular sensing (from RV tip to LV tip; the interventricular refractory period should be programmed to the patient's IVCD + 30 ms).

Automatic sensitivity controls allow accurate sensing in both the atrium and the ventricle over a wide range of signal strengths. As shown in Fig. 14.34, the threshold starts at 50% of the measured R wave (if the R wave is between 2 and 6 mV) and decays linearly until the next sensed beat or until it reaches the maximum sensitivity threshold. If the maximum R wave amplitude is greater than 6 mV or less than 2 mV, the threshold start is set to 3 mV or 1 mV, respectively. To prevent oversensing, a decay delay can be programmed: decay delay is the amount of time after the sensed or paced refractory period that the threshold remains at the threshold start value before beginning its decay (Fig. 14.35). If necessary, increasing the decay delay can prevent oversensing of P waves in the atrium and T waves in the ventricle.

The new generation of devices with independent ventricular ports allows sensing of just one ventricle, especially the right ventricle.

Far-field sensing of atrial depolarization in cardiac resynchronization therapy devices

An LV lead inserted into a coronary sinus vein may sense the far-field P wave because of the vicinity of the LV electrode and the left atrium. This phenomenon is often observed when the LV lead is dislodged towards the AV groove. Far-field sensing by the ventricular channel may inhibit biventricular

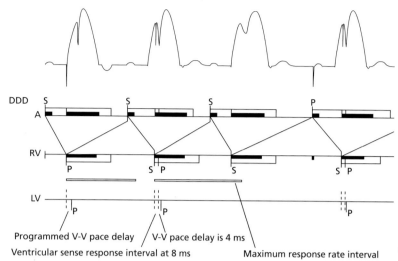

Programmed V-V pace delay / V-V pace delay is 4 ms

Ventricular sense response interval at 8 ms

Maximum response rate interval

Figure 14.32 Diagrammatic representation of the ventricular sense response (VSR) in the Medtronic InSync III pacemaker. This function is intended to provide cardiac resynchronization in the presence of ventricular sensing. A ventricular sensed event during the AV delay (initiated by a paced atrial event) triggers immediate biventricular pacing with a V–V delay of 4 ms between the ventricular stimuli. A ventricular sensed event preceded by a non-refractory atrial sensed event will also trigger immediate biventricular pacing pulses provided the stimuli do not violate the programmed upper rate interval. In the VSR function, the triggered pulse is delivered according to the programmed ventricular setting, one option being biventricular pacing. A, atrium; RV, right ventricle; LV, left ventricle; P, paced event; S, non-refractory sensed event. Note the short P–P intervals representing the V–V delay or the timing difference between LV and RV stimulation. Reprinted with the permission of Medtronic, Inc. © 2001 Medtronic, Inc.

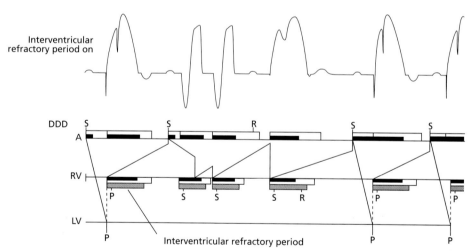

Interventricular refractory period

Figure 14.33 Diagrammatic representation of the interventricular refractory period (IRP) in the Medtronic InSync III pacemaker. The IRP prevents sensing of a second ventricular depolarization when the right and left ventricles do not depolarize simultaneously. Thus, a sensed event in the IRP (either following a ventricular paced event or a non-refractory sensed event) does not initiate new timing cycles. A, atrium; RV, right ventricle; LV, left ventricle; S, non-refractory sensed event; P, paced event; R, refractory sensed event. Note the short P–P intervals representing the V–V delay or the timing difference between LV and RV stimulation. Reprinted with the permission of Medtronic, Inc. © 2001 Medtronic, Inc.

pacing. The consequence may be much worse in a pacemaker-dependent patient, for example after AV node ablation. One solution could be to reduce ventricular sensitivity with the risk of losing normal ventricular sensing [44–46]. In some cases, the LV lead needs to be repositioned (Fig. 14.36).

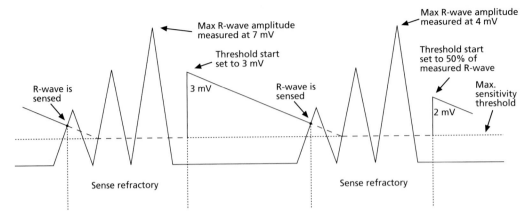

Figure 14.34 Automatic sensitivity control feature of the St Jude Atlas + HF. This feature allows accurate sensing in both the atrium and the right ventricle over a wide range of signal strengths. Threshold start begins at 50% of the measured R wave (if the R wave is between 2 and 6 mV) and decays linearly until the next sensed beat or until it reaches the maximum sensitivity threshold. If the maximum R wave amplitude is greater than 6 mV or less than 2 mV, the threshold start is set to 3 mV or 1 mV, respectively. Sensing in the atrium is identical, with the threshold start being 50% of the measured P wave if the P wave is between 0.6 and 3 mV. After a paced event, the threshold start is nominally set to 0.8 mV in the atrium and to adjust automatically based on the pacing rate in the right ventricle. Courtesy of St Jude Medical.

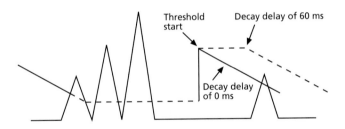

Figure 14.35 Decay delay in the St Jude Atlas + HF. Decay delay is the amount of time after the sensed or paced refractory period that the threshold remains at the threshold start value before beginning its decay. If necessary, increasing the decay delay can prevent oversensing of P waves in the atrium and T waves in the ventricle. Courtesy of St Jude Medical.

Far-field atrial sensing in biventricular implantable cardioverter defibrillators

Far-field atrial sensing can cause inappropriate therapy in a biventricular ICD with simultaneous sensing from both ventricles under certain circumstances such as: double counting of a far-field atrial near-field ventricular signal, triple counting of a far-field atrial signal with double counting of the QRS complex and repeated counting of far-field atrial fibrillation [26, 41]. In this case reprogramming the device with a decrease in ventricular sensitivity may compromise the detection of ventricular fibrillation. Other solutions are to replace the device that ignores LV activity or to reposition the LV lead or to use specific algorithms to prevent far-field atrial oversensing.

Pacemaker-mediated tachycardia

Some reports have shown that biventricular pacing, especially in patients with permanent atrial fibrillation implanted with conventional dual-chamber pacemakers, may induce pacemaker-mediated tachycardia [47]. For example, Barold and Byrd reported a case of pacemaker-mediated tachycardia in a patient with permanent atrial fibrillation and complete heart block. The LV lead was connected to the atrial port of a standard dual pacemaker and the RV lead to the ventricular port [48]. The unipolar configuration for detection of the LV lead along with a high sensitivity programmed at 1 mV on the atrial channel resulted in oversensing of T waves outside of the PVARP and induced a pacemaker-mediated tachycardia [48]. This was eliminated by

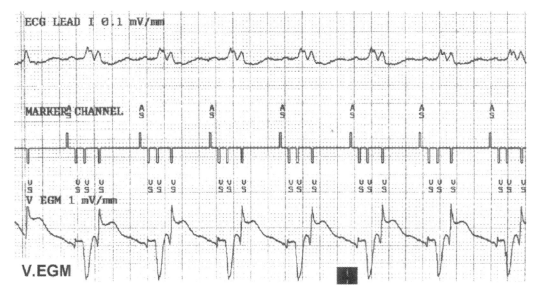

ECG LEAD I 0.1 mV/mm

MARKERS CHANNEL

V EGM 1 mV/mm

V.EGM

Figure 14.36 Far-field atrial sensing resulting in triple counting. Simultaneous recordings (from top to bottom) of the ECG, the marker channel and telemetered ventricular electrogram of a (dual cathodal) Medtronic InSync DDDR biventricular pacemaker programmed to the ODO mode (25 mm/s). There is sinus rhythm with 1:1 AV conduction with ventricular inhibition. The LV lead detects the late portion of the P wave because of its proximity to the coronary sinus and left atrium (VS follows each AS closely), resulting in complete inhibition of ventricular pacing. Every P wave is conducted and produces a wide QRS sequentially sensed by the RV lead, then by the LV lead, as a function of the distance between the leads and the long interventricular conduction time. Therefore, there are three ventricular sensed markers associated with each QRS complex: the first VS is the far-field atrial signal; the second and third VS are the two near-field components of the ventricular electrograms originating from the RV and LV leads, respectively. In the DDDR mode, the two signals generated by ventricular depolarization were recorded as VR events (refractory sensed) by the marker channel. VS, ventricular sensed event; AS, atrial sensed event. Reproduced from Barold *et al.* [26] with permission from Blackwell Publishing Ltd.

lengthening the PVARP from 250 ms to >350 ms or decreasing the ventricular sensitivity to 2 mV.

Another case of pacemaker-mediated tachycardia with biventricular pacing was reported by Van Gelder *et al.* in a patient with permanent atrial fibrillation and preserved AV conduction [49]. In this case the RV lead was connected to the atrial port of a conventional dual-chamber pacemaker and the LV lead to the ventricular port. Each intrinsic ventricular beat with LBBB was first sensed at the RV lead and followed by LV pacing with the shortest AV interval of 10 ms. To obtain the earliest RV sensing, the sensitivity was programmed at 0.15 mV. Therefore, T wave detection outside the PVARP resulted in pacemaker-mediated tachycardia. To prevent further initiation of tachycardia, atrial sensitivity was increased to 1.0 mV.

Pacemaker-mediated tachycardia due to oversensing of myopotentials in the atrial channel in permanent atrial fibrillation with a standard dual-chamber pacemaker for biventricular pacing has also been reported [50]. To avoid pacemaker-mediated tachycardia in such patients, disabling of automatic sensitivity and lengthening the PVARP or mode switch to DVIR can be proposed. An alternative solution in the presence of permanent atrial fibrillation is to implant a CRT pacemaker, sealing the atrial port by a plug and connecting the RV and the LV leads to the right and left ventricular channels.

Ventricular arrhythmias

The potential proarrhythmogenic role of biventricular pacing is questionable. In some cases biventricular pacing was associated with the occurrence of severe ventricular tachyarrhythmias [51–53] related to the LV epicardial pacing. In a rabbit wedge preparation Medina-Ravell *et al.* demonstrated the pacing site-dependent transmural propagation of phase 2 early after-depolarization (EAD). With endocardial pacing, perfusion of dofetilide led to the occurrence of EAD without transmural propagation. By contrast, during epicardial pacing, a transmural propagation of EAD was observed leading to the development of R on T extrasystoles generating torsades de pointes requiring an ICD shock [52]. However, previous studies have shown that biventricular pacing significantly decreased the number of ventricular arrhythmias [54, 55] and might also reduce the inducibility of ventricular tachyarrhythmias during electrophysiologic testing in cardiac arrest survivors with guideline-recommended CRT indications [56].

Controlled and randomized trials in patients with CRT and ICD indications did not show any significant difference in the number of appropriate or inappropriate therapies in patients with CRT off and in patients with CRT on [43, 57]. The Ventak-CHF trial showed that the number of therapeutic episodes was significantly reduced with CRT on as compared to CRT off (0.6 ± 2.1 vs. 1.4 ± 3.5; $P = 0.035$] [58]. The results of the extended CARE-HF trial yielded interesting results: biventricular pacing without ICD capabilities significantly reduced the sudden cardiac death of 46% as compared to a control group with a mean follow-up time of 37 months [8]. Interestingly, the sudden cardiac death was similar in both groups with a shorter follow-up duration of 29 months, suggesting that the beneficial effect of CRT on sudden death appears only after a long follow-up [7].

Diaphragmatic stimulation

Diaphragmatic stimulation is a complication related to LV lead implantation. In CRT patients a permanent or paroxysmal diaphragmatic stimulation may occur in up to 5–10% of patients, resulting in major discomfort for the patients [11–14]. This complication is related to the anatomical vicinity of the left phrenic nerve and the LV pacing site, especially when the LV lead is implanted into a posterior or posterolateral vein of the coronary sinus. With recent developments, producing thinner LV leads and using the over-the-wire technique, this complication seems to appear more frequently, perhaps due to the more distal position of the LV

lead in the coronary vein. During LV lead implantation phrenic nerve stimulation has to be assessed using a high voltage output at 10 V and deep breath maneuvers. When phrenic nerve stimulation occurs during LV lead implantation, it is recommended to consider another LV pacing site without phrenic nerve stimulation. However, despite this precaution a permanent or paroxysmal diaphragmatic stimulation (during upright posture or physical activity) may occur, requiring immediate action. An alternative could be to keep the same pacing site only if the LV pacing threshold is low and the phrenic nerve stimulation high, but in this case the risk of the occurrence of phrenic nerve stimulation cannot be ignored.

The occurrence of phrenic nerve stimulation early after LV lead implantation may signal an LV lead migration, sometimes without significant changes in the chest X-ray. The assessment of the LV capture threshold and of the phrenic nerve stimulation thresholds has to be performed. If the LV capture threshold falls far below the phrenic nerve stimulation threshold, the reduction in LV pacing amplitude below the phrenic nerve stimulation threshold may simply solve the problem. However, overlapping or minimally different thresholds that preclude a programmable solution mandate repositioning of the LV lead as illustrated in Fig. 14.37. Programming the LV amplitude at or barely above the LV capture may result in the loss of resynchronization, inducing a hemodynamic deterioration. One alternative solution in some cases is to decrease the LV pacing output and to increase the pulse width. With this compromise, the LV capture is still permanent but without the discomfort of the phrenic nerve stimulation.

The new generation of CRT devices with separate ventricular channels allowing independent programming of the two ventricular outputs, especially when a significant difference in impedance is observed between the two ventricular leads, decreases the need for LV lead repositioning. Recent bipolar pacing LV leads with the benefit of reducing the bipolar dipole, as well as devices allowing reprogramming of the LV lead pacing in various configurations might be useful to decrease phrenic nerve stimulation without the need of LV lead replacement (Fig. 14.38).

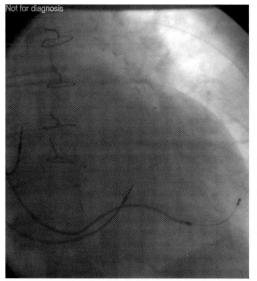
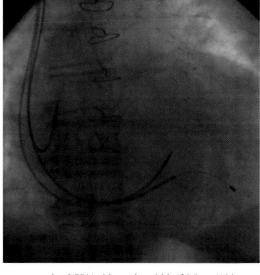

(A)

(B)

Figure 14.37 (A) Intra-operative chest X-ray showing an atrial lead placed in the right atrial appendage, an RV lead screwed in the mid interventricular septum and an LV lead inserted into the posterolateral vein of the coronary sinus. A diaphragmatic stimulation occurred even with low LV output (1 V). The LV pacing threshold was measured at 0.75 V with a pulse width of 0.5 ms. With a more proximal position of the LV lead in the posterolateral vein, diaphragmatic stimulation disappeared even at high output (10 V) with an acceptable LV pacing threshold at 1.25 V.

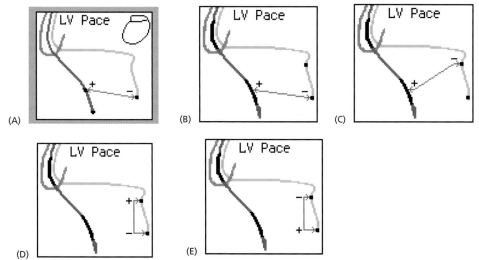

Figure 14.38 Biventricular paced configurations of the Guidant Renewal. (A) When the single (extended bipolar) configuration is programmed, the pacing stimulus is applied between the LV coronary venous lead tip and the RV distal coil electrode (Tip>>Coil). (B) When Tip>>Coil (extended bipolar) is selected for dual configuration, the pacing stimulus is applied between the LV coronary venous lead tip and the RV distal coil electrode. (C) When Ring>>Coil (extended bipolar) is selected for dual configuration, the pacing stimulus is applied between the LV coronary venous (proximal) lead ring and the RV distal coil electrode. (D) When Tip>>Ring (standard bipolar) is selected for dual configuration, the pacing stimulus is applied between the LV coronary venous lead tip and the LV coronary venous (proximal) lead ring electrode. (E) When Ring>>Tip (standard bipolar) is selected for dual configuration, the pacing stimulus is applied between the LV coronary venous (proximal) lead ring electrode and the LV coronary venous lead tip electrode. Courtesy of Guidant Corporation.

When should another left ventricular pacing site be considered?

Consideration of another LV pacing site in replacement of or in addition to an existing LV pacing site is a crucial clinical question. The answer is easy in the case of dislodgement of the LV lead associated with a high pacing threshold that cannot be corrected with technical issues from the CRT device. In this case a re-operation is needed. When there is lack of functional improvement with CRT, permanent capture of both ventricles has to be carefully assessed. An accurate echocardiographic evaluation of AV, interventricular, and left intraventricular dyssynchronies has to be performed with optimization of the AV and intraventricular delays. If, despite the attempt of the optimization of the delays, the clinical status remains unacceptable, we have to consider another LV pacing site, if the coronary sinus anatomy offers alternatives. In this case, epicardial implantation of LV leads may be considered after careful evaluation of the latest activated LV segment. However, the risk–benefit ratio of a re-operation to achieve more effective CRT has to be carefully weighed. Some patients, after an initial clinical improvement over several months or years, exhibit a hemodynamic deterioration. In these cases, implantation of a second LV pacing lead or a second RV pacing lead has been proposed. However, these options clearly require further clinical evaluation. Finally, in patients implanted with an RV apical pacing lead, another RV pacing site, for example in the RV outflow tract or in the interventricular septum, can be discussed [35].

Conclusion

Cardiac resynchronization is an effective therapy in addition to optimal drug treatment for patients with drug refractory advanced heart failure, poor LV systolic function, and ventricular dyssynchrony attested by wide QRS. The clinical follow-up of the CRT patients requires a multidisciplinary approach. Programming of the CRT devices has to be carefully evaluated to ensure permanent biventricular capture at rest as well as during exercise but also in the case of the occurrence of atrial and/or ventricular tachyarrhythmias. With the technical improvement of recent CRT devices and appropriate tuning of the devices with specific algorithms designed to improve CRT delivery, we can reasonably expect that troubleshooting should be significantly reduced. However, programming of a CRT device remains complex and has to be tailored in each individual patient.

Acknowledgements

We are grateful to Mr Mainardis from Medtronic Inc, Mr Bazillais, and Mr Serot from Guidant Corporation, and Mr Alexandre from St Jude Medical for their help with the iconography.

References

1 Swedberg K, Cleland J, Dargie H *et al.* Task Force for the Diagnosis and Treatment of Chronic Heart Failure of the European Society of Cardiology. Guidelines for the diagnosis and treatment of chronic heart failure: executive summary (update 2005). *Eur Heart J* 2005; **26**: 1115–1140.

2 Hunt S, Abraham W, Chin M *et al.* ACC/AHA 2005 guideline update for the diagnosis and management of chronic heart failure in the adult. *J Am Coll Cardiol* 2005; **46**: 1116–1143.

3 Cazeau S, Leclercq C, Lavergne T *et al.* Effects of multisite biventricular pacing in patients with heart failure and intraventricular conduction delay. *N Engl J Med* 2001; **344**: 873–880.

4 Auricchio A, Stellbrink C, Sack S *et al.* Long-term clinical effect of hemodynamically optimized cardiac resynchronization therapy in patients with heart failure and ventricular conduction delay. *J Am Coll Cardiol* 2002; **39**: 2026–2033

5 Abraham Wt, Fisher GW, Smith A *et al.* Cardiac resynchronization in heart failure. *N Engl J Med* 2002; **40**: 111–118.

6 Bristow M, Saxon L, Boehmer J *et al.* Cardiac-resynchronization therapy with or without an implantable defibrillator in advanced chronic heart failure. *N Engl J Med* 2004; **350**: 2140–2150.

7 Cleland JGF, Daubert JC, Erdmann E *et al.* The effect of cardiac resynchronization therapy on morbidity and mortality in heart failure (the CArdiac REsynchronization-Heart Failure [CARE-HF] Trial). *N Engl J Med* 2005; **352**: 1539–1549.

8 Cleland J, Tavazzi L, Freemantle N. CARE-HF: long-term effects of cardiac resynchronization therapy on mortality in the CARE-HF extension study. Clinical Trial Update

II. European Society of Cardiology meeting. Stockholm. 3 September 2005.

9 Feldmann A, de Lissovoy G, Bristow M *et al.* Cost-effectiveness of cardiac resynchronization therapy with and without a defibrillator in COMPANION heart failure patients. *J Am Coll Cardiol* 2005; **45**: 160A.

10 Bernheim A, Ammann P, Bernheim P *et al.* Right atrial pacing impairs cardiac function during resynchronization therapy: Acute effects of DDD pacing compared to VDD pacing. *J Am Coll Cardiol* 2005; **45**: 1482–1485.

11 Gassis S, Leon A. Cardiac resynchronization therapy: strategies for device programming, troubleshooting and follow-up. *J Interv Card Electrophysiol* 2005; **13**: 209–222.

12 Vardas P. Pacing follow up techniques and trouble shooting during biventricular pacing. *J Interv Card Electrophysiol* 2003; **9**: 183–187.

13 Ellery S., Paul V. Complications of biventricular pacing. *Eur Heart J* 2004; **6**(suppl D): D117–D121.

14 Bhatta L, Luck J, Wolbrette D *et al.* Complications of biventricular pacing. *Curr Opin Cardiol* 2004; **19**: 31–35.

15 Knight B, Desai A, Coman J *et al.* Long-term retention of cardiac resynchronization therapy. *J Am Coll Cardiol* 2004; **44**: 72–77.

16 Richardson K, Cook K, Wang P *et al.* Loss of biventricular pacing: what is the cause? *Heart Rhythm* 2005; **2**: 110–111.

17 Kay G. Troubleshooting and programming of cardiac resynchronization therapy. In: Ellenbogen K, Kay N, Wilkoff B, eds. *Device Therapy for Congestive Heart Failure.* Elsevier, Oxford, 2004.

18 Linde C, Leclercq C, Rex S *et al.* Long-terms benefits of biventricular pacing in congestive heart failure: results from the MUSTIC study. *J Am Coll Cardiol* 2002; **40**: 111–118.

19 Barold S. Herweg B. Giudici M. Electrocardiographic follow-up of biventricular pacemakers. *Ann Noninvasive Electrocardiol* 2005; **10**: 231–255

20 Asirvatham S. Electrocardiogram interpretation with biventricular pacing devices. In: Hayes DL, Wang PJ, Sackner-Bernstein J, Asirvatham S, eds. *Resynchronization and Defibrillation for Heart Failure: a Practical Approach.* Blackwell-Futura, Oxford, 2004.

21 Garrigue S, Barold SS, Clementy J. Electrocardiography of multisite ventricular pacing. In: Barold SS, Mugica J, eds. *The Fifth Decade of Cardiac Pacing.* Blackwell-Futura, Elmsford, NY, 2004: 84–100.

22 Steinberg J, Maniar P, Higgins S *et al.* Noninvasive assessment of the biventricular pacing system. *Ann Noninvasive Electrocardiol* 2004; **9**: 58–70.

23 Lau C, Barold S, Tse H *et al.* Advances in devices for cardiac resynchronization in heart failure. *J Interv Card Electrophysiol* 2003; **9**: 167–181.

24 Ammann P. Sticherling C. Kalusche D. An electrocardiogram-based algorithm to detect loss of left ventricular capture during cardiac resynchronization therapy. *Ann Intern Med* 2005; **142**: 968–973.

25 Diotallevi P. Ravazzi P. Gostoli E *et al.* An algorithm of verifying biventricular capture based on evoked-response morphology. *Pacing Clin Electrophysiol* 2005; **28**: 15–18.

26 Barold SS, Garrigue S, Israel C.W, Gallardo I, Clementy J. Arrhythmias of biventricular pacemakers and implantable cardioverter defibrillators. In: Barold SS, Mugica J, eds. *The Fifth Decade of Cardiac Pacing.* Blackwell-Futura, Elmsford, NY, 2004: 100–117.

27 Herweg B, Barold S. Anodal capture with second generation biventricular cardioverter-defibrillator. *Acta Cardiol* 2003; **58**: 435–436.

28 Steinhaus D, Suleman A, Vlach K *et al.* Right ventricular anodal capture in biventricular stimulation for heart failure. A look at multiple lead models. *J Am Coll Cardiol* 2002; **39A**.

29 Van Gelder B, Bracke, Pilmeyer A *et al.* Triple site ventricular pacing in a biventricular pacing system. *Pacing Clin Electrophysiol* 2001; **24**: 1165–1167.

30 Bulava A, Ansalone G, Ricci R *et al.* Triple site pacing with biventricular device. Incidence of the phenomenon and cardiac resynchronization benefit. *J Interv Card Electrophysiol* 2004; **10**: 37–45.

31 Boriani G, Biffi M, Martignani C *et al.* Electrocardiographic remodeling in cardiac resynchronization therapy. *Int J Cardiol* 2005; May 26 [Epub ahead of print].

32 Barold S. Herweg B. Upper rate response of biventricular pacing devices. *J Interv Card Electrophysiol* 2005; **12**: 129–136

33 Wang P., Kramer A., Estes III N *et al.* Timing cycles for biventricular pacing. *Pacing Clin Electrophysiol* 2002; **25**: 62–75.

34 Leclercq C, Kass DA. Retiming the failing heart: principles and current clinical status of cardiac resynchronization. *J Am Coll Cardiol* 2002; **39**: 194–201.

35 Leclercq C, Hare J. Ventricular resynchronization. Current state of the art. *Circulation* 2004; **10**: 296–299.

36 CIBIS II Investigators and Committees. The Cardiac Insufficiency Bisoprolol Study II (CIBIS II): a randomized trial. *Lancet* 1999; **353**: 9–13.

37 MERIT-HF Study Group. Effect of Metoprolol CR/XL in chronic heart failure: Metroprolol CR/XL Randomized Intervention in Congestive Heart Failure (MERIT-HF). *Lancet* 1999; **353**: 2001–2007.

38 Middelkauf HR, Stevenson WG, Stevenson LW. Prognostic significance of atrial fibrillation in advanced heart failure. A study of 390 patients. *Circulation* 1991; **84**: 40–48.

39 Leclercq C, Walker S, Linde C *et al.* Comparative effects of permanent biventricular and right-univentricular pacing in heart failure patients with chronic atrial fibrillation. *Eur Heart J* 2002; **23**: 1780–1787.

40 Brignole M, Gammage M, Puggioni E et al. Comparative assessment of right, left, and biventricular pacing in patients with permanent atrial fibrillation. *Eur Heart J* 2005; **26**: 712–722.

41 Barold S, Herweg B, Gallardo I. Double counting of the ventricular electrogram in biventricular pacemakers and ICDs. *Pacing Clin Electrophysiol* 2003; **26**: 1645–1648.

42 Chugh A, Scharf C, Hall B et al. Prevalence and management of inappropriate detection and therapies in patients with first-generation biventricular pacemaker-defibrillators. *Pacing Clin Electrophysiol* 2005; **28**: 44–50.

43 Higgins S, Hummel J, Niazi I et al. Cardiac resynchronization therapy for the treatment of heart failure in patients with intraventricular conduction delay and malignant ventricular tachyarrhythmias. *J Am Coll Cardiol* 2003; **42**: 1454–1459.

44 Lipchenca I, Garrigue S, Glikson M et al. Inhibition of biventricular pacemakers by oversensing of far-field atrial depolarization. *Pacing Clin Electrophysiol* 2002; **25**: 365–367.

45 Oguz E, Akyol A, Okmen E. Inhibition of biventricular pacing by far-field left atrial activity sensing: case report. *Pacing Clin Electrophysiol* 2002; **25**: 1517–1518.

46 Taieb J, Benchaa T, Foltzer E et al. Atrioventricular crosstalk in biventricular pacing: a potential cause of ventricular standstill. *Pacing Clin Electrophysiol* 2002; **25**: 929–935.

47 Blanc J, Fatemi M. A new cause of pacemaker-mediated tachycardia in patients implanted with a biventricular device. *Pacing Clin Electrophysiol* 2001; **24**: 1711–1712.

48 Barold S, Byrd C. Cross-ventricular endless loop tachycardia during biventricular pacing. *Pacing Clin Electrophysiol* 2001; **24**: 1821–1823.

49 Van Gelder B, Bracke F, Meijer A. Pacemaker-mediated tachycardia in a biventricular pacing system. *Pacing Clin Electrophysiol* 2001; **24**: 1819–1820.

50 Guenoun M., Hero M., Roux O et al. Cross-ventricular pacemaker-mediated tachycardia by myopotential induction during biventricular pacing. *Pacing Clin Electrophysiol* 2005; **28**: 585–587.

51 Rivero-Ayerza M. Vanderheyden M. Verstreken S et al. Polymorphic ventricular tachycardia induced by left ventricular pacing. *Circulation* 2004; **109**: 2924–2925.

52 Medina-Ravell V, Lankipalli R, Yan G et al. Effect of epicardial or biventricular pacing to prolong QT interval and increase transmural dispersion of repolarization: does resynchronization therapy pose a risk for patients predisposed to long QT or torsade de pointes? *Circulation* 2003; **107**: 740–746.

53 Mykytsez A, Maheshwari P, Dhar G et al. Ventricular tachycardia induced by biventricular pacing in patient with severe ischemic cardiomyopathy. *J Cardiovasc Electrophysiol* 2005; **16**: 655–658.

54 Walker S, Levy T, Rex S et al. Usefulness of suppression of ventricular arrhythmia by biventricular pacing in severe congestive heart failure. *Am J Cardiol* 2000; **86**: 231–233.

55 Kiès P, Bax J, Molhoeck S et al. Effect of left ventricular remodeling after cardiac resynchronization therapy on frequency of ventricular arrhythmias. *Am J Cardiol* 2004; **94**: 130–132.

56 Kiès P, Bax J, Molhoeck S et al. Effect of cardiac resynchronization therapy on inducibility of ventricular arrhythmias in cardiac arrest survivors with either ischemic or idiopathic dilated cardiomyopathy. *Am J Cardiol* 2005; **95**: 1111–1114.

57 Young J, Abraham W, Leon A et al. Combined cardiac resynchronization therapy and implantable cardioversion defibrillation in advanced chronic heart failure. *JAMA* 2002; **289**: 2685–2694.

58 Higgins S, Yong P, Scheck D et al. Biventricular pacing diminishes the need for implantable cardioverter defibrillator therapy. *J Am Coll Cardiol* 2000; **36**: 824–827.

CHAPTER 15

Device-based monitoring of heart failure by intrathoracic impedance

Jeffrey Wing-Hong Fung, MBChB(CUHK), MRCP(UK), FHKCP, FHKAM(Medicine), FRCP(Edin) *& Cheuk-Man Yu,* MBChB(CUHK), MRCP(UK), MD(CUHK), FHKCP, FHKAM(Medicine), FRACP, FRCP (Edin)

Introduction

Pulmonary congestion, as a result of elevated left atrial and left ventricular (LV) filling pressures, is the cardinal feature leading to heart failure hospitalization. The factors contributing to heart failure exacerbation leading to hospitalization are diverse, including natural progression of the disease, suboptimal regimen of medical therapy, non-compliance, inadequate follow-up, failure to seek medical attention when experiencing worsening of symptoms or inability to detect worsened heart failure.

Prevention of hospitalization due to decompensation is one of the many goals in heart failure management. In fact, within the huge health care burden for the management of heart failure, 70% of the expenses go to the treatment of acute heart failure exacerbation in the UK [1]. Prevention not only reduces health care costs but, more importantly, it improves quality of life for patients and can alter the clinical course of the heart failure, resulting in a better long-term outcome. Ideally, it should be possible precisely to predict an upcoming exacerbation and deliver appropriate intervention to prevent hospitalization. Prophylactic treatment or the adjustment of medication dosage (e.g. diuretic) given when an early warning sign appears may obviate the necessity for hospitalization. Close monitoring of symptoms, volume status, body weight, or changes in ventricular performance by means of frequent visit and physical examination for heart failure pa-

tients is recommended as part of the management program. However, none of these measures has shown a promising impact on heart failure morbidity [2, 3].

In a recent randomized study, a structured disease management program failed to reduce hospitalization rates or health care costs in patients with heart failure [4]. Symptoms leading to heart failure hospitalization usually occur only 3 days on average before hospital admission [5]. It seems that a symptom-based approach may not be "early enough" to prevent hospitalization in these patients. Physical findings of high LV filling pressures are frequently undetectable clinically even when the pressures are high [6]. Brain natriuretic peptide is a useful marker for heart failure exacerbation or volume-overloaded states. It allows physicians to differentiate between dyspnea of cardiac or non-cardiac origin [7]. However, brain natriuretic peptide as an assessment for heart failure status is rather sporadic and continuous monitoring is not feasible for ambulatory patients.

Increasing numbers of heart failure patients are now receiving device-based therapy including cardiac resynchronization therapy (CRT) and implantable cardioverter defibrillators (ICDs) [8–11]. It would be useful to be able to monitor heart failure status through these implantable devices. In our opinion, an ideal monitoring device should have the following characteristics: (1) it should provide continuous monitoring in ambulatory patients irrespective of patients' activity; (2) the parameters measured should be highly sensitive and specific to predict heart failure exacerbation; (3) it should provide a reasonable window of time or "early enough" warning sign before symptomatic heart failure exacerbation; (4) the early alert should lead to prevention of hospitalization by appropriate clinical intervention; (5) the measured parameters should facilitate the titration of medication and provide prognostic information; (6) there should be no need for additional equipment (e.g. leads) that require extra intervention apart from the conventional device implantation (i.e. it should be a built-in feature of existing heart failure devices); (7) the data stored and processed should be transferable to health care providers by an available communication channel for remote monitoring.

The main areas of device-based monitoring for heart failure status are central hemodynamic and thoracic impedance monitoring.

Central hemodynamic monitoring

Early investigations have shown that implantable sensors that allow the measurement of mixed venous oxygen saturation and pressure in the right ventricle on a beat-by-beat basis are technically feasible [12]. These hemodynamic sensors, when incorporated into device-based therapies for heart failure, can serve as a channel providing additional information or even early warning signs to predict heart failure exacerbation requiring hospitalization. In brief, optical sensors are adopted to measure the mixed venous oxygen saturation, and the hemodynamic monitoring system requires a specialized transvenous lead positioned into the right ventricular (RV) outflow tract. Absolute pressure values are obtained from the pressure sensors. The device continuously measures the RV systolic and diastolic pressures, estimates pulmonary artery diastolic pressure and maximum change in RV pressure over time.

This long-term hemodynamic monitoring has been shown to reduce hospitalization rates by more than 50% in one non-randomized study [13]. In a single-blind randomized study using the continuous intracardiac pressure monitoring device, 274 patients in New York Heart Association (NYHA) classes III and IV were recruited to receive the pres-

sure monitoring device. Patients were blinded and randomized either to care under clinicians who had access to the hemodynamic data or to care under those without access. Clinicians were allowed to titrate the medication according to volume status as reflected by the RV pressure data. Although the event rates were lower than expected, patients with the hemodynamic data monitoring available had significantly lower hospitalization rates, especially for those in NYHA class III [14].

However, mixed venous oxygen saturation and RV pressure monitoring has several limitations. Although there is no report about the technological problems in the use of optical sensors, fibrin deposition or fibrous encapsulation were observed with the sensors and this sensor was removed from the subsequent monitoring systems [12].

With regard to the RV pressure monitoring device, the information is derived from a stand-alone device. Technology may allow the incorporation of this monitoring system into the currently available devices (e.g. ICDs or CRT) in the future. However, the issue of an additional specialized transvenous lead containing the sensors or transducers positioned in the RV outflow tract requires special attention. The safety, maneuverability, electrical stability and bio-interface properties of this extra lead need to be evaluated in a large-scale trial, like conventional pacemaker or ICD leads [12].

Despite using a solid-state transducer to measure pressure, patients are required to carry an external pressure reference device at all times to collect barometric pressure changes and calculate the RV pressures. Patient compliance therefore may be a challenge. At least one pressure measured by the system had a sustained increase 4 ± 2 days before heart failure hospitalization and marked increase in all these parameters occurred only 24 h before clinical intervention in one study [13]. These warning signs may still not be "early enough" or optimal to prevent hospitalization.

Principles of thoracic impedance monitoring

Thoracic impedance refers to the hindrance to flow of the current carried by ions across the chest. When an electrical current is passed across the lung, accumulation of intrathoracic fluid during pulmonary edema results in a decrease of impedance because fluid is a better electrical conductor than air. Thus, in theory, thoracic impedance should be related to the total volume of fluid in the electric field of interest. The factors that affect measured thoracic impedance during heart failure are as follows:

- *Lung conductivity*: In general, fluid accumulates when heart failure is developing. Pulmonary vascular congestion progresses into interstitial congestion and eventually pulmonary edema. As fluid is a better conductor than air in the alveoli, the impedance decreases as heart failure worsens. Similarly, chest consolidation would also lead to a drop in the impedance measured. On the other hand, pulmonary edema significantly increases the resistance of small airways in an animal study [15] and subsequently increases the end-expiratory lung volume. The increase in lung volume thus becomes a counteracting force, resulting in a rise of thoracic impedance. Another factor that may affect the degree of pulmonary fluid accumulation during heart failure is lymphatic drainage. Prolonged increased in left atrial pressure may lead to a 20-fold increase in lymph flow to protect further accumulation of fluid in the lung [16]. Thus a non-linear relationship may exist between the progression of heart failure decompensation and measured impedance. In a canine heart failure model, however, the overall trend of intrathoracic impedance seems to decrease with increasing pulmonary congestion [17].

- *Fluid redistribution*: Heart chamber dilatation is commonly observed during heart failure. Venous congestion and occurrence of pleural effusion contribute to the decrease in the measured impedance. However, RV failure may develop as a result of LV failure progression and pulmonary fluid may be redistributed to the systemic circulation [16].

- *Soft tissue resistance*: Reduced perfusion to skeletal muscle and other soft tissues surrounding the electrodes for impedance measurement due to decreased cardiac output increases resistivity. On the other hand, trauma, infection, or swelling of the muscle and soft tissues decreases the impedance measured. Skin resistance is a real concern for transthoracic impedance via surface electrodes. Different electrode placements or skin contacts can result in significant changes in impedance measured [18, 19].

Transthoracic impedance

Measurement of thoracic impedance as a reflection of the severity of pulmonary edema has been under investigation for many years [20]. The concept has been evaluated in a non-invasive transthoracic setting in animal studies. For example, one study showed that induction of pulmonary edema by alloxan or sucrose infusion in canines resulted in a small decrease in transthoracic impedance [21]. Another animal study demonstrated that transthoracic impedance was proportional to the amount of pulmonary extravascular volumes in dogs [22]. In human studies, transthoracic impedance measured by surface electrodes has been shown to correlate well with the changes in clinical and radiological indices of severe pulmonary edema [23]. Other studies have also shown that a reduction in transthoracic impedance closely correlates with positive fluid balance during vascular and chest surgery. It has been suggested that transthoracic impedance measurement may be an additional tool for earlier diagnosis of fluid overload in the emergency room [24].

Several factors limit the role of transthoracic impedance as an ideal monitoring tool for pulmonary fluid accumulation in the ambulatory patient. In the early human study, there were significant changes in the measured impedance when patients adopted different body postures [23]. The significance of a single measurement of transthoracic impedance by surface electrodes is doubtful. Variations in transthoracic impedance are observed when there are slight differences in placement of surface electrodes or skin contact [18, 19]. Moreover, the measured impedance may also be affected by respiratory movement. Therefore, transthoracic impedance cannot fulfill the primary aim as a monitoring tool to provide continuous measurement of fluid status unless the patients are hospitalized and the electrodes are kept in the same position throughout their stay.

In order to solve the problem of variations in the measured impedance due to different placements of the electrodes, a new external device to estimate skin electrode impedance has been introduced [25]. The effect of skin impedance related to the use of surface electrodes could be eliminated by a special algorithm. Thus the measured transthoracic impedance becomes a more reliable surrogate measure of thoracic impedance. In one study it was shown to correlate well with cardiogenic pulmonary edema in the critical care unit [25]. However, the clinical usefulness of this device has not yet been evaluated in ambulatory patients.

Intrathoracic impedance

To overcome the problems associated with transthoracic impedance, intrathoracic measurement may be the solution. In an animal study, the question of whether the measured intrathoracic impedance by means of implanting a modified pacemaker in a heart failure canine model would correlate with the level of pulmonary congestion and LV end-diastolic pressure was examined [17]. A tripolar ICD lead was positioned into the right ventricle and connected to a modified pacemaker capable of measuring impedance. The proximal connection pin of the ICD lead was modified for connection to the atrial ring port of the pacemaker. The pacemaker was able to measure impedance with a resolution of 0.3 Ω at a range of 0–100 Ω. Impedance was measured from the ICD lead using a pathway from RV ring electrode to device case for current stimulation and RV coil to device case for voltage measurement. The LV end-diastolic pressure in the canine was measured by the pressure sensor lead in the LV, which was connected to an implantable hemodynamic device as mentioned before. Both the intrathoracic impedance and LV end-diastolic pressure data were

collected during the stabilization phase over a period of 4–6 weeks after the implantation procedure and followed by a seven-day control period. Heart failure was then induced by rapid RV pacing at 240–250 bpm for 3–4 weeks.

During the early stabilization phase there was an initial drop in the intrathoracic impedance while the LV end-diastolic pressure remained unchanged. A diurnal variation of measured intrathoracic impedance was also observed. Figure 15.1 shows the relationship between the measured intrathoracic impedance and the LV end-diastolic pressure during pacing and recovery. There was a significant rise of LV end-diastolic pressure, while a decrease in measured impedance was observed. The close inverse relationship between the two parameters is shown in Fig. 15.2 during the control, pacing, and recovery periods.

The key findings of this study are as follows: (1) The measurement of intrathoracic impedance is technically feasible with an implanted device and it provides continuous impedance monitoring on an ambulatory basis. (2) The measured intrathoracic impedance by the pacemaker correlated significantly with the degree of pulmonary congestion as reflected by the changes in the LV end-diastolic pressure. (3) The impedance measured was relatively stable with only small variation within and between

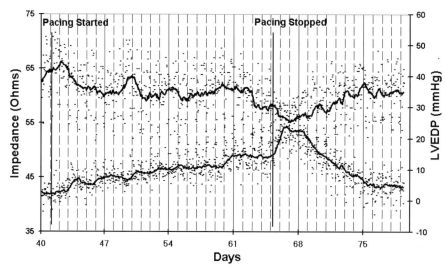

Figure 15.1 Hourly (dots) and 24-h average (solid line), impedance (upper trace), and left ventricular end-diastolic pressure (LVEDP, lower trace) from one of the dogs during pacing and recovery. The LVEDP was rising and impedance was decreasing during pacing. The reverse was observed after pacing was stopped. From Wang *et al.* [17] with permission.

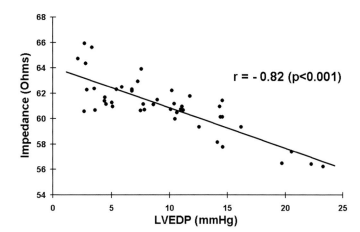

Figure 15.2 Correlation between impedance and left ventricular end-diastolic pressure in the same dog as in Fig. 15.1. From Wang *et al.* [17] with permission.

canines. The most obvious disadvantage of this approach is its invasive nature when compared with transthoracic measurement. On the other hand, intrathoracic impedance measurement by implanted device has several advantages. The implanted device eliminates the problems of variable skin impedance by external electrodes in different positions. Although there is an initial decrease in the impedance after implantation due to pocket swelling, the pattern is consistent, predictable, and reversible in all canines. Moreover, the stability of the measured impedance over time on a continuous and ambulatory basis is demonstrated. For a sensitive monitoring system, spontaneous fluctuations in the measured parameters should be minimal.

Unlike transthoracic measurement, which may only be useful in a hospital or clinic setting, impedance measurement by implanted device provides continuous monitoring with a relatively stable reference. There was a clear trend for impedance to decrease when heart failure developed and to rise when heart failure was resolved in this study. The results of this animal study established the foundation that chronic ambulatory impedance measured by an implanted device may be a potentially useful clinical tool to monitor fluid status in heart failure patients.

Disease progression and exacerbation of heart failure in patients, however, is different from the pacing-induced heart failure model in canines under a controlled environment. The relationship between measured intrathoracic impedance and degree of pulmonary congestion in human must be

established before such devices can be applied clinically. In the first human clinical study, 34 patients who were in NYHA functional class III or IV with an average 2.7 ± 1.7 heart failure hospitalizations in one year were recruited [26]. A conventional ICD lead was inserted transvenously into the RV apex and was connected to a modified pacemaker. The device was able to measure intrathoracic impedance with a resolution of 0.4 Ω and a range of 0–107 Ω. A constant current was sent through the tissue between the RV coil electrode and device case and the voltage was then measured to calculate the intrathoracic impedance. To eliminate the effect of cardiac and respiratory movements, more than 2000 impedance measurements were averaged over 2 min to provide a mean impedance value. To evaluate the relationship between intrathoracic impedance and pulmonary congestion, pulmonary capillary wedge pressure was determined by transvenous Swan–Ganz catheter once patients were hospitalized for decompensated heart failure. Other hemodynamic parameters, including systemic blood pressure, heart rate, and input/output fluid balance were measured as well.

There were 24 hospitalizations in nine patients in this study [26]. Intrathoracic impedance started to decrease and provided early warning with a mean lead time of 18 days prior to admission while symptoms of dyspnea only occurred 3 days ahead. A 12.3% reduction of impedance from the reference baseline was noted on the day before hospitalization. One of the examples is shown in Fig. 15.3. During the hospitalization period, intrathoracic impedance

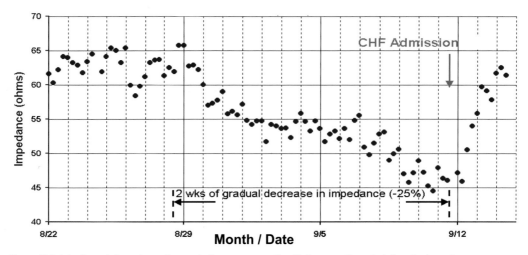

Figure 15.3 Intrathoracic impedance changes before and after admission for congestive heart failure (CHF). The initial drop in intrathoracic impedance was noted as early as 14 days before hospitalization. With intravenous diuretic therapy after admission, the impedance was increased and close to the reference baseline. Courtesy of CM Yu with permission.

correlated significantly with pulmonary capillary wedge pressure ($r = -0.61$, $P < 0.001$) and net fluid loss with diuretic therapy ($r = -0.70$, $P < 0.001$) (Fig. 15.4). Thus, the intrathoracic impedance may serve as a surrogate measure of pulmonary fluid status in heart failure patients.

Interestingly, impedance in one patient was elevated while he was dehydrated and it returned to the reference range after fluid administration. In the same study, a special algorithm of heart failure prediction based on reduction of intrathoracic impedance below the reference impedance was developed (Fig. 15.5). Using 60 Ω-day as the nominal threshold, the device has a sensitivity of 76.9% at the cost of 1.5 false-positives per patient-year of monitoring and gives an early warning of 13.4 ± 6.2 days before heart failure hospitalization (Fig. 15.6). Figure 15.7 is an example of successful prediction of heart

failure event and Fig. 15.8 demonstrates a patient without heart failure hospitalization who has had no false alarm. Though labeled as false-positives as no hospitalization occurred after a drop in impedance, these events may actually represent diuretic changes, chest infections, or fluid non-compliance, which would require medical attention (Fig. 15.9).

The feasibility of an implanted device that measures intrathoracic impedance in humans has been demonstrated in this study. The relationship between intrathoracic impedance and the severity of heart failure as reflected by filling pressure was also firmly established. Early warning by intrathoracic impedance monitoring 15 days ahead of the symptom onset may allow clinical intervention, such as fluid restriction or medication adjustment, to prevent hospital admission. In addition, the measurement may also serve as a guide for therapy after hos-

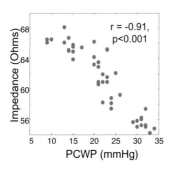

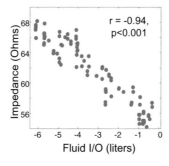

Figure 15.4 Correlation between intrathoracic impedance and pulmonary capillary wedge pressure (PCWP) and fluid input/output (I/O) balance in a patient admitted for acute heart failure. He was treated with intravenous diuretics for 4 days. The correlation coefficient are shown.

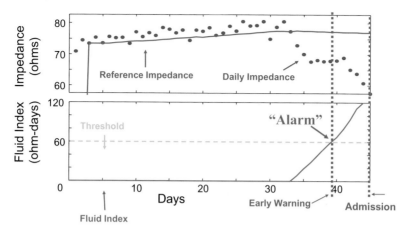

Figure 15.5 Algorithm of predicting heart failure. An automated algorithm for detection of transient decreases in impedance before heart failure admission was developed on a randomly selected portion of the available data and then validated on the remaining data. On days when the measured impedance was less than the reference impedance, the difference between the measured impedance and the reference impedance was accumulated to produce the output of the algorithm, the fluid index. If the measured impedance was consistently greater than the reference impedance, the fluid index was set to 0. The fluid index was compared with a threshold to detect a sustained transient decrease in impedance.

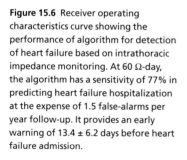

Figure 15.6 Receiver operating characteristics curve showing the performance of algorithm for detection of heart failure based on intrathoracic impedance monitoring. At 60 Ω-day, the algorithm has a sensitivity of 77% in predicting heart failure hospitalization at the expense of 1.5 false-alarms per year follow-up. It provides an early warning of 13.4 ± 6.2 days before heart failure admission.

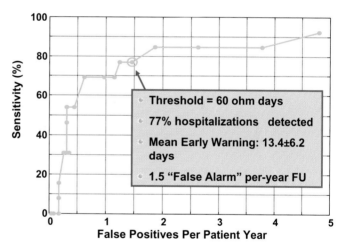

pitalization to ensure optimal volume status and to prevent over-diuresis. From the technical point of view, intrathoracic impedance can be measured via the conventional ICD or CRT system without the need for additional lead implantation.

The idea of intrathoracic impedance in device therapy has become a key feature in the cutting-edge model of CRT-D. One of the examples is shown in Fig. 15.10. There are at least two multicenter clinical trials being conducted to assess the efficacy of intrathoracic impedance monitoring with the alert algorithm on the prediction of heart failure events in patients with ICD indication. One method is to download the software into those patients who have already received the ICD and the other is a prospective study on new implantations of CRT-D. The two studies together will include more than 1000 patients. Of course, the potential clinical utility of intrathoracic impedance monitoring in the management of heart failure should be explored further, to include reduction of heart failure events with early incorporation of interventional measures.

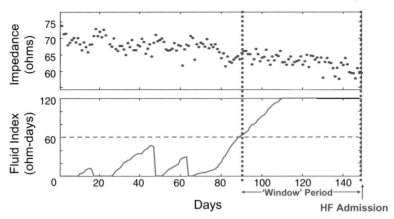

Figure 15.7 An example of successful prediction of heart failure hospitalization by intrathoracic impedance monitoring. This patient had progressive decrease in impedance value with cumulated increase in fluid index until it crossed the threshold of 60 Ω-day. The interval between supra-threshold crossing and admission for heart failure (HF) is the window period for potential intervention (e.g. increase in dose of diuretics).

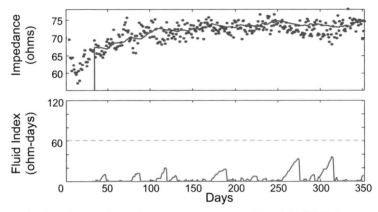

Figure 15.8 An example of a patient who has no heart failure hospitalization during the follow-up period with intrathoracic impedance monitoring. The impedance value was stable and the fluid index never exceeded the threshold of 60 Ω-day.

Comparison between two systems

The differences between the two modalities of heart failure monitoring systems are summarized in Table 15.1. There are no clinical data comparing the efficacy of both systems to predict and prevent heart failure exacerbation leading to hospitalization. Technically, intrathoracic impedance monitoring seem to be simpler than hemodynamic systems as no specialized leads are required. The central hemodynamic monitoring focuses on the change of RV pressure and estimated pulmonary diastolic pressure. Strictly speaking, it does not directly measure the degree of pulmonary congestion. From a pathophysiological point of view, elevation in LV and left atrial pressures results in pulmonary congestion and subsequently symptoms of dyspnea and hospitalization. The elevation of RV pressure may not occur in the early stages of heart failure or well in advance of symptom onset. On the other hand, impedance monitoring has been shown to correlate with LV end-diastolic pressure in canines and with pulmonary capillary wedge pressure in humans. It reflects the degree of pulmonary congestion as fluid accumulation in the lung decreases the resistance of current flow.

When comparing the early alert capabilities of the two systems, in intrathoracic impedance meas-

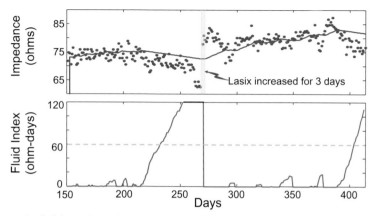

Figure 15.9 An example of "false-positive" detection of heart failure. This event was labeled as false-positive since there was no hospitalization for heart failure despite reduction of intrathoracic impedance and increase in fluid index above the threshold value. However, at clinic follow-up the patient was found to have clinical signs of increasing fluid overload. Based on clinical judgment, the physician decided to increase the dose of oral frusemide (Lasix) from 40 to 80 mg for 3 days. This led to the rapid rise of impedance above the reference line, and the fluid index is reset to baseline value.

urements a drop occurs around 18 days before hospitalization but in the case of hemodynamic monitoring the warning is only 4 days. Nevertheless, data from randomized study have confirmed the benefits of hemodynamic monitoring in reducing hospitalization rates but such information is still lacking in intrathoracic impedance measurements. Clinical applications of impedance monitoring still require large-scale investigation to confirm its role in heart failure management. On the other hand, the two systems may in fact be complementary to each other with regard to monitoring of heart failure status. It may be desirable to have both systems incorporated into the currently used heart failure devices if technology allows.

Telemonitoring

There is growing evidence that organized heart failure care can have a favorable impact on hospitalization and mortality [27, 28]. Lack of qualified health care workers (e.g. nurse specialists for heart failure) may be one of the main obstacles to provide quality care to the growing heart failure population. Much attention has been paid to the adoption of advanced technology to provide telemonitoring or remote patient care in recent years. The idea of home telemonitoring allows frequent assessment of patients' clinical status and provides diagnostic information. Early signs of heart failure exacerbation may be de-

tected by telemonitoring. Health care providers can then deliver appropriate interventions (e.g. an extra clinic visit or titration of medication) to reduce the risk of hospitalization. The mean duration of hospital stay has been shown to be reduced by this approach in a recent study [29].

Application of remote patient management by modern technology may further enhance the efficacy of hemodynamic and impedance monitoring systems in implantable devices to improve the quality of life, reduce hospitalization, and even mortality rate in patients with heart failure. Such an application has been tested in the implantable hemodynamic monitoring system. The stored hemodynamic data in the device were read out by radiofrequency transmission to a secure centralized server where the data are maintained and reviewed by clinicians through internet-based websites [30]. There are several requirements to be fulfilled before telemonitoring can be implemented in the general heart failure population. The template used must be patient-friendly and patients must be motivated to upload the information to the central server. Transmission, security, and storage of raw data and conversion into a meaningful format for assessment are technical challenges, though it has gained preliminary success by some vendors. Further exploration and evaluation of the telemonitoring concept in impedance monitoring for heart failure management program are needed.

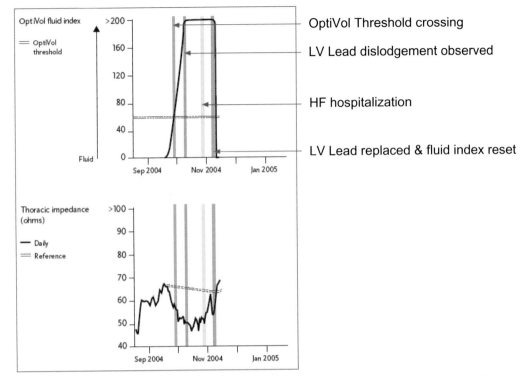

OptiVol Threshold crossing

LV Lead dislodgement observed

HF hospitalization

LV Lead replaced & fluid index reset

Figure 15.10 The patient is a 65-year-old male who has a history of myocardial infarction, sick sinus syndrome, and ventricular tachycardia, and the left ventricular ejection fraction was 28%. Cardiac resynchronization therapy (CRT) with defibrillator function was implanted in August 2004. Red bar: The time when there was a drop in intrathoracic impedance and the OptiVol fluid index crossed the threshold value. The alarm will be activated at this point onwards. Green bar: At regular follow-up LV lead dislodgement was noted but the patient remained asymptomatic. He was scheduled to have repositioning four weeks later. Yellow bar: The patient was hospitalized for heart failure. His body weight was 96 kg on admission and brain naturetic peptide (BNP) level was 1960 pg/mL. Blue bar: After intravenous diuretic therapy, heart failure was resolved and the LV lead was explanted and replaced. The intrathoracic impedance increased above the reference impedance value and therefore the OptiVol fluid index was reset automatically to baseline value. The patient's body weight was 80 kg and BNP level was 786 pg/mL. This case illustrates that lack of CRT therapy due to LV lead dislodgement resulted in heart failure decompensation. The fall in impedance was anticipated 29 days before hospitalization and even earlier than the LV lead dislodgement was detected. Moreover, the effect of diuresis on the impedance was demonstrated. Reproduced with permission from Medtronic Inc., Minnesota with courtesy of Dr T. Lavergne, Hôpital Européen Georges Pompidou, France.

The future

Despite the improved survival in patients with heart failure by means of neurohormonal blockade in the last two decades [31], hospitalization rates and health care expenditures related to heart failure are still increasing. Accurate prediction of heart failure exacerbation and prevention of hospitalization by prompt clinical intervention may be the way to reduce health care costs and improve the quality of life in those with heart failure. Ambulatory heart failure monitoring by the currently available heart failure devices (e.g. CRT-D) may be a valuable tool to prevent hospitalization. In the future with advancing technology, there may be a device that can provide, in addition to resynchronization and defibrillation therapy, information including intrathoracic impedance, RV pressures changes, peak oxygen consumption, oxygen saturation, cardiac output, heart rate variability, brain naturetic peptide level, patients' activity level, etc. All this information could be transmitted to the doctors' office or health care organization by telemetry. Appropriate intervention may then be given to prevent hospitalization,

Table 15.1 Comparison between central hemodynamic and intrathoracic impedance monitoring for heart failure

	Central hemodynamic	Intrathoracic impedance
Parameters measured	RV systolic and diastolic pressures; estimated pulmonary diastolic pressure	Intrathoracic impedance between RV apex and left pectoral device case across the left lung
Specialized lead requirement	Yes, pressure sensor lead in RV outflow tract	No, conventional ICD lead at RV apex
Stand alone device	Yes	No, in CRT-D
External accessory requirement	Yes, external pressure reference device to measure barometric pressure changes	No
Early alert capability	4 ± 2 days [13]	18.3 ± 10.1 days [26]
Conditions other than HF that may potentially affect the measurement	Chronic lung disorder, pulmonary embolism, RV infarction	Chronic lung disorder, chest infection, pocket infection, pulmonary embolism
Reduction in hospitalization rates demonstrated in randomized study	Yes, 21% risk reduction in first HF-hospitalization and 24% risk reduction in NYHA class III from COMPASS-HF[a]	No, large clinical trial result pending

RV, right ventricular; ICD, implantable cardioverter defibrillator; CRT-D, cardiac resynchronization therapy with defibrillator; HF, heart failure.

[a]COMPASS-HF: Chronicle Offers Management to Patients with Advanced Signs and Symptoms of Heart Failure study, presented in annual scientific congress of American College of Cardiology, March 2005.

improve quality of life, or even increase the chance of survival of high-risk patients with heart failure.

References

1 Stewart S, Jenkins A, Buchan S, McGuire A, Capewell S, McMurray JJ. The current cost of heart failure to the National Health Service in the UK. *Eur J Heart Failure* 2002; **4**: 361–371.

2 Goldberg LR, Piette JD, Walsh MN, Frank TA, Jaski BE, Smith AL, Rodriguez R, Mancini DM, Hopton LA, Orav EJ, Loh E. Randomized trial of a daily electronic home monitoring system in patients with advanced heart failure: The weight monitoring in heart failure (WHARF) trial. *Am Heart J* 2003; **46**: 705–712.

3 Louis AA, Turner T, Gretton M, Baksh A, Cleland JGF. A systematic review of telemonitoring for the management of heart failure. *Eur J Heart Failure* 2003; **5**: 583–590.

4 Galbreath AD, Krasuski RA, Smith B, Stajduhar KC, Kwan MD, Ellis R, Freeman GL. Long-term healthcare and cost outcomes of disease management in a large, randomized, community-based population with heart failure. *Circulation* 2004; **110**: 3518–3526.

5 Friedman MM. Older adults' symptoms and their duration before hospitalization for heart failure. *Heart Lung* 1997; **26**: 169–176.

6 Stevenson LW, Perloff JK. The limited reliability of physical signs for estimating hemodynamics in chronic heart failure. *JAMA* 1989; **261**: 884–888.

7 Maisel AS, Krishnaswamy P, Nowak RM, McCord J, Hollander JE, Duc P. Rapid measurement of B-type natriuretic peptide in the emergency diagnosis of heart failure. *N Engl J Med* 2000; **34**: 161–167.

8 Abraham WT, Fisher WG, Smith AL *et al.* MIRACLE Study Group. Multicenter InSync Randomized Clinical Evaluation. *N Engl J Med* 2002; **346**: 1845–1853,

9 Bristow MR, Saxon LA, Boehmer J *et al.* Comparison of Medical Therapy, Pacing, and Defibrillation in Heart Failure (COMPANION) Investigators: Cardiac-Resynchronization Therapy with or without an Implantable Defibrillator in Advanced Chronic Heart Failure. *N Engl J Med* 2004; **350**: 2140–2150.

10 Young JB, Abraham WT, Smith AL *et al.* Multicenter In-Sync ICD Randomized Clinical Evaluation (MIRACLE ICD) Trial Investigators: Combined cardiac resynchronization and implantable cardioversion defibrillation in advanced chronic heart failure. *JAMA* 2003; **289**: 2685–2694.

11 Cleland JG, Daubert JC, Erdmann E *et al.* Cardiac Resynchronization-Heart Failure (CARE-HF) Study Investigators: The effect of cardiac resynchronization on morbid-

ity and mortality in heart failure. *N Engl J Med* 2005; **352**: 1539–1549.

12 Bennett T, Kjellstrom B, Taepke R, Ryden L. Development of implantable devices for continuous ambulatory monitoring of central hemodynamic values in heart failure patients. *Pacing Clin Electrophysiol* 2005; **28**: 573–584.

13 Adamson PB, Magalski A, Braunschweig F *et al.* Ongoing right ventricular hemodynamics in heart failure: clinical value of measurements derived from an implantable monitoring system. *J Am Coll Cardiol* 2003; **41**: 565–571.

14 Cleland JG, Coletta AP, Freemantle N, Velavan P, Tin L, Clark AL. Clinical trials update from the American College of Cardiology meeting: CARE-HF and the Remission of Heart Failure, Women's Health Study, TNT, COMPASS-HF, VERITAS, CANPAP, PEECH and PREMIER. *Eur J Heart Failure* 2005; **7**: 931–936.

15 Hogg JC, Agarawal JB, Gardiner JS, Palmer WH, Macklem PT. Distribution of airway resistance with developing pulmonary edema in dogs. *J Appl Physiol* 1972; **32**: 20–24.

16 Guyton AC. The Pulmonary Circulation. In *Textbook of Medical Physiology*. WB Saunders Company, Philadelphia, PA, 1986.

17 Wang L, Lahtinen S, Lentz L *et al.* Feasibility of using an implantable system to measure thoracic congestion in an ambulatory chronic heart failure canine model. *Pacing Clin Electrophysiol* 2005; **28**: 404–411.

18 Ramos MU, LaBree JW, Remole W, Kubicek WG. Transthoracic electric impedance. A clinical guide of pulmonary fluid accumulation in congestive heart failure. *Minn Med* 1975; **58**: 671–676.

19 Yamamoto T, Yamamoto Y, Ozawa T. Characteristics of skin admittance for dry electrodes and the measurement of skin moisturisation. *Med Biol Eng Comput* 1986; **24**: 71–77.

20 Pomerantz M, Baumgartner R, Lauridson J, Eiseman B. Transthoracic electrical impedance for the early detection of pulmonary edema. *Surgery* 1969; **66**: 260–268.

21 Luepker RV, Michael JR, Warbasse JR. Transthoracic electrical impedance; quantitative evaluation of a non-invasive measure of thoracic fluid volume. *Am Heart J* 1973; **85**: 83–93.

22 Baker LE, Denniston JC. Noninvasive measurement of intrathoracic fluids. *Chest* 1974; **65**: suppl-37S.

23 Fein A, Grossman RF, Jones JG, Goodman PC, Murray JF. Evaluation of transthoracic electrical impedance in the diagnosis of pulmonary edema. *Circulation* 1979; **60**: 1156–1160.

24 Saunders CE. The use of transthoracic electrical bioimpedance in assessing thoracic fluid status in emergency department patients. *Am J Emerg Med* 1988; **6**: 337–340.

25 Charach G, Rabinovich P, Grosskopf I, Weintraub M. Transthoracic monitoring of the impedance of the right lung in patients with cardiogenic pulmonary edema. *Crit Care Med* 2001; **29**: 1137–1144.

26 Yu CM, Wang L, Chau E, Chan RH, Kong SL, Tang MO, Christensen J, Stadler RW, Lau CP. Intrathoracic impedance monitoring in patients with heart failure: correlation with fluid status and feasibility of early warning preceding hospitalization. *Circulation* 2005; **112**: 841–848.

27 Stewart S, Marley JE, Horowitz JD. Effects of a multidisciplinary, home-based intervention on unplanned readmissions and survival among patients with chronic congestive heart failure a randomised trial. *Lancet* 1999; **354**: 1077–1083.

28 McAlister FA, Stewart S, Ferrua S, McMurray JJV. Multidisciplinary strategies for the management of heart failure patients at high risk for readmission. *J Am Coll Cardiol* 2004; **44**: 810–819.

29 Cleland JGF, Louis AA, Rigby AS, Janssens U, Balk AHMM, on behalf of the TEN-HMS Investigators. Noninvasive home telemonitoring for patients with heart failure at high risk of recurrent admission and death: the Trans-European Network-Home-Care Management System (TEN-HMS) study. *J Am Coll Cardiol* 2005; **45**: 1654–1664.

30 Kjellstrom B, Igel D, Abraham J, Bennett T, Bourge R. Trans-telephonic monitoring of continuous haemodynamic measurements in heart failure patients. *J Telemed Telecare* 2005; **11**: 240–244.

31 Roger VL, Weston SA, Redfield MM, Hellermann-Homan JP, Killian J, Yawn BP, Jacobsen SJ. Trends in heart failure incidence and survival in a community-based population. *JAMA* 2004; **292**: 344–350.

CHAPTER 16

Continuous heart rate variability from a cardiac resynchronization device – prognostic value and clinical application

Philip B. Adamson, MD, FACC

Introduction

The paradigm of hospital versus outpatient management of patients with heart failure has evolved with each therapy demonstrating a positive effect on health care utilization in the populations studied [1–3]. This is important since acute decompensation of chronic heart failure is a dangerous event associated with 4% in-hospital mortality [4]. Continuously acquired physiologic information in patients with heart failure has demonstrated that changes in right ventricular pressures [5], heart rate variability [6, 7], and intrathoracic impedance [8] occur long before patients have symptoms that they deem significant enough to be brought to the health care provider's attention. It is therefore logical to conclude that earlier intervention may be important to reduce progression of an exacerbation to a level serious enough to require hospitalization, which not only would be beneficial from a morbidity and economic standpoint, but would also have long-term mortality implications.

As previously noted, the continuously acquired data stream from implantable devices holds valuable information that may be useful in the longitudinal clinical management and assessment of the incidence of atrial or ventricular arrhythmias. Heart rate responses to atrial tachycardia or atrial fibrillation, patient activity, average heart rate during the daytime or nighttime and percentage of atrial or ventricular pacing are all parameters that have direct impact on patient management and may influence important outcomes.

This chapter will review the basis for continuously acquired heart rate variability measured from sensed atrial cycle lengths in devices with an atrial lead. Clinical evidence will be presented outlining potential for predicting physiologic decline in patients with chronic heart failure who require hospitalization. Finally, practical suggestions for applying this information to clinical practice will be presented, including acquisition and impact on clinical decision making.

Physiologic basis of heart rate variability

Heart rate variability (HRV) arises from complex interactions between multiple cardiac control systems and serves to augment cardiac output to meet the individual's physiologic needs [9]. Even though many cardiac regulatory systems are involved, HRV primarily arises from interactions between the sympathetic and parasympathetic branches of the autonomic nervous system at the sinoatrial node [10]. Autonomic interactions adjust the atrial activation interval in response to input from cardiopulmonary and baroreceptor afferent signals. Other control systems also influence HRV, such as angiotensin II, which may have a direct heart rate effect or one mediated through facilitation of norepinephrine release.

Parasympathetic control of the heart is mediated through muscarinic receptor stimulation by acetylcholine released from post-ganglionic neurons arising from the cardiac vagus (cranial nerve X) and from intracardiac neural reflexes in the intrinsic cardiac nervous system. Parasympathetic control exerts a high-frequency adjustment of the atrial cycle length in response to cardiopulmonary afferent input to central respiratory centers [11]. Therefore, strong vagal control of the heart produces a greater degree of beat-to-beat heart rate variability with periodic influences entrained to the prevailing respiratory rate (usually 0.15–0.25 Hz) [11–13]. Sympathetic nervous control influences cardiac function by accelerating heart rate with an increase in inotropy and lusitropy mediated by stimulation of beta-adrenergic receptors throughout the heart. However, sympathetic influence at the sinoatrial node tends to have a lower frequency effect and is not entrained by the prevailing respiratory rate. Lower frequency sympathetic control of the heart rate (usually <0.15 Hz) results in reduced overall variability [12]. Therefore, HRV measurements summate the status of various cardiac control systems, in particular the two limbs of the autonomic nervous system.

Changes in autonomic control of the heart, particularly an increase in sympathetic input and/or parasympathetic withdrawal, occur in response to physiologic stressors, which may signal a general decline in stability over time. HRV measurements then may provide insight into how the neural control system perceives the status and stability of the cardiovascular system. Gaining access to this information in a continuous manner may be more effective in managing patients with heart failure than standard tools available to heart failure practitioners.

Since HRV measurements reflect the overall condition of the cardiovascular system, differences in HRV measurements between populations have been exploited to estimate the relative risk for cardiovascular events, particularly total cardiovascular mortality or sudden death risk [14–22]. This approach is based on the hypothesis that individuals with low HRV are characterized by a relative autonomic imbalance favoring sympathetic control of the heart which represents a stressed, high-risk system. In contrast, subjects with high HRV are characterized by relatively strong vagal control of the heart representing lower risk for arrhythmias or death. Individual differences in HRV may also arise from events that influence autonomic nervous control of the heart, such as upright posture, exercise, or differences in angiotensin II activation.

These influences are minimized when variability measurements are made over short periods in which environmental conditions are standardized and controlled, but shorter sampling of heart rate may not capture meaningful variability events. Therefore, measurement techniques and duration of heart rate sampling are important to understand as they may determine the clinical utility of HRV.

Heart rate variability in clinical practice

Basic science evidence and large clinical trials conducted with patients following myocardial infarction or with chronic heart failure demonstrate that reduced RR interval variability is associated with increased mortality risk [14–22]. Subsequent investigation, also relying on RR interval variability measurements, led to the clear understanding that individual neural control of the heart has inherent characteristics that predate overt cardiovascular disease and may contribute to the risk of unheralded sudden death [19, 20]. Cardiovascular disease further alters cardiac neural control, with some individuals responding to myocardial injury with sympathetic activation and vagal withdrawal, while others respond with preserved autonomic balance [18, 19]. The neural response to myocardial injury is an important determinant for eventual outcome, with sympathetic activation increasing the risk of total cardiovascular mortality and sudden death compared with those that respond to injury with preserved vagal control [18]. When heart failure follows myocardial injury, the degree of clinical decompensation is directly related to both circulating catecholamines and decline in heart rate variability.

Until recently, HRV was measured exclusively from short-term continuous ECG recordings by measuring and storing RR intervals and then analyzing the interval time series either using statistical methods such as standard deviation of the RR interval or other "time-domain" methods. Even more information about influences on heart rate from individual limbs of the autonomic nervous system can be obtained from "frequency-domain" measurements that rely on fast Fourier transformation or autoregressive analysis of heart rate time series. Frequency domain methods can capture periodic events at lower frequency to determine the power associated with a particular autonomic input [22]. Traditional HRV measurements, however, are limited to quantifying variability or frequency events during the time of surface ECG acquisition and therefore provide a "baseline" of information that can be used to stratify risk for subsequent events. Such measurements are based on short ECG acquisition (e.g. 512 beats) or 24–48 h Holter recordings. Dynamic changes that may occur over longer periods of time, when physiologic events influence neural control of the heart, cannot be determined by shorter term HRV measurements. Short-term HRV corresponds to NYHA classification of heart failure symptoms and stratifies subsequent mortality risks with reasonable predictive accuracy.

Clinical utility of continuously acquired heart rate variability

Continuous monitoring of HRV as a physiologic marker was not practical until recently when measured from the signal generated from the atrial lead of a biventricular pacing system. Device-based HRV is quantified by measuring the standard deviation of the 5 min median A–A interval (SDAAM) continuously [6, 7]. Initial evidence demonstrated that CRT with biventricular pacing improved long-term HRV when compared with a group that had the device implanted, but did not receive therapy [6]. Higher HRV in patients with CRT suggested that the physiologic impact of improving cardiac function associated with CRT resulted in less sympathetic activation and more vagal control of the heart over time. This improvement in autonomic function is likely a marker of improved clinical status, but may also be a part of the long-term mechanism involved in the benefits of CRT. Other interventions that reduce cardiac adrenergic effect, for example beta blocker therapy, are very important components of the

standard of care, resulting in a significant reduction in mortality and morbidity associated with chronic heart failure. In fact, preliminary data suggests that beta blocker therapy may further enhance the beneficial autonomic effects of CRT.

Continuous HRV measurements add the advantage of comparing day-to-day autonomic assessments in hopes of detecting changes that accompany, or ideally precede, clinical decompensation. This hypothesis was tested in a group of patients implanted with a CRT device and followed for 18 months [7]. HRV was measured at baseline and quantified as the standard deviation of the atrial-to-atrial depolarization interval averaged over 7 days of continuous acquisition. The predictive value of this measurement was then examined longitudinally to compare the measurement with previous HRV applications [7].

Baseline HRV measurements were significantly lower in patients who eventually required hospitalization for heart failure exacerbation in the 18-month follow-up period. In fact, patients who required hospitalization in the follow-up period were much more likely to have NYHA class IV heart failure symptoms coupled with low HRV (suggesting significant sympathetic activation). These findings have implications for CRT use and underscore the significance of the fact that CRT clinical trial experience was mostly in patients with NYHA class III heart failure symptoms. Additionally, baseline SDAAM values less than 50 ms were associated with a significantly increased cardiovascular mortality risk (hazard ratio of 3.2, $P < 0.02$) [7]. These data support the hypothesis that SDAAM measurements can identify a group of patients at higher mortality risk, which is important but certainly not helpful in day-to-day clinical management of heart failure patients.

Changes in continuously acquired heart rate variability and clinical events

Optimal heart failure management in specialized treatment programs relies on frequent patient assessment either with office visits or by patient-initiated monitoring such as daily weight measurements [23]. These systems are effective in reducing the need for inpatient treatment by reducing the number of hospitalizations in severely symptomatic patients. Multiple heart failure caregivers are required to provide frequent patient contact and currently there is no tested means to triage follow-up in patients who have not had recent medication or device changes. This is especially true of care outside of specialized treatment programs where the daunting challenge of follow-up becomes a major issue. Therefore, a means to predict risk for heart failure decompensation is needed to allow more patients with this chronic disease to be evaluated at appropriate intervals.

Sympathetic activation and vagal withdrawal characterize chronic heart failure patients who experience clinical decompensation and these neural changes in cardiac control should alter continuously measured HRV as the decompensation worsens. This hypothesis was tested in 288 patients who received a CRT device and follow-up for 18 months. During the follow-up period, 34 patients experienced clinical decompensation requiring hospitalization. When considered as a group, the patients with decompensation during follow-up had persistently lower SDAAM measurements (74 ± 22 ms) than their counterparts who either had no clinical adverse event (90 ± 22 ms) or had need of changes in outpatient diuretics, but no need for hospitalization (88 ± 25 ms) [7]. Therefore, the SDAAM value holds important prognostic information and can be used to triage follow-up in clinical heart failure management systems.

Significant reductions in SDAAM were detected as early as three weeks before patients decompensated and required hospitalization. The pathophysiologic implications of the early change in HRV prior to hospitalization suggest that the cardiac neural control system detects cardiovascular system decline long before patients feel ill enough to seek medical care. These data are similar in timing to those found with intrathoracic impedance measurements, but changes in HRV and impedance occur long before intracardiac pressures increase. Therefore, monitoring patients with insight from the cardiac neural control system provides information that would not be apparent when relying on the history and physical examination alone, which may allow more accurate identification of impending clinical decompensation.

Strategy for clinical use of continuous heart rate variability

Currently, HRV measurements are available during device interrogation while the patient is present in the examination room or, for certain vendor systems, remotely from internet-based information systems that receive device data from patient-initiated download from their home. Therefore, there are generally two possible strategies to utilize device-based monitoring information. First, for sites or device systems without internet-based data transmission, either a device technician or the heart failure practitioner can obtain physiologic data acquisition by device interrogation. The automatic printout of device diagnostics does not require programming or a change in device settings, which minimizes the training needed for data acquisition, and can be produced using a standard printer connected to the programmer.

Once printed, device-based diagnostics can then be used in a manner similar to vital signs with review of actual and trended data in the report (Fig. 16.1). If the point estimate HRV value is less than 75 ms, patients are at higher risk for subsequent need for hospitalization and represent a group with frequent follow-up needs. In contrast, if the SDAAM value is greater than 100 ms, patients have a very low risk for acute decompensation and can be followed up at longer intervals. Trend analysis is also very important and can provide clues about patient stability. For example, consider the 75-year-old man with an ischemic dilated cardiomyopathy, ejection fraction of 20%, with clinically stable NYHA class III heart failure, whose information is displayed in Fig. 16.2. The patient presented for routinely scheduled follow-up and had no new complaints. However, the patient's SDAAM on the day of follow-up was approximately 75 ms, which was substantially lower than the 90 ms seen at the previous interrogation. Inspection of the trend analysis suggests that the patient's HRV decline was fairly recent, occurring over the previous week. This patient was followed at weekly intervals until the HRV values returned to baseline and eventually required an increase in diuretics for a 0.9 kg (2 pound) weight gain and the appearance of elevated jugular venous pressures on physical examination. Whether this approach re-

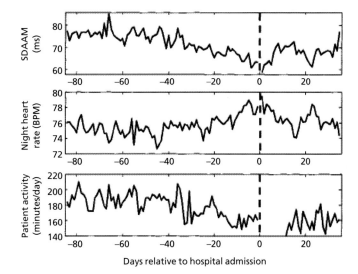

Figure 16.1 Decline in heart rate variability, increase in night heart rate, and reduction in patient activity continuously measured by a CRT device in 34 patients hospitalized for a heart failure exacerbation at day 0. Sensitivity and specificity measurements were better for heart rate variability compared with the other physiologic parameters. Used with permission from Adamson *et al.*, *Circulation* 2004; **110**: 2389–2394 [7].

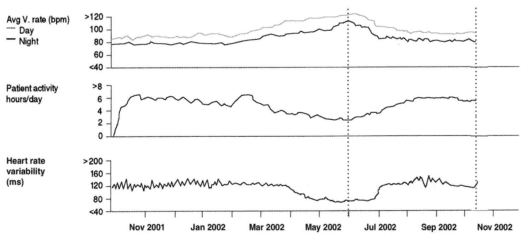

Figure 16.2 Continuously acquired day and nighttime heart rate (top panel), patient activity (middle panel), and heart rate variability (bottom panel) in a patient with chronic heart failure implanted with a cardiac resynchronization device. Note the progressive decline in heart rate variability associated with an increase in daytime and nighttime heart rate and slight decrease in patient activity. The patient presented with decline in clinical status with associated signs and symptoms of acute volume overload (dotted line June 2002). Outpatient medical therapy successfully restored optimal volume and heart rate variability returned to baseline values.

duces hospitalizations has not been prospectively validated in clinical trials, but an automated detection algorithm was developed to scan data streams to capture meaningful HRV changes with 70% sensitivity associated with 2.4 false-positive notifications per patient-year of follow-up.

With the advent of internet-based information systems, monitoring data can be sent from the patient's home at specific intervals or when concerns arise. Automatic scanning of downloaded data is still being validated and may be robust enough to automatically notify patients of problems, which would then lead to the patient contacting the heart failure provider for instructions. Until patient notification systems are in place, an effective strategy is for patients to download information from home immediately prior to follow-up visits so the internet-based data can be available immediately to the heart failure practitioner in the clinic. This approach obviates the need to interrogate the de-

Table 16.1 Suggested clinical application of continuously measured heart rate variability derived from an implanted device

Heart rate variability (measured as SDAAM) value	Predicted hospitalization risk	Suggested follow-up
Less than 50 ms	High	Every 2–4 weeks
50–100 ms	Intermediate	Every 6–8 weeks with remote monitoring monthly
Greater than 100 ms	Low	Every 12–16 weeks with remote monitoring every 6 weeks
Persistent decline for 7 days	High	Institute frequent follow-up protocols with adjustment of medical therapies

SDAAM, standard deviation of the 5 min median atrial to atrial depolarization interval. Remote monitoring can be obtained from Internet-based information systems in which patients download device information at regular intervals.
Adapted from Adamson PB: *Congestive Heart Failure* 2005 (in press).

vice in a busy office practice. Device downloads can also be initiated in the event of patient concerns or problems, but to avoid missing important information it remains the patient's responsibility to notify the heart failure practitioner that a data download occurred. (See Table 16.1.)

Limitations of continuous device-based heart rate variability

Measurements of the standard deviation of the median atrial-to-atrial depolarization intervals (SDAAM) are possible when patients have sinus rhythm at least 20% of the 24-h period. Therefore, patients with atrial fibrillation or atrial pacing that exceeds 80% of the day will not have HRV measurements available. In order to obtain HRV diagnostics, the pacing parameters used in the MIRACLE trial should be used (lower rate limit 40 bpm) if possible. Differences in activity over the long term can have a significant effect on HRV measurements, but the end-organ effect of activity is mediated through the autonomic nervous system. Additionally, activity alone was not as predictive of heart failure hospitalizations when compared head-to-head with HRV. Therefore, HRV incorporates individual autonomic characteristics and differences in activity levels to produce a predictive algorithm useful in clinical management of heart failure patients.

Conclusions

Continuous HRV is a marker of cardiac autonomic control that reflects the clinical status of patients with chronic heart failure. Incorporation of this di-

agnostic feature of an implanted device can triage follow-up and detect impending clinical decompensation. Continuous HRV data can be downloaded from the patient's home and accessed using internet-based information systems or obtained from direct interrogation of the device in an office setting. Diagnostic information obtained from implanted therapeutic devices is an important component of the data matrix available to maximize outcomes of outpatient management strategies for patients with chronic heart failure. Appropriate use of and reliance on physiologic insight into patient's status has promise for early intervention strategies designed to reduce the need for hospitalizations and dangerous heart failure exacerbations.

References

1 Abraham WT, Wagoner LE. Medical management of mild-to-moderate heart failure before the advent of beta-blockers. *Am J Med* 2001; **7A**: 47S–62S.

2 Yancy CW. Comprehensive treatment of heart failure: state-of-the-art medical therapy. *Rev Cardiovasc Med* 2005; **6**: S43–S57.

3 Adamson PB, Germany R. Therapy interactions in chronic heart failure: synergies and asynergies of medication and device interventions. *Drug Discov Today Ther Strategies* 2004; **1**: 135–141.

4 Adams KF Jr, Fonarow GC, Emerman CL *et al*. Characteristics and outcomes of patients hospitalized for heart failure in the United States: rationale, design, and preliminary observations from the first 100,000 cases in the Acute Decompensated Heart Failure National Registry (ADHERE). *Am Heart J* 2005; **149**: 209–216.

5 Adamson PB, Magalski A, Braunschweig F *et al*. Ongoing right ventricular hemodynamics in heart failure: Clini-

cal value of measurement derived from an implantable monitoring system. *J Am Coll Cardiol* 2003; **41**: 563–567.

6 Adamson PB, Kleckner K, VanHout WL *et al.* Cardiac resynchronization therapy improves heart rate variability in patients with symptomatic heart failure. *Circulation* 2003; **108**: 266–269.

7 Adamson PB, Smith AL, Abraham WT *et al.* Continuous autonomic assessment in patients with symptomatic heart failure: Prognostic value of heart rate variability measured by an implanted cardiac resynchronization device. *Circulation* 2004; **110**: 2389–2394.

8 Yu CM, Wang L, Chau E *et al.* Intrathoracic impedance monitoring in patients with heart failure: correlation with fluid status and feasibility of early warning preceding hospitalization. *Circulation* 2005; **112**: 841–848.

9 Lanfranchi PA, Somers VK. Arterial baroreflex function and cardiovascular variability: interactions and implications. *Am J Physiol Regul Integr Comp Physiol* 2002; **283**: R815–R826.

10 Lombardi F. Clinical implications of present physiological understanding of HRV components. *Card Electrophysiol Rev* 2002; **6**: 245–249.

11 Bernardi L, Porta C, Gabutti A *et al.* Modulatory effects of respiration. *Auton Neurosci* 2001; **90**: 47–56.

12 Pagani M, Malliani A. Interpreting oscillations of muscle sympathetic nerve activity and heart rate variability. *J Hypertens* 2000; **18**: 1709–1719.

13 Katona PG, Jih F. Respiratory sinus arrhythmia: noninvasive measure of parasympathetic cardiac control. *J Appl Physiol* 1975; **39**: 801–805.

14 Huikuri HV, Makikallio T, Airaksinen KE *et al.* Measurement of heart rate variability: a clinical tool or a research toy? *J Am Coll Cardiol* 1999; **34**: 1878–1883.

15 La Rovere MT, Pinna GD, Hohnloser SH *et al.* Baroreflex sensitivity and heart rate variability in the identification of patients at risk for life-threatening arrhythmias: implications for clinical trials. *Circulation* 2001; **103**: 2072–2077.

16 Malik M, Camm AJ, Janse MJ *et al.* Depressed heart rate variability identifies postinfarction patients who might benefit from prophylactic treatment with amiodarone: a substudy of EMIAT (The European Myocardial Infarct Amiodarone Trial). *J Am Coll Cardiol* 2000; **35**: 1263–1275.

17 Malik M, Camm AJ. Heart rate variability. *Clin Cardiol* 1990; **13**: 570–576.

18 Adamson PB, Vanoli E. Early autonomic and repolarization abnormalities contribute to lethal arrhythmias in chronic ischemic heart failure: characteristics of a novel heart failure model in dogs with postmyocardial infarction left ventricular dysfunction. *J Am Coll Cardiol* 2001; **37**: 1741–1748.

19 Adamson PB, Huang MH, Vanoli E *et al.* Unexpected interaction between beta-adrenergic blockade and heart rate variability before and after myocardial infarction. A longitudinal study in dogs at high and low risk for sudden death. *Circulation* 1994; **90**: 976–982.

20 Hull SS Jr, Evans AR, Vanoli E *et al.* Heart rate variability before and after myocardial infarction in conscious dogs at high and low risk of sudden death. *J Am Coll Cardiol* 1990; **16**: 978–985.

21 La Rovere MT, Bigger JT Jr, Marcus FI *et al.* Baroreflex sensitivity and heart rate variability in prediction of total cardiac mortality after myocardial infarction. ATRAMI (Autonomic Tone and Reflexes After Myocardial Infarction) Investigators. *Lancet* 1998; **351**: 478–484.

22 Task force of the European Society of Cardiology and the North American Society of Pacing and Electrophysiology. Heart rate variability: standards of measurement, physiological interpretation and clinical use. *Circulation* 1996; **93**: 1043–1065.

23 Fonarow GC, Stevenson LW, Walden JA *et al.* Impact of a comprehensive heart failure management program on hospital readmission and functional status of patients with advanced heart failure. *J Am Coll Cardiol* 1997; **20**: 725–732.

CHAPTER 17

Optimization of cardiac resynchronization therapy: the role of echocardiography in atrioventricular, interventricular and intraventricular delay optimization

Stephane Garrigue, MD, PhD

Introduction

As noted in earlier chapters, heart failure is a remarkably common but quite complex syndrome and a large and growing worldwide population suffers from this disease. Prognosis is still poor, particularly in the presence of conduction disorders [1–4] and associated inter- and/or intra-left ventricular (LV) conduction delays [4–6], which may lead to intra-LV mechanical dyssynchrony, delayed LV wall systolic motion, non-uniform wall stress, increase in mitral regurgitation, and reduced diastolic filling times [5, 6]. Despite significant progress in pharmacologic treatment of heart failure, its effect on regional LV conduction abnormalities remains limited. Cardiac resynchronization therapy (CRT) has been considered in these patients as a revolutionary non-pharmacological treatment to counteract electromechanical consequences of ventricular conduction abnormalities [7–9]. This has resulted in considering the pacing device as a true hemodynamic treatment option for heart failure patients with conduction disorders [10, 11]. However, several pathophysiologic aspects remain to be clarified in order to better understand CRT mechanisms and to optimize selection of patients for CRT.

Indeed, it remains still unclear whether CRT-induced hemodynamic benefits are mainly due to major improvements in inter- or intraventricular synchronization [12–16], and furthermore, should simultaneous CRT or sequential CRT be preferred. In other words, since the LV lead is usually positioned in the lateral or posterior LV wall and the RV lead is close to the septal wall, it seems logical to consider LV or RV pre-excitation after taking into account the latest point of mechanical or electrical activation and the relative positioning of the leads. Indeed, it has already been demonstrated that the RV lead located at the apex is responsible for at least 40% of the LV activation area [17]. Accordingly, one may suggest that CRT results in LV resynchronization rather than interventricular (VV) resynchronization. Non-invasive techniques such as echocardiography have brought precious information on short- and long-term follow-up of resynchronized patients in terms of ventricular dyssynchrony [12, 15, 16, 18, 19]. Several echocardiographic measures have been proposed to assess and even quantify CRT effects.

Even though this research field is fascinating, we should not forget the long accepted concept of "simple" atrioventricular delay optimization that still has a role in CRT patients.

This chapter discusses this evolving field and current methods for assessing the impact of AV and VV delays on CRT patients.

Why optimize cardiac resynchronization therapy?

Most CRT studies have reported a non-responder rate of 20 to 35% with simultaneous CRT [11, 20–22]. This leads to at least three hypotheses:

1 Simultaneous biventricular pacing has no effect in a specific "yet-to-be-defined" population of heart failure patients which might represent 20–30% of heart failure patients.

2 The LV lead has not been positioned at the optimal site so that cardiac function cannot be improved.

3 Only tailored sequential biventricular pacing can improve all patients with severe heart failure and ventricular conduction disturbances because the LV lead cannot be located at the optimal site for every candidate for CRT.

Patients who are candidates for CRT are usually those that have severe heart failure retractory to usual medical management due, at least in part, to major ventricular conduction disturbances and/or intra- and/or interventricular electromechanical dyssynchrony [6, 11, 13]. It is easy to hypothesize that non-responders occur primarily because of our limited knowledge in the field of electromechanical coupling in heart failure. If simultaneous biventricular pacing fails to improve an otherwise "ideal" candidate for CRT, it suggests that a significant area of LV myocardium remains dyssynchronous compared with the other LV segments (assuming that this LV area is still contracting, i.e. not infarcted). If this is true, pre-excitation of this singular asynchronous ventricular region or increasing LV filling could result in more synchronous LV contraction and improved cardiac function along with improved clinical status [15, 19]. This is the hypothesis that will be discussed in this chapter.

Tailored sequential biventricular pacing might be a reliable solution to decrease the numbers of non-responders. Indeed, sequential CRT with individually optimized interventricular delay has been shown to result in additional significant increase in diastolic filling time and a further reduction in intra-LV dyssynchrony [19].

Role of atrioventricular optimization

Although the importance of AV delay optimization for patients with AV conduction disease requiring dual-chamber pacing is unquestioned (Fig. 17.1), the impact in the heart failure population with spontaneous conduction remains more difficult to assess. Early reports suggested that AV synchronization in patients with end-stage heart failure receiving

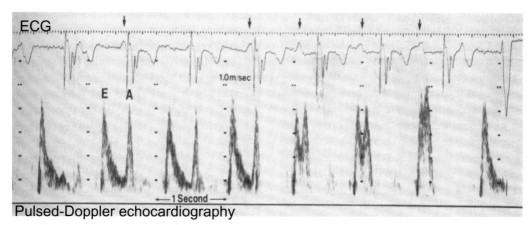

Pulsed-Doppler echocardiography

Figure 17.1 VVI pacing asynchronous to the atrial activity (obvious P waves on the surface ECG, see arrows). The ECG is recorded simultaneously with the LV filling pattern (E and A waves) obtained by pulsed-Doppler echocardiography. This patient presents with a complete AV block, so that the seven ventricular stimuli give a large panel of different timings between the P wave and ventricular activation. This results in different patterns of LV filling and then in varying levels of contributive filling to the systolic phase.

dual-champer pacing significantly improved cardiac function by employing short AV delays [23, 24].

However, further studies did not corroborate such beneficial effects by systematically programming short AV delays [25, 26]. Instead the authors demonstrated important patient-to-patient variations in optimal AV delay. In some patients, even changing the AV delay did not significantly improve cardiac function. In the latter case, if LV filling cannot be directly improved, other therapies, such as CRT, have to be tested in order to improve the systolic phase, which by feedback would improve diastolic function [13, 27, 28].

Some authors have speculated that improvement in patients with heart failure by optimizing the AV delay results from changes in the AV mechanical sequence as well as the ventricular activation sequence. Thus, it seems reasonable to speculate that optimization of AV delay is definitely an important factor in patients benefiting from CRT. Several studies have examined this impact [28–30]. Auricchio *et al.* [30] showed that AV delay does positively influence hemodynamics even though the paced ventricular chamber (right or left ventricle) seems to play a more important role for cardiac function improvement. The other studies that have evaluated the effects of CRT on LV diastolic function have relied upon pulsed wave Doppler-derived transmitral filling parameters, with variable results. It is well established that LV diastolic filling time increases after CRT [31–34]. However, the mitral E wave velocity or E/A ratio may not be significantly improved [32–35]. Accordingly, the timing between the P wave sensed by the CRT device and the ventricular stimulus should be optimized in order to maximize potential diastolic filling improvement. Interestingly, the increase in mitral E wave deceleration time was observed mainly in those patients who demonstrate significant reductions in LV volumes and/or increases in LV ejection fraction (LVEF) > 5% [12, 33–35]. It may be postulated that increases in deceleration time after CRT may reflect improvements in LV compliance [16, 18].

Consequently, optimizing the AV delay in CRT patients is crucial for at least two reasons:
1 An optimal LV filling time improves cardiac function in most cases.
2 In patients with normal AV conduction (i.e. normal PR interval on the surface ECG), we have to ensure complete biventricular capture and then shorten the AV delay compared with the spontaneous PR interval.

This leads to the following: the AV delay should be optimized for every CRT patient.

When should we optimize the atrioventricular delay?

It seems reasonable to initially optimize the AV delay before the patient is discharged from the hospital following CRT implantation. Since biventricular stimulation will change the ventricular activation sequence, we know that electromechanical changes will counteract LV remodeling; the end-diastolic and end-systolic volumes will decrease over time. Consequently, diastolic and systolic pressures will also change along with LV filling. Due to these changes, the cardiologist should periodically assess the LV filling pattern and readjust the AV delay in order to ensure the patient has an optimal LV filling sequence. Since several studies have already shown that early changes in the LV geometry generally occur within three months after CRT [10–12], AV delay optimization should be reassessed at this time and then periodically. Further studies are needed to determine how often the AV delay should be optimized.

How to optimize the atrioventricular delay

Carlton *et al.* [36] were the first to highlight the importance of AV synchrony in paced patients with high-degree AV block. Furthermore, Ronaszecki [37] demonstrated the impact of optimal AV delay in minimizing LV filling pressures and mitral regurgitation. Rey *et al.* [38] noted that the longest ventricular filling time without interruption of the A wave resulted in the highest cardiac outputs (Fig. 17.2). Ritter *et al.* [39, 40] subsequently reported on a method based on Doppler echocardiography to assess electromechanical intervals, whereby AV timing could be optimized with the use of a relatively simple and clinically practical protocol.

The "Ritter" technique has been described in detail in many echocardiographic manuals and has several important advantages. For example, it is based on echocardiography, which has the advantage of being non-invasive and readily available for every cardi-

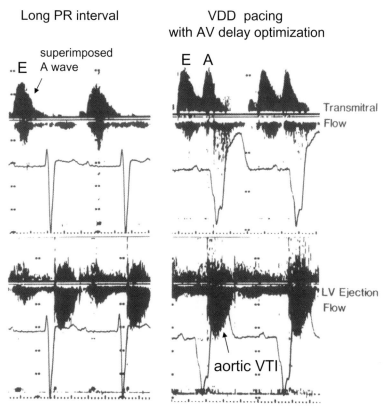

Long PR interval

VDD pacing
with AV delay optimization

Figure 17.2 Pulsed wave Doppler echocardiography coupled with the surface ECG in a patient with a long PR interval. Left panel: The E and A waves are superimposed due to the very late diastole resulting from a very delayed ventricular activation from the atrial activity (P wave on the surface ECG). Right panel: ventricular stimulation has tremendously shortened the delay between the sensed P wave and ventricular activation, so that the ventricular end-systolic phase terminates much earlier, enabling the E wave to appear far before atrial contraction (A wave). This results in important prolongation of the LV filling time and induces an increase in aortic velocity–time integral (VTI).

ologist with some knowledge of hemodynamics. The method requires programming the AV delay to a short interval and a long interval while testing each setting for its impact on end-diastolic filling with Doppler echocardiography (Fig. 17.3). The interval is first set inappropriately short (e.g. 50 ms) so that mitral valve closure is postponed until end-diastolic filling is prematurely terminated by the onset of ventricular contraction. This provides the longest time interval between the ventricular pacing artifact and mitral valve closure (Q–A interval for a short AV delay). In some patients, the A wave can be truncated because of sub-optimal Doppler acquisition, and careful extrapolation from the downslope of the Doppler profile to the baseline. This is done with a potential degree of measurement error. Following this, the AV delay is set inappropriately long

(e.g. 250 ms), which shortens the time interval between the V pacing artifact and mitral valve closure that generates the Q–A interval for a long AV delay (found generally as a negative value). The optimal AV delay is then determined by adding the short AV delay to the time shift from "a" to "b" (Fig. 17.3), so that the calculated optimal AV delay is derived from the following: short AV delay + ("a"–"b"). The goal is to allow for completion of end-diastolic filling precisely at the onset of ventricular contraction.

Limitations of the Ritter method are mainly related to the lack of data in CRT patients along with technical issues related to the acquisition of Doppler information. This method was originally reported and previously validated among patients with a dual-chamber pacemaker for conduction system disease [41]. Moreover, identifying the onset of the

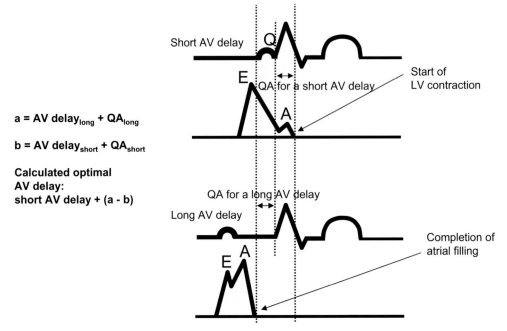

Figure 17.3 AV delay optimization mechanics according to the Ritter method. The AV interval is set short (50–60 ms) so that mitral valve closure is postponed until end-diastolic filling is prematurely terminated by the onset of ventricular contraction. The Q–A interval is then measured at this setting. The AV interval is then set inappropriately long (250 ms), which shortens the Q–A time interval and may even generate a negative value (as above). The optimal AV delay is determined by the value : short AV delay + (a–b). Adapted from Kindermann *et al.* [41].

QRS complex (recorded on an echocardiography device) when measuring the Q–A interval may be quite difficult, in addition to the potentially poor quality of the A wave signal. Finally, in patients who benefit from CRT and with a normal or short (<150 ms) PR interval, it can be very difficult to ensure biventricular pacing with a long AV delay, which has to be considered for the second part of the Ritter method.

A more empirical method consists of considering the variations of the aortic velocity–time integral values with different AV delays. The optimal AV delay goes with the highest value of aortic velocity–time integral (Fig. 17.2). The main limitation is the extreme variability of the aortic velocity–time integral which can be a source of measurement error.

Another method is to consider only the echocardiographic LV filling pattern; the optimal AV delay is the one providing the longest LV filling time without truncating the A wave and without changing the LV filling pattern. The advantage of this technique is that it avoids the variability of the aortic velocity–time integral measurement and is less time consuming [12, 15, 29, 41].

Although echocardiography has become a popular way to assess LV filling, a non-invasive AV delay optimization via an external device has been proposed to automatically quantify and assess LV filling. Two encouraging studies have shown that plethysmography can easily and automatically calculate variations in cardiac output [28, 42]. The optimal AV delay should result in the highest cardiac output value recorded. Butter *et al.* [28] compared measurements obtained by finger photoplethysmography and those by invasive aortic pressure simultaneously collected from 57 heart failure patients during intrinsic rhythm alternating with very brief periods of pacing at 4–5 AV delays (Fig. 17.4). The finger sensor was a conventional pulse oximetry probe (model 8000K2, Nonin Medical Inc., Plymouth, MN, USA). Plethysmography correctly identified positive aortic pulse pressure responses with 71% sensitivity and 90% specificity and negative aortic pulse pres-

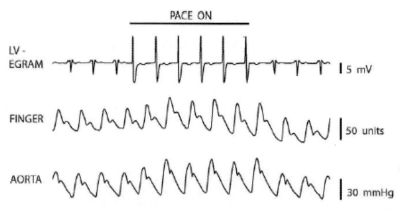

Figure 17.4 Example of cardiac resynchronization therapy pacing effects on ascending aortic pressure and finger photoplethysmogram signal from one patient. Adapted from Butter *et al.* [28].

sure responses with 57% sensitivity and 96% specificity. The magnitude of plethysmographic changes was strongly correlated with positive aortic pulse pressure changes ($r^2 = 0.73$; $P < 0.0001$) but less well correlated with negative aortic pulse pressure changes ($r^2 = 0.43$; $P < 0.001$). Plethysmography selected 78% of the patients having positive aortic pulse pressure changes to CRT and identified the AV delay giving maximum aortic pulse pressure change in all selected patients. Accordingly, plethysmography can provide a simple non-invasive method for identifying significant changes in aortic pulse pressure in CRT patients and the optimal AV delay giving the maximum aortic pulse pressure.

Role of interventricular optimization

CRT improves systolic and diastolic functions by restoring a more synchronized ventricular mechanical activation pattern [12–15]. However, several pathophysiological aspects remain to be clarified in order to better understand CRT mechanisms and to optimize patient selection for this non-pharmacological treatment. Indeed, it remains unclear whether CRT-induced hemodynamic benefits are mainly due to major improvement in inter- or intraventricular synchronization. The availability of separate activation of the ventricular leads offers multiple configurations of ventricular activation sequences (various levels of RV or LV pre-activation) and consequently, permits more in-depth investigation of the relationships between the different degrees and types of ventricular dyssynchrony with hemodynamic parameters.

Why consider a new parameter such as the VV delay which corresponds to the delay between RV and LV pacing (positive or negative delay)? Preliminary studies have suggested greater hemodynamic improvement if the LV lead was positioned in the region of greatest LV mechanical delay. If this could not be achieved, pre-exciting the lead closer to this particular area with slow conduction could improve cardiac function beyond that provided with simultaneous RV and LV stimulation [43].

Sogaard *et al.* [19] performed one of the first studies dedicated to VV delay in heart failure patients who were candidates for CRT. The authors defined a new parameter, the extent of delayed LV longitudinal contraction (DLC) (Fig. 17.5). DLC is calculated using tissue Doppler imaging (TDI) coupled with strain rate analysis. A segment was considered to have DLC if the strain rate analysis demonstrated motion reflecting true contraction and if the end of the segmental contraction occurred after the aortic valve closure [44, 45]. They found that the extent of myocardium with DLC predicted improvement in LV systolic performance and reversion of LV remodeling during short- and long-term CRT [44, 45]. Their observations indicate that DLC represents mechanical LV dyssynchrony and thus a contractile reserve, which can be recruited by means of CRT [45] (Fig. 17.5). However, in patients with heart failure and ventricular conduction disturbances, the location of myocardium displaying DLC may vary. Like Greenberg *et al.* [43], Sogaard *et*

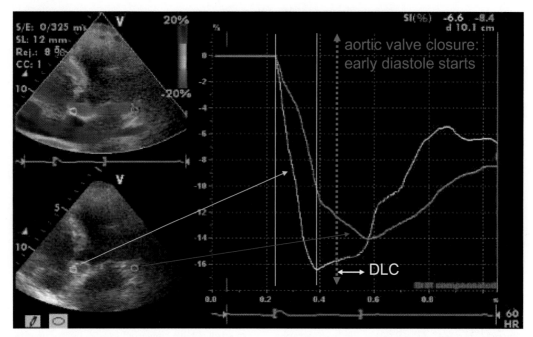

Figure 17.5 Apical long-axis view in patient with dilated cardiomyopathy and left bundle branch block. One Doppler sample (yellow) is positioned at base of the septal LV wall, and another (green) is at base of lateral wall. In each of the two points, strain analysis is carried out in the range of 10 mm around the center of the cursor. First vertical line (right) shows onset of negative strain (yellow curve), indicating active contraction in systole. Second vertical line indicates cessation of septal systole where strain (yellow curve) becomes positive. Third vertical line (red) represents the aortic valve closure. Note that negative strain is still observed in the lateral wall (green curve), and this phenomenon persists, indicating active shortening in early diastole until strain becomes positive (i.e. delayed longitudinal contraction (DLC)).

al. [19] hypothesized that individually tailored pre-activation of myocardium displaying DLCs could further improve the overall response to CRT.

This study examined patients with left bundle branch block (LBBB), a QRS width >130 ms, and a New York Heart Association (NYHA) functional class III or IV heart failure with DTI techniques specifically before and after implantation (i.e. CRT). Post-implantation studies were performed during simultaneous CRT at 12-, 20-, 40-, 60-, and 80-ms delay intervals with either LV or RV pre-excitation. The study population consisted of 11 patients with ischemic cardiomyopathy and nine patients with idiopathic dilated cardiomyopathy. As noted in prior studies, DLC was identified in the lateral and posterior LV walls. In contrast, patients with ischemic cardiomyopathy exhibited DLC in the septal and inferior walls. Echocardiographic parameters improved during sequential CRT, with LV pre-activation being superior in nine patients and RV pre-activation being superior in 11 patients (Fig. 17.6). Compared with simultaneous CRT, tailored sequential CRT reduced the extent of segments with DLC in the base from $23 \pm 13\%$ to $11 \pm 7\%$ ($P < 0.05$). Ejection fraction increased from $30 \pm 5\%$ to $33.6 \pm 6\%$ ($P < 0.01$). Additionally, the diastolic filling time increased even without any AV delay optimization.

Finally, the authors concluded that the location of DLC predicted the optimal sequential CRT, as posterior lateral wall-DLC was associated with optimal sequential CRT via LV pre-activation and septal and inferior wall-DLC was associated with optimal sequential CRT via RV pre-activation. The optimal VV delay determined by the investigators ranged between 12 and 20 ms.

A second important study confirmed the value of sequential CRT for further improvement in cardiac function compared with simultaneous CRT in heart failure patients. Perego *et al.* [46] maintained that simultaneous CRT was not physiologic. Indeed, sev-

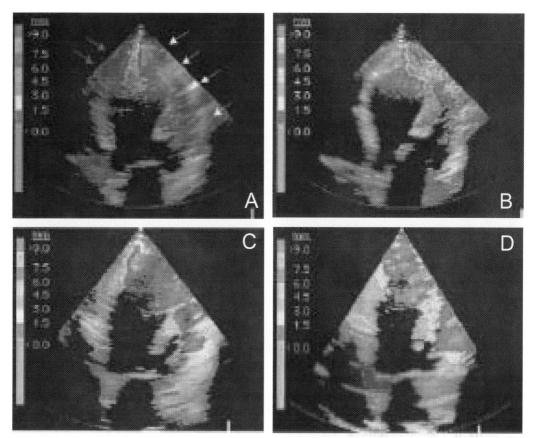

Figure 17.6 (A) Transthoracic tissue tracking echocardiographic images in apical four-chamber view in systole in patient with idiopathic dilated cardiomyopathy before implantation of CRT device. Most of the lateral wall, posterior wall, and distal parts of anterior wall are gray, indicating lack of systolic motion toward the apex (white arrows). Color-coded scaling at left side of each image indicates regional motion amplitude. Mechanical function of interventricular septum and inferior walls is abnormal, with greater motion amplitude in segments adjacent to apex (green arrows). (B) Extent of myocardium (colored segments) with delayed longitudinal contraction (DLC) in diastole (mitral valve open) present in the lateral wall. Note that remaining part of LV is gray, indicating no motion (the rest of the LV entered the relaxation phase). (C) Same patient with simultaneous CRT resulting in contraction of larger proportion of lateral wall. In addition, each segment shows improved systolic shortening as seen from color coding. Moreover, abnormal distribution of myocardial motion in interventricular septum has been normalized. (D) Impact of sequential CRT with LV activated by 20 ms before RV. Compared with simultaneous CRT, sequential CRT yields further improvement in overall proportion of contracting myocardium in the lateral wall. In addition, each segment shows further improvement in systolic shortening amplitude. Adapted from Sogaard P et al. [19].

eral pathophysiologic considerations support the hypothesis that the best mechanical efficiency is not necessarily achieved by the simultaneous delivery of stimuli to both ventricles. First, in normal hearts, the activation of the two ventricles does not occur simultaneously (i.e. epicardial RV depolarization starts a few milliseconds earlier than LV depolarization) [47]. Second, in CRT, the left ventricle is paced from the epicardial side, and this could account for a delay in the transmission of the stimulus that needs to reach the subendocardial conduction system before spreading to the remaining ventricle. Third, in advanced cardiomyopathy, right ventricle to left ventricle interactions can be different from those in normal hearts. As a consequence, the best mechanical efficiency might be achieved with different patterns of ventricular activation. Fourth, the baseline ventricular conduction defect differs considerably from case to case: in patients with a QRS duration longer than 150 ms [48], the conduction delay is possibly due not only to an isolated bundle branch block, but also to more global anisotropic disturbances of the conduction system and/or myocardial scars. Finally, the ventricular leads (particularly LV leads) are placed in quite different anatomical positions, depending on the operator's choice and coronary sinus anatomy, leading to ventricular activation patterns during pacing that differ from patient to patient.

Perego *et al.* [46] performed a particularly robust study (even though the sample size remained rather small) that compared simultaneous and sequential CRT via the variations in LV and RV dP/dt. In 12 patients, LV pressure, RV pressure and respective rates of change of pressure (dP/dt) were acutely measured during biventricular pacing with different AV and VV delays ranging from –60 (LV pre-activation) to +40 ms (RV pre-activation). It is interesting to observe changes in the QRS morphology on the surface

ECG according to the degree of LV or RV pre-activation (Fig. 17.7). The average increase versus baseline in maximum LV dP/dt was higher for sequential than for simultaneous biventricular pacing (VDD mode: 35 ± 20 vs. $29 \pm 18\%$, $P < 0.01$; DDD mode: 38 ± 23 vs. $34 \pm 25\%$, $P < 0.01$), with a minority of patients accounting for most of the difference. The mean optimal VV delay was -25 ± 21 ms in VDD mode and -25 ± 26 ms in DDD mode. With these settings, RV dP/dt was not significantly different from baseline. QRS shortening was not predictive of an increase in LV dP/dt. The authors concluded that a significant increase of LV dP/dt with no change in RV dP/dt can be obtained by sequential biventricular pacing compared to simultaneous biventricular pacing (Fig. 17.8). The highest LV dP/dt was achieved with LV pre-activation.

Sogaard *et al.* [19] and Perego *et al.* [46], respectively, performed a tremendous task when they sug-

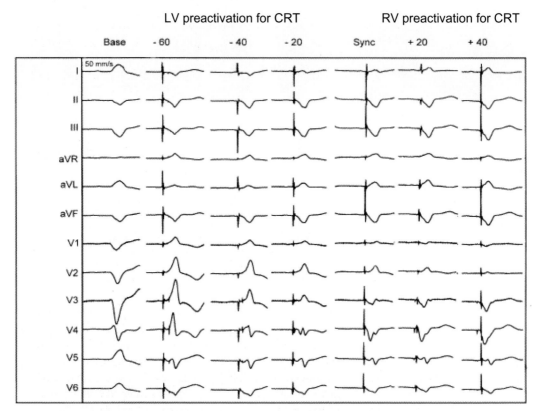

Figure 17.7 Gradual transition from a right bundle branch block to a left bundle branch block pattern due to progressive increase in interventricular interval from negative (left ventricle pacing before right ventricle stimulation) to 0 ms (simultaneous CRT) to positive (right ventricle before left ventricle stimulation). Adapted from Perego *et al.* [46].

% LV dP/dt versus baseline

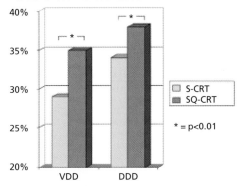

Figure 17.8 Average maximum rate of change of LV pressure (LV d*P*/d*t*) for simultaneous (S-CRT) and sequential (SQ-CRT) biventricular pacing. Data are expressed as % variations from baseline. Adapted from Perego *et al.* [46].

gested a relationship between better LV synchronous contraction and sequential CRT, and by demonstrating that sequential CRT could result in further hemodynamic improvement in CRT patients.

However, it is unreasonable to have all CRT patients undergo repetitive invasive procedures such as LV and RV d*P*/d*t* measurements with the aim of optimizing the VV delay. Sogaard *et al.* have demonstrated how to use non-invasive techniques such as echocardiography for VV optimization. Therefore, one question remains: which is the most reliable and reproducible echo technique to use to optimize sequential CRT? Also, should one give greater consideration to interventricular electromechanical dyssynchrony as suggested by Cazeau *et al.* [49], or LV intraventricular dyssynchrony?

Besides echo-Doppler techniques, Pitzalis *et al.* [50] proposed a simple method to quantify the degree of intra-LV dyssynchrony. They utilized standard M-mode echocardiography to take full advantage of the excellent temporal resolution and the widespread familiarity of this technique. Aligning the M-mode cursor orthogonal to the short axis of the mid-LV at the base of the heart in the parasternal long axis view, one can determine the earliest point of activation in the anterior septum as well as the latest point of activation and anterior movement in the posterior wall (Fig. 17.9). This method is called "septal-to-posterior wall motion mechanical delay" (SPWMD). At one month following initiation of CRT, the SPWMD decreased from an average of 192 ± 92 ms to 14 ± 67 ms ($P < 0.001$). Not only did SPWMD have a higher specificity with the QRS width (63% versus 13%) with use of 130 and 150 ms as cutoffs, but the positive predictive value was also significantly greater. The weakest point of this technique is that SPWMD is a regional index dedicated only to two segments of a 16-segment ventricle. Consequently, this can lead to a dangerous underestimation in heart failure patients that may be candidates for CRT.

In order to quantify the degree of inter- and intra-LV asynchrony between the different ventricular segments, TDI technique appears to be the most promising tool because all the ventricular segments can be studied and assessed. Yet, several technical issues remain to be clarified. For instance, should one consider ventricular dyssynchrony from the onset, the peak or the end of the systolic motion of the dif-

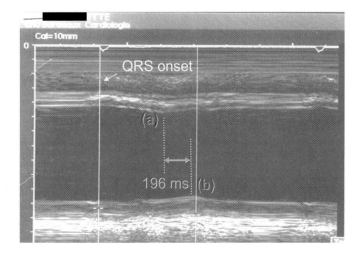

Figure 17.9 Mono-dimensional short-axis view of the echocardiographic image taken at the level of the papillary muscles. Calculation of septal-to-posterior wall motion delay (SPWMD) obtained by measuring the shortest interval between the maximal posterior displacement of the septum (a) and the posterior wall (b).

ferent ventricular walls in order to quantify at best the degree of dyssynchrony and its hemodynamic consequences? Some studies suggested that the main role of CRT is to reduce the number of ventricular segments contracting after the aortic valve closure (delayed longitudinal contraction assessed by Sogaard *et al.* [19, 44–45]) leading to contractile reserve recruitment. Accordingly, any measure of cardiac dyssynchrony should consider motion in segments exhibiting post-systolic contraction. Others identified ventricular dyssynchrony from measurements of the delay between the onset or the peak of contraction of 12 ventricular segments [12, 33]. From those values, the standard deviation can be calculated and provide the index of dyssynchrony.

The different techniques will be described in order to identify those that would provide the greatest accuracy in reflecting hemodynamic changes. Such a tool would permit determination of the optimal sequential CRT without requiring invasive procedures and with a good reproducibility. We performed a study [15] with the aim of identifying such an echocardiographic parameter.

Forty-one patients with drug-resistant heart failure undergoing implantation of a CRT device were prospectively enrolled. Patients were selected for biventricular pacing on the following basis: (1) LV ejection fraction <40%; (2) QRS duration >120 ms, LBBB; and (3) NYHA functional class III or IV, despite optimal medical treatment. To ensure ventricular pacing and allow optimization of the AV delay during the study protocol, patients were selected with a PR interval 200 ms. Patients with a history of atrial arrhythmias, primary mitral regurgitation, or ongoing symptoms of myocardial ischemia were excluded from the study protocol. In addition, to limit the variations among the LV pacing site, patients were excluded if the LV lead could not be positioned in a lateral or posterolateral vein.

All pacemaker leads were positioned transvenously. The atrial lead was positioned at the right atrial appendage and the RV lead at the apex. All devices implanted had two separate ventricular channels for RV and LV pacing with a programmable interventricular stimulation delay of 0–80 ms.

After implantation of a CRT device, the study protocol was performed. For the study protocol, different predetermined pacing configurations were assessed using spontaneous atrial synchronized pacing. To ensure complete ventricular capture during the different pacing configurations, the QRS morphology and width were verified to be similar between the non-atrial synchronized (VVI mode) and atrial synchronized (VDD mode) ventricular pacing configurations. The AV delay was modified and optimized for each tested configuration in order to provide the longest transmitral filling time without truncation of the A wave from pulsed Doppler analysis of the LV filling [41]. Cardiac output, severity of mitral regurgitation, and parameters of inter- and intraventricular dyssynchrony were evaluated using echocardiography at the following predetermined configurations of ventricular pacing: (1) RV pacing; (2) LV pacing; (3) simultaneous CRT; (4) sequential CRT with RV pre-activation with interventricular intervals of 12, 20, 40, and 80 ms; and (5) sequential CRT with LV pre-activation with interventricular intervals of 12, 20, 40, and 80 ms. These configurations were performed in random order with baseline data being determined during simultaneous CRT at the start and completion of the protocol to control for the effects of the study duration. After the study protocol, patients were maintained in the individually optimized sequential CRT configuration. The optimal pacing configuration for a given patient was identified as that achieving the maximal increase in cardiac output during the study protocol.

Echocardiography was performed before and on the day after pacemaker implantation, using a 2.5–5.0 MHz imaging probe connected to a Vingmed-General Electric ultrasound system (System 5; Horten, Norway) and performed in accordance with the American Society of Echocardiography guidelines. Each parameter was measured and averaged over three consecutive beats during sinus rhythm. The off-line analysis was performed by a different observer and was blinded to the pacing mode. The LV filling time was determined by pulsed wave Doppler transmitral flow as the time between the onset of the E wave and the end of the A wave. Cardiac output was determined by the LV outflow method [51]. The severity of mitral regurgitation was assessed by the proximal isovelocity surface area, as previously described [52, 53].

At each predetermined interval, features of interventricular and intra-LV dyssynchrony were evaluated as previously described. Interventricular dyssynchrony was defined as the difference between the aortic and pulmonary pre-ejection delays and determined as the time from the onset of the QRS complex to the beginning of each respective systolic ejection by pulsed wave Doppler imaging [49].

LV intraventricular dyssynchrony was determined using TDI to assess segmental wall motion, as previously described [12, 33]. In brief, TDI was applied by placing the sample volume in the middle of the basal and mid-segmental portions of the septal, lateral, inferior, anterior, posterior, and anteroseptal walls.

The following were determined off-line:

- Variation in the onset of segmental LV contraction (intra-LV delay-onset) was evaluated by determining the electromechanical delay-onset for each segment by measuring the interval between the onset of the QRS complex and the onset of each segmental contraction. The intra-LV delay-onset was then calculated as the difference between the shortest and longest of the 12 segmental electromechanical delay-onset values [12, 33] (Fig. 17.10).

- Variation in the peak of segmental LV contraction (intra-LV delay-peak) was evaluated by determining the electromechanical delay-peak for each segment by measuring the interval between the onset of the QRS complex and the peak of each segmental contraction. The intra-LV delay-peak was then calculated as the difference between the shortest and longest of the 12 segmental electromechanical delay-peak values.

- The index of systolic dyssynchrony first described by Yu *et al.* [12] was defined as the standard deviation of the 12 LV segmental electromechanical delay-peak values already cited (the lower, the better).

- Delayed longitudinal contraction (DLC) first described by Sogaard *et al.* [19] was calculated using TDI coupled with strain rate analysis. A segment was considered to present with DLC if the strain rate analysis demonstrated motion reflecting true contraction and if the end of the segmental contraction occurred after the aortic valve closure (Fig. 17.5). DLC is presented as the number of segments demonstrating DLC, expressed as a per-

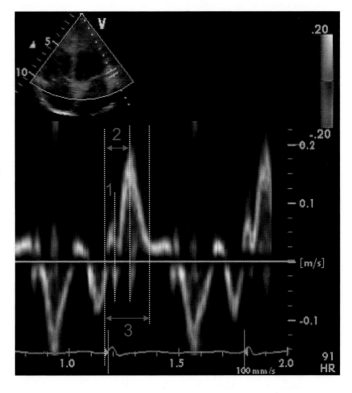

Figure 17.10 Transthoracic pulsed Doppler tissue imaging echocardiographic images in apical four-chamber view in systole in a patient with idiopathic dilated cardiomyopathy before implantation of a CRT device. The cursor is located at the base of the lateral LV wall. Time interval "1" is the respective electromechanical delay between the onset of the QRS complex and the onset of the wall systolic motion. Time interval "2" is the respective electromechanical delay between the onset of the QRS complex and the peak of the wall systolic motion. Time interval "3" (data not published) is the respective electromechanical delay between the onset of the QRS complex and the end of the wall systolic motion.

centage of the total number of segments evaluated [19]. In addition, the SPWMD was determined as a marker of intraventricular delay. The SPWMD was defined as the shortest interval between the maximal displacement of the LV septum and that of the posterior LV wall, as determined by M-mode echocardiography in the short-axis view at the papillary muscle level [50].

- Finally, interventricular dyssynchrony was defined as the difference between the aortic and pulmonary pre-ejection delays and determined as the time from the onset of the QRS complex to the beginning of each respective systolic ejection by pulsed wave Doppler imaging [49].

All patients underwent clinical evaluation at baseline before biventricular pacing implantation and at three months after individually optimized biventricular pacing. During clinical evaluation, a 6-Minute Hall-Walk Test and quality-of-life assessment using the Minnesota Living with Heart Failure were performed. The results were as follows:

Variations in intra-LV delay-peak, intra-LV delay-onset, and index of LV dyssynchrony measured by pulsed DTI were highly correlated with those of the cardiac output ($r = -0.67$, $r = -0.64$, $r = -0.67$ respectively; $P < 0.001$) and mitral regurgitation ($r = 0.68$, $r = 0.63$, $r = 0.68$ respectively; $P < 0.001$), while variations in extent of myocardium displaying delayed longitudinal contraction ($r = -0.48$ and $r = 0.51$ respectively; $P < 0.05$) and the variations in SPWMD ($r = -0.41$; $P < 0.05$ and $r = 0.24$; $P =$ ns, respectively) were less well correlated (Table 17.1). The changes in interventricular dyssynchrony were not significantly correlated ($P =$ ns), suggesting that interventricular dyssynchrony might not be

considered as a major marker of CRT-induced improvement in heart failure patients. Compared with simultaneous biventricular pacing, individually optimized sequential biventricular pacing significantly increased cardiac output ($P < 0.01$), decreased mitral regurgitation ($P < 0.05$), and improved all parameters of intra-LV dyssynchrony ($P < 0.01$). At three months, a significant reverse mechanical LV remodeling was observed with significantly decreased LV volumes ($P < 0.01$) associated with an increased LVEF ($P = 0.035$).

Interestingly, presence of DLC was significantly but poorly correlated with hemodynamic parameters. This may be explained by the fact that DLC represents the proportion of LV segments (among the 12 studied LV segments) contracting after aortic valve closure. Accordingly, for each segment, the DLC analysis is dichotomic (presence or absence of DLC) without calculating the time spent in DLC for each LV segment.

In addition, when looking for a reliable and simple tool for guiding sequential CRT optimization, this tool should not be time-consuming. The index of systolic dyssynchrony first described by Yu *et al.* [12] and other indices derived from 12 LV segments, for example, are accurate but time consuming for routine use. Pulsed TDI applied to the base of the four LV walls appeared to be strongly correlated with hemodynamic changes and feasible in routine practice. However, this method cannot quantify dyssynchrony for the LV mid-segments and is even less feasible for the apical segments. Newer three-dimensional automatic algorithms that consider the entire LV are expected to add significantly to the methods already discussed.

Table 17.1 Correlations between the markers of ventricular dyssynchrony and those of hemodynamic status

Markers of ventricular dyssynchrony	Cardiac output (% changes)		Mitral regurgitation (% changes)	
	r	P-value	r	P-value
Intra-LV delay$_{peak}$	−0.67	<0.001	0.68	<0.001
Intra-LV delay$_{onset}$	−0.64	<0.001	0.63	<0.001
Index of LV dyssynchrony	−0.67	<0.001	0.68	<0.001
SPWMD	−0.41	<0.05	0.24	ns
% of DLC	−0.48	<0.05	0.51	<0.05
Inter-V dyssynchrony	−0.24	ns	0.06	ns

ns, not significant; SPWMD, septal-to-posterior wall motion mechanical delay; DLC, delayed LV longitudinal contraction. Adapted from Bordachar P *et al.* [15].

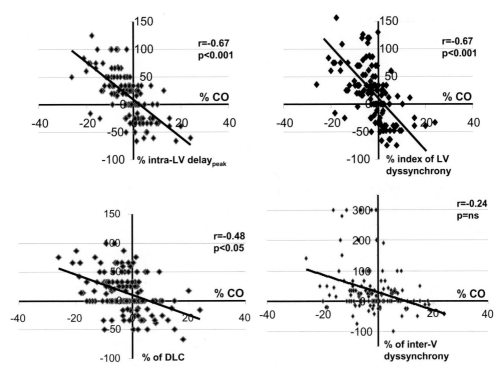

Figure 17.11 Correlation between the changes in the parameters of ventricular dyssynchrony and those of cardiac output (CO). A high correlation is shown between the changes in the index of dyssynchrony, the intraventricular delay peak, and the changes in CO; lower correlation for the extent of myocardium displaying delayed longitudinal contraction (DLC); no correlation for the interventricular delay. Adapted from Bordachar *et al.* [15].

According to these data, it can be seen that specific echocardiographic measurements of ventricular dyssynchrony are highly correlated with hemodynamic changes and may be a useful adjunct in CRT optimization (Figs 17.11 and 17.12).

The findings of this work also suggest that the optimal sequence of CRT might be difficult to predict from patient to patient. Although in some individuals, CRT with LV pre-activation results in a significant cardiac output increase (compared with simultaneous CRT), in others, the greatest improvements were observed with RV pre-activation (Fig. 17.13). Unfortunately, we could not identify pre-implant parameters predictive of the best sequential CRT configuration. Interestingly, in only 15% of patients was simultaneous CRT found to be the optimal configuration. These observations underscore the importance of individually tailored optimized sequential CRT at pre-discharge with the aim of providing the greatest optimization of cardiac output and minimization of mitral regurgitation. However, the definite benefits of VV optimization need to be confirmed by large, randomized follow-up studies that compare sequential and simultaneous CRT.

Potential for device-based "auto" optimization

Available non-invasive techniques and more specifically echocardiography with or without TDI to optimize sequential CRT require experienced physicians, and measurement variability should be determined in every heart failure center. The ideal tool would be a pacemaker equipped with a specific sensor able to record and monitor cardiac function via software independent of the variability of "human touch." Such a sensor is likely to represent the future with the aim of permanently optimizing CRT and avoiding periodic and repetitive outpatient visits. Different sensors are being assessed. The Peak Endocardial Acceleration (PEA, SORIN Group; Milan, Italy) sensor has been evaluated for almost 10 years and several studies have already suggested that data recorded by this sensor could be highly

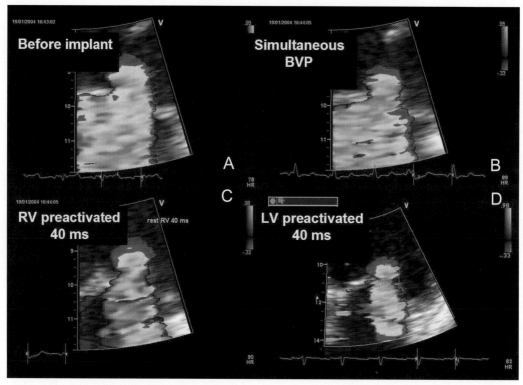

Figure 17.12 Reduction of mitral regurgitation with optimized sequential CRT. Pre-implant effective regurgitant orifice area (EROA): 31 mm²; simultaneous CRT EROA: 22 mm²; sequential CRT with RV pre-activation of 40 ms EROA: 21 mm²; optimized sequential CRT with LV pre-activation of 40 ms EROA: 10 mm². Adapted from Bordachar *et al.* [15].

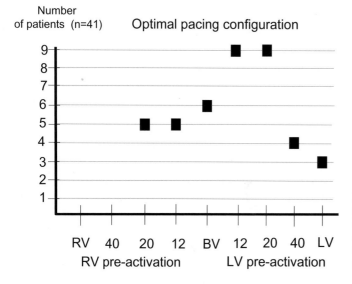

Figure 17.13 Distribution of the best sequential CRT configurations, patient by patient. Only 15% of patients were optimized at best with simultaneous CRT while 61% of patients required LV pre-activation.

correlated to LV function. Signals measured by the sensor are based on the amplitude of the first heart sound vibrations and identified as the variations of the PEA at each systole [54–56]. These variations are collected via a micromass accelerometer sensor located at the tip of an endocardial RV pacing lead and connected to the pacemaker. This has the advantage that no material needs to be implanted in the left heart cavities. Rickards *et al.* [57] demonstrated by temporarily occluding the pulmonary artery in a sheep model that the PEA signal variations remained highly correlated to the LV dP/dt rather than the RV dP/dt (Fig. 17.14). Even though

pulmonary artery occlusion in a sheep model is far from the situation in humans, the data are encouraging.

Variations of the LV dP/dt in heart failure patients and comparison to PEA variations have also been studied. The first results seem to be promising, having exhibited a correlation coefficient reaching 0.87 [58] (Fig. 17.15).

Because CRT optimization is time-consuming and sensitive to intra- and interobserver variability, pacemakers providing not only electrical stimulation to the heart but also precious information to the physician on cardiac function, will greatly im-

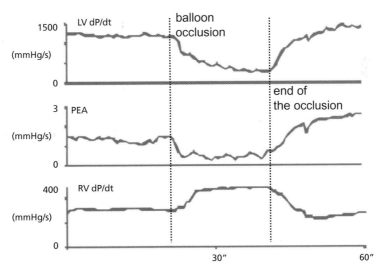

Figure 17.14 Peak endocardial acceleration (PEA) versus LV dP/dt_{max} and RV dP/dt_{max} during pulmonary artery balloon occlusion in a sheep model.

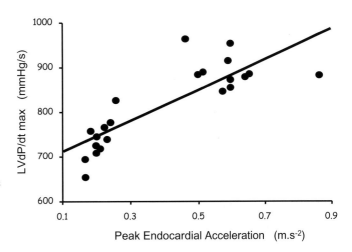

Figure 17.15 Correlation between variations of the LV dP/dt_{max} and PEA in a severe heart failure patient (LV ejection fraction: 28%) in whom 22 combinations of acute sequential CRT (3 min for each combination) at different LV and RV pacing sites were hemodynamically assessed.

prove the clinical status and life expectancy in our drug-resistant heart failure patients.

There is a definite need for sensors able to monitor instantaneous changes in left atrial and/or ventricular pressure. This new research field in cardiac pacing will result in tremendous change in our daily practice since preclinical signals provided by the device would require data analysis and potential modification of the treatment and/or programming of the CRT device. Such a mutation to "electronic cardiology" will represent a paradigm shift in practice as a result of device capabilities.

References

1 Schoeller R, Andersen D, Buttner P et al. First- or second-degree atrioventricular block as a risk factor in idiopathic dilated cardiomyopathy. Am J Cardiol 1993; **71**: 720–726.

2 Aaronson KD, Schwartz JM, Chen TM et al. Development and prospective validation of a clinical index to predict survival in ambulatory patients referred for cardiac transplant evaluation. Circulation 1997; **95**: 2660–2667.

3 Wilensky RL, Yudelman P, Cohen AI et al. Serial electrocardiographic changes in idiopathic dilated cardiomyopathy confirmed at necropsy. Am J Cardiol 1988; **62**: 276–283.

4 Xiao HB, Roy C, Fujimoto S, Gibson DG. Natural history of abnormal conduction and its relation to prognosis in patients with dilated cardiomyopathy. Int J Cardiol 1996; **53**: 163–170.

5 Grines CL, Bashore TM, Boudoulas H et al. Functional abnormalities in isolated left bundle branch block. The effect of interventricular asynchrony. Circulation 1989; **79**: 845–853.

6 Xiao HB, Brecker SJ, Gibson DG et al. Effects of abnormal activation on the time course of the left ventricular pressure pulse in dilated cardiomyopathy. Br Heart J 1992; **68**: 403–407.

7 Bakker P, Chin A, Sen K et al. Biventricular pacing improves functional capacity in patients with end-stage congestive heart failure. [abstract] Pacing Clin Electrophysiol 1995; **18**: 825.

8 Cazeau S, Ritter P, Bakdach S et al. Four chamber pacing in dilated cardiomyopathy. Pacing Clin Electrophysiol 1994; **17**: 1974–1979.

9 Blanc JJ, Etienne Y, Gilard M et al. Evaluation of different ventricular pacing sites in patients with severe heart failure. Results of an acute hemodynamic study. Circulation 1997; **96**: 3273–3277.

10 Cazeau S, Leclercq C, Lavergne T et al. Effects of multisite biventricular pacing in patients with heart failure and intraventricular conduction delay. N Engl J Med 2001 ; **344**:

873–880.

11 Abraham WT, Fisher WG, Smith AL et al. Cardiac resynchronization in chronic heart failure. The MIRACLE prospective study. N Engl J Med 2002; **346**: 1845–1853.

12 Yu CM, Chau E, Sanderson JE et al. Tissue Doppler echocardiographic evidence of reverse remodeling and improved synchronicity by simultaneously delaying regional contraction after biventricular pacing therapy in heart failure. Circulation 2002; **105**: 438–445.

13 Leclercq C, Kass DA. Retiming the failing heart: principles and current clinical status of cardiac resynchronization. J Am Coll Cardiol 2002; **39**: 194–201.

14 Cazeau S, Bordachar P, Jauvert G et al. Echocardiographic modeling of cardiac dyssynchrony before and during multisite stimulation: a prospective study. Pacing Clin Electrophysiol 2003; **26**: 137–143.

15 Bordachar P, Lafitte S, Reuter S et al. Echocardiographic parameters of ventricular dyssynchrony validation in patients with heart failure using sequential biventricular pacing. J Am Coll Cardiol 2004; **44**: 2154–2165.

16 Penicka M, Bartunek J, De Bruyne B et al. Improvement of left ventricular function after cardiac resynchronization therapy is predicted by tissue Doppler imaging echocardiography. Circulation 2004; **109**: 978–983.

17 Garrigue S, Reuter S, Efimov IR et al. Optical mapping technique applied to biventricular pacing: potential mechanisms of ventricular arrhythmias occurrence. Pacing Clin Electrophysiol 2003; **26**: 197–205.

18 Bax JJ, Molhoek SG, Marwick TH et al. Usefulness of myocardial tissue Doppler echocardiography to evaluate left ventricular dyssynchrony before and after biventricular pacing in patients with idiopathic dilated cardiomyopathy. Am J Cardiol 2003; **91**: 94–97.

19 Sogaard P, Egleblad H, Pedersen AK et al. Sequential versus simultaneous biventricular resynchronization for severe heart failure. Evaluation by tissue Doppler imaging. Circulation 2002; **106**: 2078–2084.

20 Reuter S, Garrigue S, Barold SS et al. Comparison of characteristics in responders versus non-responders with biventricular pacing for drug resistant congestive heart failure. Am J Cardiol 2002; **89**: 346–350.

21 Gras D, Leclercq C, Tang AS et al. Cardiac resynchronization therapy in advanced heart failure; The multicenter InSync clinical study. Eur J Heart Fail 2002; **4**: 311–320.

22 Cleland JGF, Daubert JC, Erdmann E et al. The effect of cardiac resynchronization on morbidity and mortality in heart failure. N Engl J Med 2005; **352**: 1539–1549.

23 Hochleitner M, Hortnagl H, Fridich L et al. Uselulness of physiologic dual-chamber pacing in drug-resistant idiopathic dilated cardiomyopathy. Am J Cardiol 1990; **66**: 198–202.

24 Brecker S., Xiao H., Sparrow J, Gibson G. Effects of dual-chamber pacing with short atrioventricular delay in di-

lated cardiomyopathy. *Lancet* 1992; **340**: 1308–1312.

25 Nishimura RA, Hayes DL, Holmes DR, *et al.* Mechanisms of hemodynamic improvement by dual chamber pacing for severe left ventricular dysfunction: an acute Doppler and catheterization study. *J Am Coll Cardiol* 1995; **25**: 281–288.

26 Heyndrickx GR, Paulus WJ. Effect of asynchrony on left ventricular relaxation. *Circulation* 1990; **81**(suppl III): 41–47.

27 Mehra MR, Greenberg BH. Cardiac resynchronization therapy: Caveat medicus! *J Am Coll Cardiol* 2004; **43**: 1145–1148.

28 Butter C, Stellbrink C, Belalcazar A *et al.* Cardiac resynchronization therapy optimization by finger plethysmography. *Heart Rhythm* 2004; **1**: 568–575.

29 Sawhney NS, Waggoner AD, Garhwal S *et al.* Randomized prospective trial of atrioventricular delay programming for cardiac resynchronization therapy. *Heart Rhythm* 2004; **1**: 562–567.

30 Auricchio A, Stellbrink C, Block M *et al.* Effect of pacing chamber and atrioventricular delay on acute systolic function of paced patients with congestive heart failure. The Pacing Therapies for Congestive Heart Failure Study Group. The Guidant Congestive Heart Failure Research Group. *Circulation* 1999; **99**: 2993–3001.

31 Lau CP, Yu CM, Chau E *et al.* Reversal of left ventricular remodeling by synchronous biventricular pacing in heart failure. *Pacing Clin Electrophysiol* 2000; **23**: 1722–1725.

32 Porcianai MC, Puglisi A, Colella A *et al.* Echocardiographic evaluation of the effect of biventricular pacing: the In-Sync Italian Registry. *Eur Heart J* 2000; Suppl J: J23–30.

33 Yu C, Fung W, Lin H, Zhang Q, Sanderson JE, Lau C. Predictors of left ventricular reverse remodeling after cardiac resynchronization therapy for heart failure secondary to idiopathic dilated or ischemic cardiomyopathy. *Am J Cardiol* 2002; **91**: 684–688.

34 St. John Sutton M, Plappert T, Abraham WT *et al.* Effect of cardiac resynchronization therapy on left ventricular size and function in chronic heart failure. *Circulation* 2003; **107**: 1985–1990.

35 Saxon LA, De Marco T, Schafer J *et al.* Effects of long-term biventricular stimulation for resynchronization of echocardiographic measure of remodeling. *Circulation* 2002; **105**: 1304–1310.

36 Carlton RA, Rassovoy M, Graettinger JS. The importance and timing of left atrial systole. *Chem Sci* 1969; **30**: 151–159.

37 Ronaszecki A. Hemodynamic consequences of the timing of atrial contraction during complete AV block. *Acta Biomed Lovaniensia* 1989; **15**.

38 Rey JL, Slama MA, Tribouilloy C *et al.* Etude par echo-Doppler des variations hemodynamiques entre modes

double stimulation et detection de l'oreillette chez des patients porteurs d'un stimulateur double chambre. *Arch Mal Cœur* 1990; **83**: 961–966.

39 Ritter P, Dib JC, Lelievre T *et al.* Quick determination of the optimal AV delay at rest in patients paced in DDD mode for complete AV block. [abstract] *Eur J Cardiac Pacing Electrophysiol* 1994; **4**: A163.

40 Ritter P, Padeletti L, Gillio-Meina L, Gaggini G. Determination of the optimal atrioventricular delay in DDD pacing: Comparison between echo and peak endocardial acceleration measurements. *Europace* 1999; **1**: 126–130.

41 Kindermann M, Frohlig G, Doerr T, Schieffer H. Optimizing the AV delay in DDD pacemaker patients with high degree AV block: mitral valve Doppler vs impedance cardiography. *Pacing Clin Electrophysiol* 1997; **20**: 2453–2462.

42 Hayes DL, Hayes SN, Hyberger LK *et al.* Atrioventricular interval optimization after biventricular pacing: echo-doppler vs. impedance plethysmography. *Pacing Clin Electrophysiol* 2000; **23**: 590.

43 Greenberg J, Delurgio DBM, Mera F. Left ventricular lead location in biventricular pacing with variable RV-LV timing does not affect optimal stroke volume. [abstract] *Pacing Clin Electrophysiol* 2002; **24**: 191.

44 Sogaard P, Kim WY, Jensen HK *et al.* Impact of acute biventricular pacing on left ventricular performance and volumes in patients with severe heart failure: a tissue Doppler and three-dimensional echocardiographic study. *Cardiology* 2001; **95**: 173–182.

45 Sogaard P, Egeblad H, Kim Y, *et al.* Tissue Doppler imaging predicts improved systolic performance and reversed left ventricular remodeling during long-term cardiac resynchronization therapy. *J Am Coll Cardiol* 2002; **40**: 723–730.

46 Perego GB, Chianca R, Facchini M *et al.* Sequential versus simultaneous biventricular pacing in heart failure: an acute hemodynamic study. *Eur J Heart Fail* 2003; **5**: 305–313.

47 Auricchio A, Salo RW. Acute hemodynamic improvements by pacing in patients with severe congestive heart failure. *Pacing Clin Electrophysiol* 1997; **20**: 313–324.

48 Nelson GS, Curry CW, Wyman BT *et al.* Predictors of systolic augmentation from left ventricular preexcitation in patients with dilated cardiomyopathy and intraventricular conduction delay. *Circulation* 2000; **101**: 2703–2709.

49 Cazeau S, Gras D, Lazarus A, Ritter P, Mugica J. Multisite stimulation for correction of cardiac asynchrony. *Heart* 2000; **84**: 579–581.

50 Pitzalis MV, Iacoviello M, Romito R *et al.* Cardiac resynchronization therapy tailored by echocardiographic evaluation of ventricular asynchrony. *J Am Coll Cardiol* 2002; **40**: 1615–1622.

51 Dubin J, Wallerson DC, Cody RJ *et al.* Comparative accuracy of Doppler echocardiography methods for clinical stroke volume determination. *Am Heart J* 1990; **120**: 116–123.

52 Enriquez-Sarano M, Seward JB, Bailey KR *et al.* Effective regurgitant orifice area: a non invasive Doppler development of an old hemodynamic concept. *J Am Coll Cardiol* 1994; **23**: 443–451.

53 Breithardt OA, Sinha AM, Schwammenthal E *et al.* Acute effects of resynchronization therapy on functional mitral regurgitation in advanced systolic heart failure. *J Am Coll Cardiol* 2003; **41**: 765–770.

54 Wood JC, Festen MP, Lim MJ *et al.* Regional effects of myocardial ischemia on epicardially recorded canine first heart sound. *J Appl Physiol* 1994; **76**: 291–302.

55 Bongiorni MG, Soldati E, Arena G *et al.* Is local myocardial contractility related to endocardial acceleration signals detected by a transvenous pacing lead? *Pacing Clin Electrophysiol* 1996; **19**: 1682–1688.

56 Occhetta E, Perucca A, Rognoni G *et al.* Experience with a new myocardial acceleration sensor during dobutamine infusion and exercise test. *Eur J Cardiac Pacing Electrophysiol* 1995; **5**: 204–209.

57 Rickards AF, Bombardini T, Corbucci G *et al.* An implantable intracardiac accelerometer for monitoring myocardial contractility. *Pacing Clin Electrophysiol* 1996; **19**: 2066–2071.

58 Ritter P, Padeletti L, Delnoy PP, *et al.* Device based AV delay optimization by peak endocardial acceleration in cardiac resynchronization therapy. [abstract] *Heart Rhythm* 2004; **1**: 120.

Index

329